Endoscopic Cranial Base and Pituitary Surgery

Editors

RAJ SINDWANI
TROY D. WOODARD
PABLO F. RECINOS

OTOLARYNGOLOGIC CLINICS OF NORTH AMERICA

www.oto.theclinics.com

February 2016 • Volume 49 • Number 1

ELSEVIER

1600 John F. Kennedy Boulevard • Suite 1800 • Philadelphia, Pennsylvania, 19103-2899

http://www.oto.theclinics.com

OTOLARYNGOLOGIC CLINICS OF NORTH AMERICA Volume 49, Number 1
February 2016 ISSN 0030-6665, ISBN-13: 978-0-323-41763-1

Editor: Jessica McCool
Developmental Editor: Alison Swety

Otolaryngologic Clinics of North America (ISSN 0030-6665) is published bimonthly by Elsevier, Inc., 360 Park Avenue South, New York, NY 10010-1710. Months of issue are February, April, June, August, October, and December. Business and Editorial Offices: 1600 John F. Kennedy Blvd., Suite 1800, Philadelphia, PA 19103-2899. Customer Service Office: 6277 Sea Harbor Drive, Orlando, FL 32887-4800. Periodicals postage paid at New York, NY and additional mailing offices. Subscription prices are $370.00 per year (US individuals), $765.00 per year (US institutions), $100.00 per year (US student/resident), $485.00 per year (Canadian individuals), $969.00 per year (Canadian institutions), $540.00 per year (international individuals), $969.00 per year (international institutions), $270.00 per year (international & Canadian student/resident). Foreign air speed delivery is included in all *Clinics'* subscription prices. All prices are subject to change without notice. **POSTMASTER:** Send address changes to *Otolaryngologic Clinics of North America*, Elsevier Health Sciences Division, Subscription Customer Service, 3251 Riverport Lane, Maryland Heights, MO 63043. **Telephone: 1-800-654-2452 (U.S. and Canada); 314-447-8871 (outside U.S. and Canada). Fax: 314-447-8029. E-mail: journalscustomerservice-usa@elsevier.com (for print support); journalsonlinesupport-usa@elsevier.com (for online support).**

Reprints. For copies of 100 or more of articles in this publication, please contact the Commercial Reprints Department, Elsevier Inc., 360 Park Avenue South, New York, NY 10010-1710. Tel.: 212-633-3874; Fax: 212-633-3820; E-mail: reprints@elsevier.com.

Otolaryngologic Clinics of North America is also published in Spanish by McGraw-Hill Interamericana Editores S.A., P.O. Box 5-237, 06500 Mexico D.F., Mexico.

Otolaryngologic Clinics of North America is covered in *MEDLINE/PubMed (Index Medicus), Current Contents/Clinical Medicine, Excerpta Medica, BIOSIS, Science Citation Index,* and *ISI/BIOMED*.

PROGRAM OBJECTIVE
The goal of the *Otolaryngologic Clinics of North America* is to provide information on the latest trends in patient management, the newest advances; and provide a sound basis for choosing treatment options in the field of otolaryngology.

LEARNING OBJECTIVES
Upon completion of this activity, participants will be able to:
1. Review the anatomy and physiology of the skull base and pituitary gland.
2. Discuss imaging, reconstruction techniques, and possible complications of endoscopic surgery of the skull base.
3. Recognize innovations in management and treatment of sinonasal and endonasal malignancies.

ACCREDITATION
The Elsevier Office of Continuing Medical Education (EOCME) is accredited by the Accreditation Council for Continuing Medical Education (ACCME) to provide continuing medical education for physicians.

The EOCME designates this enduring material for a maximum of 15 *AMA PRA Category 1 Credit*(s)™. Physicians should claim only the credit commensurate with the extent of their participation in the activity.

All other health care professionals requesting continuing education credit for this enduring material will be issued a certificate of participation.

DISCLOSURE OF CONFLICTS OF INTEREST
The EOCME assesses conflict of interest with its instructors, faculty, planners, and other individuals who are in a position to control the content of CME activities. All relevant conflicts of interest that are identified are thoroughly vetted by EOCME for fair balance, scientific objectivity, and patient care recommendations. EOCME is committed to providing its learners with CME activities that promote improvements or quality in healthcare and not a specific proprietary business or a commercial interest.

The planning committee, staff, authors and editors listed below have identified no financial relationships or relationships to products or devices they or their spouse/life partner have with commercial interest related to the content of this CME activity:
Mahmoud Abbassy, MD; Ana Lorena Abello, MD; AbdulAziz AlQahtani, MD; Muhamad Amine, MD; Vijay Anand, MD; Paolo Antognoni, MD; Leonardo Balsalobre, MD; Paolo Battaglia, MD; André Beer-Furlan, MD; Paolo Bossi, MD; Damien Bresson, MD; Ricardo L. Carrau, MD; Paolo Castelnuovo, MD; Anthony G. Del Signore, MD; Vincent DiNapoli, MD, PhD; Charles S. Ebert, MD, MPH; Matthew G. Ewend, MD; Alexander A. Farag, MD; Christopher J. Farrell, MD; Juan C. Fernandez-Miranda, MD; Anjali Fortna; Sébastien Froelich, MD; Gary L. Gallia, MD, PhD; Ashleigh Halderman, MD; Philippe Herman, MD; Gregory K. Hong, MD, PhD; Peleg M. Horowitz, MD, PhD; Benjamin Y. Huang, MD, MPH; Masaru Ishii, MD, PhD; John A. Jane Jr, MD; Cristine N. Klatt-Cromwell, MD; Varun R. Kshettry, MD; Davide Locatelli, MD; João Mangussi-Gomes, MD; Jessica McCool; Piero Nicolai, MD; Renato Hoffmann Nunes, MD; Gurston G. Nyquist, MD; Chirag R. Patel, MD; Spencer C. Payne, MD; Marc Polivka, MD; Daniel M. Prevedello, MD; Santha Priya; Shaan M. Raza, MD; Pablo F. Recinos, MD; Douglas D. Reh, MD; Marc R. Rosen, MD; Christopher R. Roxbury, MD; Deanna Sasaki-Adams, MD; Theodore H. Schwartz, MD; Michael F. Shriver, BS; Raj Sindwani, MD, FACS; Aldo C. Stamm, MD, PhD; Janalee K. Stokken, MD; Shirley Y. Su, MD; Megan Suermann; Brian D. Thorp, MD; Duc A. Tien, MD; Mario Turri-Zánoni, MD; Eduardo A.S. Vellutini, MD, PhD; Eric W. Wang, MD, FACS; Wei-Hsin Wang, MD; Troy D. Woodard, MD, FACS; Brad E. Zacharia, MD, MS; Adam M. Zanation, MD.

The planning committee, staff, authors and editors listed below have identified financial relationships or relationships to products or devices they or their spouse/life partner have with commercial interest related to the content of this CME activity:
James J. Evans, MD is a consultant/advisor for Styker, and receives royalties/patents from Mizuho.

UNAPPROVED/OFF-LABEL USE DISCLOSURE
The EOCME requires CME faculty to disclose to the participants:
1. When products or procedures being discussed are off-label, unlabelled, experimental, and/or investigational (not US Food and Drug Administration [FDA] approved); and
2. Any limitations on the information presented, such as data that are preliminary or that represent ongoing research, interim analyses, and/or unsupported opinions. Faculty may discuss information about pharmaceutical agents that is outside of FDA-approved labelling. This information is intended solely for CME and is not intended to promote off-label use of these medications. If you have any questions, contact the medical affairs department of the manufacturer for the most recent prescribing information.

TO ENROLL

To enroll in the *Otolaryngologic Clinics of North America* Continuing Medical Education program, call customer service at 1-800-654-2452 or sign up online at http://www.theclinics.com/home/cme. The CME program is available to subscribers for an additional annual fee of USD 260.

METHOD OF PARTICIPATION

In order to claim credit, participants must complete the following:

1. Complete enrolment as indicated above.
2. Read the activity.
3. Complete the CME Test and Evaluation. Participants must achieve a score of 70% on the test. All CME Tests and Evaluations must be completed online.

CME INQUIRIES/SPECIAL NEEDS

For all CME inquiries or special needs, please contact elsevierCME@elsevier.com.

Contributors

EDITORS

RAJ SINDWANI, MD, FACS
Vice Chairman and Section Head, Rhinology, Sinus and Skull Base Surgery, Head and Neck Institute; Co-Director, Minimally Invasive Cranial Base and Pituitary Surgery Program, Burkhardt Brain Tumor and Neuro-Oncology Center, Neurological Institute, Cleveland Clinic, Cleveland, Ohio

TROY D. WOODARD, MD, FACS
Section of Rhinology, Sinus and Skull Base Surgery, Head and Neck Institute; Minimally Invasive Cranial Base and Pituitary Surgery Program, Burkhardt Brain Tumor and Neuro-Oncology Center, Neurological Institute, Cleveland Clinic, Cleveland, Ohio

PABLO F. RECINOS, MD
Section of Rhinology, Sinus and Skull Base Surgery, Head and Neck Institute; Co-Director, Minimally Invasive Cranial Base and Pituitary Surgery Program, Burkhardt Brain Tumor and Neuro-Oncology Center, Neurological Institute, Cleveland Clinic, Cleveland, Ohio

AUTHORS

MAHMOUD ABBASSY, MD
Rosa Ella Burkhardt Brain Tumor and Neuro-Oncology Center, Cleveland Clinic, Cleveland, Ohio; Department of Neurosurgery, Faculty of Medicine, Alexandria University, Alexandria, Egypt

ANA LORENA ABELLO, MD
Radiologist, Department of Radiology, University of North Carolina at Chapel Hill, Chapel Hill, North Carolina; Department of Radiology, Universidad del Valle, Valle del Cauca, Colombia

ABDULAZIZ ALQAHTANI, MD
Department of Otolaryngology–Head and Neck Surgery, Prince Sultan Military Medical City, Riyadh, Saudi Arabia

MUHAMAD AMINE, MD
Department of Otolaryngology–Head and Neck Surgery, New York Presbyterian Hospital, Weill Medical College of Cornell University, New York, New York

VIJAY ANAND, MD
Department of Otolaryngology–Head and Neck Surgery, New York Presbyterian Hospital, Weill Medical College of Cornell University, New York, New York

PAOLO ANTOGNONI, MD
Division of Radiation Oncology, University of Insubria, Varese, Italy

LEONARDO BALSALOBRE, MD
São Paulo Skull Base Center; São Paulo ENT Center, Edmundo Vasconcelos Hospital, São Paulo, Brazil

PAOLO BATTAGLIA, MD
Unit of Otorhinolaryngology, Department of Biotechnology and Life Sciences (DBSV), Ospedale di Circolo e Fondazione Macchi; Department of Biotechnology and Life Sciences (DBSV), Head and Neck Surgery and Forensic Dissection Research Center (HNS&FDRc), University of Insubria, Varese, Italy

ANDRÉ BEER-FURLAN, MD
São Paulo Skull Base Center; DFVneuro Neurosurgical Group, São Paulo, Brazil

PAOLO BOSSI, MD
Head and Neck Cancer Medical Oncology Unit, Fondazione IRCCS Istituto Nazionale dei Tumori, Milano, Italy

DAMIEN BRESSON, MD
Neurosurgery Department, Assistance Publique-Hôpitaux de Paris, Paris, France

RICARDO L. CARRAU, MD
Departments of Neurosurgery and Otolaryngology–Head and Neck Surgery, Wexner Medical Center at the Ohio State University, Columbus, Ohio

PAOLO CASTELNUOVO, MD
Unit of Otorhinolaryngology, Department of Biotechnology and Life Sciences (DBSV), Ospedale di Circolo e Fondazione Macchi; Department of Otorhinolaryngology; Department of Biotechnology and Life Sciences (DBSV), Head and Neck Surgery and Forensic Dissection Research Center (HNS&FDRc), University of Insubria, Varese, Italy

ANTHONY G. DEL SIGNORE, MD
Fellow Physician, Department of Otolaryngology—Head and Neck Surgery, University of North Carolina at Chapel Hill, Chapel Hill, North Carolina

VINCENT DINAPOLI, MD, PhD
Department of Neurosurgery, The University of Texas M.D. Anderson Cancer Center, Houston, Texas; Department of Neurosurgery, The Mayfield Clinic, University of Cincinnati, Cincinnati, Ohio

CHARLES S. EBERT, MD, MPH
Assistant Professor, Department of Otolaryngology—Head and Neck Surgery, University of North Carolina at Chapel Hill, Chapel Hill, North Carolina

JAMES J. EVANS, MD
Department of Neurological Surgery, Thomas Jefferson University, Philadelphia, Pennsylvania

MATTHEW G. EWEND, MD
Professor and Chair, Department of Neurosurgery, University of North Carolina at Chapel Hill, Chapel Hill, North Carolina

ALEXANDER A. FARAG, MD
Department of Otolaryngology, Thomas Jefferson University, Philadelphia, Pennsylvania

CHRISTOPHER J. FARRELL, MD
Department of Neurological Surgery, Thomas Jefferson University, Philadelphia, Pennsylvania

JUAN C. FERNANDEZ-MIRANDA, MD
Associate Director, Center for Cranial Base Surgery; Director, Surgical Neuroanatomy Lab; Associate Professor, Department of Neurological Surgery, University of Pittsburgh Medical Center, Pittsburgh, Pennsylvania

SÉBASTIEN FROELICH, MD
Neurosurgery Department, Assistance Publique-Hôpitaux de Paris, Lariboisière Hospital, Université Paris VII - Diderot, Paris, France

GARY L. GALLIA, MD, PhD
Associate Professor, Department of Neurosurgery, Johns Hopkins University School of Medicine, Baltimore, Maryland

ASHLEIGH HALDERMAN, MD
Section of Rhinology, Sinus and Skull Base Surgery, Head and Neck Institute, Cleveland Clinic Foundation, Cleveland, Ohio

PHILIPPE HERMAN, MD
ENT Department, Lariboisière Hospital, Université Paris VII - Diderot, Paris, France

GREGORY K. HONG, MD, PhD
Assistant Professor, Division of Endocrinology, Department of Medicine, University of Virginia Health System, Charlottesville, Virginia

PELEG M. HOROWITZ, MD, PhD
Department of Neurosurgery, The University of Texas M.D. Anderson Cancer Center, Houston, Texas

BENJAMIN Y. HUANG, MD, MPH
Associate Professor, Department of Radiology, University of North Carolina at Chapel Hill, Chapel Hill, North Carolina

MASARU ISHII, MD, PhD
Associate Professor, Department of Otolaryngology–Head and Neck Surgery, Johns Hopkins University School of Medicine, Baltimore, Maryland

JOHN A. JANE Jr, MD
Professor, Department of Neurosurgery, University of Virginia Health System, Charlottesville, Virginia

CRISTINE N. KLATT-CROMWELL, MD
Resident Physician, Department of Otolaryngology—Head and Neck Surgery, University of North Carolina at Chapel Hill, Chapel Hill, North Carolina

VARUN R. KSHETTRY, MD
Rosa Ella Burkhardt Brain Tumor and Neuro-Oncology Center, Cleveland Clinic, Cleveland, Ohio

DAVIDE LOCATELLI, MD
Department of Biotechnology and Life Sciences (DBSV), Head and Neck Surgery and Forensic Dissection Research center (HNS&FDRc); Department of Neurosurgery, University of Insubria, Varese, Italy

JOÃO MANGUSSI-GOMES, MD
São Paulo Skull Base Center; São Paulo ENT Center, Edmundo Vasconcelos Hospital, São Paulo, Brazil

PIERO NICOLAI, MD
Department of Otorhinolaryngology, University of Brescia, Brescia, Italy

RENATO HOFFMANN NUNES, MD
Department of Radiology, University of North Carolina at Chapel Hill, Chapel Hill, North Carolina; Radiology Program Coordinator; Radiologist, Division of Neuroradiology, Fleury Medicina e Saúde, Serviço de Diagnostico por Imagem, Santa Casa de Misericórdia de São Paulo, São Paulo, São Paulo, Brazil

GURSTON G. NYQUIST, MD
Department of Otolaryngology, Thomas Jefferson University, Philadelphia, Pennsylvania

CHIRAG R. PATEL, MD
Clinical Instructor, Department of Otolaryngology; Center for Cranial Base Surgery, University of Pittsburgh Medical Center, Pittsburgh, Pennsylvania

SPENCER C. PAYNE, MD
Associate Professor, Department of Otolaryngology - Head and Neck Surgery, University of Virginia Health System, Charlottesville, Virginia

MARC POLIVKA, MD
Department of Pathology, Lariboisière Hospital, Paris, France

DANIEL M. PREVEDELLO, MD
Departments of Neurosurgery and Otolaryngology–Head and Neck Surgery, Wexner Medical Center at the Ohio State University, Columbus, Ohio

SHAAN M. RAZA, MD
Departments of Neurosurgery and Head and Neck Surgery, The University of Texas M.D. Anderson Cancer Center, Houston, Texas

PABLO F. RECINOS, MD
Section of Rhinology, Sinus and Skull Base Surgery, Head and Neck Institute; Co-Director, Minimally Invasive Cranial Base and Pituitary Surgery Program, Burkhardt Brain Tumor and Neuro-Oncology Center, Neurological Institute, Cleveland Clinic, Cleveland, Ohio

DOUGLAS D. REH, MD
Associate Professor, Department of Otolaryngology–Head and Neck Surgery, Johns Hopkins University School of Medicine, Baltimore, Maryland

MARC R. ROSEN, MD
Department of Otolaryngology, Thomas Jefferson University, Philadelphia, Pennsylvania

CHRISTOPHER R. ROXBURY, MD
Department of Otolaryngology–Head and Neck Surgery, Johns Hopkins University School of Medicine, Baltimore, Maryland

DEANNA SASAKI-ADAMS, MD
Assistant Professor, Department of Neurosurgery, University of North Carolina at Chapel Hill, Chapel Hill, North Carolina

THEODORE H. SCHWARTZ, MD
Departments of Neurosurgery, Otolaryngology–Head and Neck Surgery, and Neuroscience, New York Presbyterian Hospital, Weill Medical College of Cornell University, New York, New York

MICHAEL F. SHRIVER, BS
Case Western Reserve University School of Medicine, Cleveland, Ohio

RAJ SINDWANI, MD, FACS
Vice Chairman and Section Head, Rhinology, Sinus and Skull Base Surgery, Head and Neck Institute; Co-Director, Minimally Invasive Cranial Base and Pituitary Surgery Program, Burkhardt Brain Tumor and Neuro-Oncology Center, Neurological Institute, Cleveland Clinic, Cleveland, Ohio

ALDO C. STAMM, MD, PhD
São Paulo Skull Base Center; São Paulo ENT Center, Edmundo Vasconcelos Hospital, São Paulo, Brazil

JANALEE K. STOKKEN, MD
Assistant Professor, Department of Otolaryngology, Head and Neck Surgery, Mayo Clinic, Rochester, Minnesota

SHIRLEY Y. SU, MD
Department of Head and Neck Surgery, The University of Texas M.D. Anderson Cancer Center, Houston, Texas

BRIAN D. THORP, MD
Fellow Physician, Department of Otolaryngology—Head and Neck Surgery, University of North Carolina at Chapel Hill, Chapel Hill, North Carolina

DUC A. TIEN, MD
Resident Physician, Section of Rhinology, Sinus and Skull Base Surgery, Head and Neck Institute, Cleveland Clinic Foundation, Cleveland, Ohio

MARIO TURRI-ZANONI, MD
Unit of Otorhinolaryngology, Department of Biotechnology and Life Sciences (DBSV), Ospedale di Circolo e Fondazione Macchi; Department of Biotechnology and Life Sciences (DBSV), Head and Neck Surgery and Forensic Dissection Research Center (HNS&FDRc), University of Insubria, Varese, Italy

EDUARDO A.S. VELLUTINI, MD, PhD
São Paulo Skull Base Center; DFVneuro Neurosurgical Group, São Paulo, Brazil

ERIC W. WANG, MD, FACS
Associate Professor, Department of Otolaryngology; Center for Cranial Base Surgery, University of Pittsburgh Medical Center, Pittsburgh, Pennsylvania

WEI-HSIN WANG, MD
Visiting Research Fellow, Surgical Neuroanatomy Lab, Department of Neurological Surgery, University of Pittsburgh Medical Center, Pittsburgh, Pennsylvania; Department of Neurosurgery, Neurological Institute, Taipei Veterans General Hospital, National Yang-Ming University, Taipei, Taiwan

TROY D. WOODARD, MD, FACS
Section of Rhinology, Sinus and Skull Base Surgery, Head and Neck Institute; Minimally
Invasive Cranial Base and Pituitary Surgery Program, Burkhardt Brain Tumor and
Neuro-Oncology Center, Neurological Institute, Cleveland Clinic, Cleveland, Ohio

BRAD E. ZACHARIA, MD, MS
Department of Neurosurgery, Penn State Hershey Medical Center, Hershey, Pennsylvania

ADAM M. ZANATION, MD
Associate Professor, Departments of Otolaryngology—Head and Neck Surgery and
Neurosurgery, University of North Carolina at Chapel Hill, Chapel Hill, North Carolina

Contents

Building an endoscopic cranial base practice can be challenging and is predicated on the right team. Successful outcomes stem from an efficient and talented team that improves its skills experientially in a supportive environment. As with most new endeavors that are beyond the traditional approach, there is a great deal of up-front effort and investment required. This article explores some of the key building blocks necessary for a successful endoscopic cranial base and pituitary program and highlights some of the lessons learned during the authors' journey at the Cleveland Clinic.

The anatomy of the skull base is complex with multiple neurovascular structures in a small space. Understanding all of the intricate relationships begins with understanding the anatomy of the sphenoid bone. The cavernous sinus contains the carotid artery and some of its branches; cranial nerves III, IV, VI, and V1; and transmits venous blood from multiple sources. The anterior skull base extends to the frontal sinus and is important to understand for sinus surgery and sinonasal malignancies. The clivus protects the brainstem and posterior cranial fossa. A thorough appreciation of the anatomy of these various areas allows for endoscopic endonasal approaches to the skull base.

The pituitary gland functions prominently in the control of most endocrine systems in the body. Diverse processes such as metabolism, growth, reproduction, and water balance are tightly regulated by the pituitary in conjunction with the hypothalamus and various downstream endocrine organs. Benign tumors of the pituitary gland are the primary cause of pituitary pathology and can result in inappropriate secretion of pituitary hormones or loss of pituitary function. First-line management of clinically significant tumors often involves surgical resection. Understanding of normal pituitary physiology and basic testing strategies to assess for pituitary dysfunction should be familiar to any skull base surgeon.

Endoscopic endonasal approaches are widely accepted techniques for managing benign and malignant processes along the ventral skull base, providing similar or better results compared with open procedures with lower rates of complication. Evaluating and managing pathology affecting the skull base can be challenging because of the region's complex anatomy and proximity to critical neurovascular structures. Furthermore, postoperative assessment can be challenging because of surgical alterations of normal anatomy and complex reconstruction techniques currently being employed. Understanding the normal imaging appearance of skull base reconstruction is important for accurate postoperative interpretation and delineation between normal reconstructive tissue and recurrent neoplasm.

The sellar region is a tiny anatomic compartment in which many lesions and developmental diseases can be found. If pituitary adenomas represent most of the sellar mass, it is important to recognize other pathologic conditions before any surgical procedure, because the optimal treatment may differ considerably from one lesion to another. A careful clinical evaluation followed by neuroimaging studies and an endocrinologic and ophtalmologic workup will lead, in most cases, to a diagnosis with near certainty. This article provides an overview of sellar diseases with emphasis on their most useful characteristics for clinical practice.

Since the description of a transnasal approach for treatment of pituitary tumors, transsphenoidal surgery has undergone continuous development. Hirsch developed a lateral endonasal approach before simplifying it to a transseptal approach. Cushing approached pituitary tumors using a transsphenoidal approach but transitioned to the transcranial route. Transsphenoidal surgery was not "rediscovered" until Hardy introduced the surgical microscope. An endoscopic transsphenoidal approach for pituitary tumors has been reported and further advanced. We describe the principles of pituitary surgery including the key elements of surgical decision making and discuss the technical nuances distinguishing the endoscopic from the microscopic approach.

Endoscopic endonasal skull base surgery has dramatically changed and expanded over recent years due to significant advancements in instrumentation, techniques, and anatomic understanding. With these advances, the need for more robust skull base reconstructive techniques was vital. In this article, reconstructive options ranging from acellular grafts to vascular flaps are described, including the strengths, weaknesses, and common uses.

Before the vascularized pedicled nasoseptal flap was popularized, lumbar drains (LDs) were routinely used for cerebral spinal fluid (CSF) diversion in endoscopic skull base reconstruction. LDs are not necessary in most CSF leaks encountered during skull base surgery. The use of an LD is considered in select high-risk settings in which a high-flow leak is anticipated and the patient has significant risk factors that make closure of the leak more challenging. Evidence for the use of LDs in preventing postoperative after endoscopic skull base reconstruction is reviewed and a rational framework for their use is proposed.

The nasal cavity has a robust vascular supply, and bleeding is a primary obstacle to the minimally invasive skull base technique. Venous bleeding, including the cavernous sinus, can be managed with various techniques using hemostatic materials and pressure. A thorough understanding of the skull base vascular anatomy is vital for avoiding injury to major arteries and having confidence to control venous bleeding to optimize the endoscopic view and tumor resection.

Meningiomas represent 30% of all primary brain tumors. Anterior skull base meningiomas represent 8.8% of all meningiomas. Surgical resection is a main treatment option for tumors that are symptomatic and/or growing. Recurrence is directly related to the extent of resection of the tumor, the dural attachment, and pathologic bone. Endoscopic endonasal approaches represent an important addition to the treatment armamentarium for skull base meningiomas. This article provides an overview of meningiomas, with a focus on those of the anterior skull base and their management.

Esthesioneuroblastoma is a rare malignant tumor of sinonasal origin. These tumors typically present with unilateral nasal obstruction and epistaxis, and diagnosis is confirmed on biopsy. Over the past 15 years, significant advances have been made in endoscopic technology and techniques that have made this tumor amenable to expanded endonasal resection. There is growing evidence supporting the feasibility of safe

> The endoscopic endonasal approach provides a direct surgical trajectory to anteriorly located lesions at the craniovertebral junction. The inferior limit of surgical exposure is predicted by the nasopalatine line, and the lateral limit is demarcated by the lower cranial nerves. Endoscopic endonasal odontoidectomy allows greater preservation of the soft palate, and patients can restart an oral diet on the first postoperative day. Treating pathologies at the craniovertebral junction using this approach requires careful preoperative planning and endoscopic endonasal surgical experience with a 2-surgeon 4-handed approach combining expertise in otolaryngology and neurosurgery.

> Endoscopic endonasal approaches to the skull base pathology have developed and evolved dramatically over the past 2 decades, particularly with collaboration between neurosurgery and otolaryngology physicians. These advances have increased significantly the use of such approaches beyond just resection of pituitary adenomas, including a variety of skull base pathologies. As the field has evolved, so has our understanding of the complications accompanying endoscopic skull base surgery, as well as techniques to both avoid and manage these complications. These are discussed here.

> Injury of the internal carotid artery during endoscopic endonasal skull base surgery is a feared and perilous scenario. This article discusses perioperative strategies to prevent or manage an internal carotid artery injury to optimize outcomes. Meticulous preoperative planning is crucial in preventing its occurrence and minimizing its consequences. An effective plan of action relies on a well-prepared protocol, availability of proper instruments and devices, and an experienced multidisciplinary team. Intraoperative control of hemorrhage and stabilization of the patient's cardiovascular status is followed by an angiography and endovascular treatment whenever possible. Close clinical and radiologic monitoring of the patient prevents early and late complications.

> To maximize outcomes from endoscopic skull base surgery, careful early postoperative management is critically important. Standardized postoperative regimens are lacking. The type of reconstruction and presence and type of cerebrospinal fluid leak dictate management. If a leak is

encountered intraoperatively, patients should avoid maneuvers that increase intracranial pressures for at least 1 month. Early postoperative care focuses on minimizing and managing nasal crusting. This article reviews the evidence in the literature on postoperative management, complications, and quality of life after surgery, and outlines our experience in the management of patients after endoscopic skull base surgery.

OTOLARYNGOLOGIC CLINICS
OF NORTH AMERICA

RELATED INTEREST

Endocrinology and Metabolism Clinics of North America
March 2015 (Vol. 44, Issue 1)
Pituitary Disorders
Anat Ben-Shlomo and Maria Fleseriu, *Editors*
Available at: http://www.endo.theclinics.com/

THE CLINICS ARE AVAILABLE ONLINE!
Access your subscription at:
www.theclinics.com

OTOLARYNGOLOGIC CLINICS
OF NORTH AMERICA

FORTHCOMING ISSUES

April 2017
Comprehensive Management of Parotid Disorders
Babak Larian and Babak Azizzadeh, Editors

June 2016
Hemostasis in Head and Neck Surgery
Carl H. Snyderman and Harshita Pant, Editors

August 2016
Frontal Sinus and Skull Base Disease
Editors

RECENT ISSUES

December 2015
Hearing Loss in Children
Bradley W. Kesser and Margaret A. Kenna, Editors

October 2015
Medical and Surgical Complications in the Treatment of Chronic Rhinosinusitis
James A. Stankiewicz, Editor

August 2015
Function Preservation in Laryngeal Cancer
Babak Sadoughi, Editor

RELATED INTEREST

Otolaryngologic Clinics of North America
Month/Volume, Year Issue XX
Pituitary Diseases
Author Name and Name, Guest Editors
Available at: http://www.xxxxxxx.theclinics.org

THE CLINICS ARE AVAILABLE ONLINE
Access your subscription at:
www.theclinics.com

Preface

Endoscopic Cranial Base and Pituitary Surgery

 CrossMark

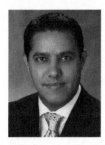 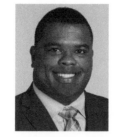 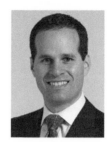

Raj Sindwani, MD, FACS   Troy D. Woodard, MD, FACS   Pablo F. Recinos, MD
Editors

Over the past two decades, there has been a dramatic evolution in the manner through which cranial base pathologies are approached and managed. The development of the endoscope, stereotactic navigation systems, and innovative surgical techniques has facilitated the transition from traditional open surgeries to minimally invasive endoscopic approaches. Not only does this expansion in practice translate into an exciting time for skull-base surgeons, but it also offers the promise of a more streamlined approach to comprehensive patient care, improved patient satisfaction and experience, and superior outcomes. The modern era of endoscopic skull-base surgery has also witnessed an unparalleled partnership between the specialties of otolaryngology and neurosurgery. Beyond even this core dyad, however, the complex nature of endoscopic skull-base surgery necessitates a cohesive multidisciplinary team consisting of otolaryngologists, neurosurgeons, ophthalmologists, endocrinologists, medical and radiation oncologists, and pathologists. Successful implementation of a skull-base program and management of these patients require a collaborative approach and valuable contributions from several medical and surgical disciplines.

Along this central theme of partnership, the articles in this unique issue of *Otolaryngologic Clinics of North America* are coauthored by tandems of experienced otolaryngologists and neurosurgeons who each bring their perspectives to bear on the foundational topics of 2-surgeon endoscopic skull-base surgery. Infused with the knowledge and wisdom of global thought leaders in the field, it was our mission to provide a conglomerate of articles that could serve as an authoritative resource to practitioners performing endoscopic skull-base procedures. The outcome is this insightful text, which explores key topics ranging from programmatic issues such as team-building and coordinated billing to clinical pearls on the management of internal carotid artery injury and nuances of complex skull-base reconstruction. We are

Otolaryngol Clin N Am 49 (2016) xix–xx
http://dx.doi.org/10.1016/j.otc.2015.09.017
0030-6665/16/$ – see front matter © 2016 Published by Elsevier Inc.

immensely grateful to our distinguished colleagues and friends for their contributions to this important project—your time and dedication are very much appreciated.

The whole is greater than the sum of its parts.
—Aristotle

Raj Sindwani, MD, FACS
Head and Neck Institute
Cleveland Clinic
9500 Euclid Avenue, A-71
Cleveland, OH 44195, USA

Troy D. Woodard, MD, FACS
Head and Neck Institute
Cleveland Clinic
9500 Euclid Avenue, A-71
Cleveland, OH 44195, USA

Pablo F. Recinos, MD
Head and Neck Institute
Cleveland Clinic
9500 Euclid Avenue, S-73
Cleveland, OH 44195, USA

E-mail addresses:
sindwar@ccf.org (R. Sindwani)
woodart@ccf.org (T.D. Woodard)
recinop@ccf.org (P.F. Recinos)

Building a Successful Endoscopic Skull Base and Pituitary Surgery Practice

Raj Sindwani, MD[a,b,]*, Troy D. Woodard, MD[a,b],
Pablo F. Recinos, MD[a,b]

KEYWORDS

- Endoscopic skull base surgery • Cranial base surgery
- Minimally invasive skull base surgery • Building a practice • 2-surgeon approach
- Lessons learned

KEY POINTS

- Building an endoscopic cranial base practice can be challenging and is predicated on the right team of neurosurgeon and rhinologist.
- Requisites for a successful program include a dedicated multidisciplinary team of people and institutional and departmental support.
- Endoscopic cranial base programs can greatly enhance resident and fellow training by offering a broader surgical experience and perspective with the management of multiple disease entities and also allowing the acquisition of novel technical skills, such as bimanual endoscopic surgery through the nose.
- Successful outcomes stem from an attentive, efficient, and dedicated team that improves its skills experientially in a supportive environment.
- The advantages of endoscopic approaches to the skull base are becoming more established, and interest in offering an endoscopic skull base experience to patients in medical centers is growing.

INTRODUCTION

Endoscopic approaches to the skull base have become a central component in providing comprehensive care to patients with skull base pathologic conditions. Although early pioneers of endoscopic skull base surgery focused on establishing

Funding Sources: None.
[a] Section of Rhinology, Sinus and Skull Base Surgery, Head and Neck Institute, Cleveland Clinic, 9500 Euclid Avenue, A71, Cleveland, OH 44195, USA; [b] Minimally Invasive Cranial Base and Pituitary Surgery Program, Rose Ella Burkhardt Brain Tumor & Neuro-Oncology Center, Cleveland Clinic, 9500 Euclid Avenue, S73, Cleveland, OH 44195, USA
* Corresponding author. Head and Neck Institute, Cleveland Clinic Foundation, 9500 Euclid Avenue, A-71, Cleveland, OH 44195.
E-mail address: sindwar@ccf.org

the feasibility and safety of these approaches,[1–4] the challenge of contemporary skull base practices is not *if* but *how* to integrate endoscopic techniques into their paradigm of patient care. Setting up a multidisciplinary skull base practice that incorporates endoscopy, however, comes with greater challenges than those encountered by a single surgeon offering a new service. On the other hand, the increased options available to treat complex skull base pathology and the resultant benefit to patients provided by a team that successfully integrates both open and endoscopic skull base techniques far exceed the practice-building challenges that are initially faced. This article explores some of the key building blocks (the *who, what, when, where,* and *how*) necessary for a successful endoscopic cranial base and pituitary program and highlights some of the lessons learned during the authors' journey at the Cleveland Clinic.

WHO

The key ingredient to building a successful endoscopic skull base program, or any program for that matter, is the people. In the case of endoscopic skull base surgery, this relationship centers on the partnership between the otolaryngologist and the neurosurgeon. The team must have a unified vision of what a successful program looks like. At its foundation, the partners must have mutual respect for one another and understand how each person contributes to the team. A clear example of this team approach is demonstrated in the operating room (OR) during pituitary surgery. Traditionally, this surgery was performed in a sequential manner via a transseptal, transnasal, or sublabial approach, which was subsequently followed by microscopic resection of the tumor.[5–7] These two roles were clearly defined and performed by each surgical team with minimal overlap. While the otolaryngologist opened and closed the surgical defect, the neurosurgeon resected the tumor. This procedure is in stark contrast to the way surgery is currently performed in a growing number of centers. Endoscopic skull base surgery involves constant overlap of the disciplines and frequent simultaneous 2-surgeon surgery using 3- and 4-handed techniques. This model only works with partners who are both committed to using a team approach.

Of course the skull base team extends far beyond the dyad of neurosurgeon and rhinologist (**Fig. 1**). Close interplay with many other specialty and hospital services, both on the outpatient and inpatient sides, is necessary. Additionally, the skull base neurosurgeon generally will initially evaluate referrals of primary intracranial pathology (pituitary tumors, meningiomas, chordomas, and so forth), whereas the skull base rhinologist will contribute referrals of primary sinonasal pathology (complex

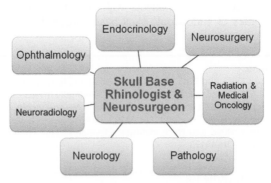

Fig. 1. Multidisciplinary network of specialists that support a robust endoscopic skull base program.

cerebrospinal fluid leaks, sinonasal tumors, and so forth). However, as the joint skull base practice develops, patients are often referred to a skull base surgeon, irrespective of their subspecialty (eg, sinonasal referrals to the neurosurgeon and pituitary tumors to the rhinologist); significant cross-pollination and a melding of practices begins to occur. As a result, close communication and interaction is required between both disciplines. This communication allows the team to more easily and effectively manage these patients. The benefits from the joint management of these patients transcend the typical limitations of each individual specialty.[8] Both the skull base rhinologist and neurosurgeon should also strive to increase interaction and collaboration with other otolaryngologists, neurosurgeons, endocrinologists, ophthalmologists, radiation, and medical oncology in order to increase awareness and collaborate together in care of patients with skull base pathology.[9]

Other requirements for a successful program include institutional and departmental support and tireless multispecialty teamwork. The interplay between departments must happen seamlessly at all levels: from leadership to midlevel providers, from residents to schedulers, from OR support staff to nursing staff, from anesthesiologists to primary care providers, and even among billing staff. All personnel must understand the importance of the team approach. The authors advise spending time getting to know the other players on the team through a variety of face-to-face methods, including having trainees, nursing staff, and midlevel providers spend time in the neurosurgery and otolaryngology clinics, doing team-building exercises/retreats, having OR in-service educational sessions, and attending one another's grand rounds. In fact, the authors think it is equally important to have *joint appointments* for the professional staff in one another's departments to overtly show the intricate partnership that is being forged. This newly formed partnership may also become a model that could help foster other relationships between department members. A prime example has occurred at the Cleveland Clinic. The authors' endoscopic neurosurgeon also works very closely with the lateral skull base surgeons, and their rhinologists are called on to manage anterior cranial fossa cerebrospinal fluid leaks endoscopically that occur in the setting of open approaches by other neurosurgeons.

WHAT

Adequate planning and a thorough understanding of resource requirements and their allocation are critical because they will make the difference between a successful joint skull base practice and one that struggles. In the operating suite, an up-front investment in purchasing equipment is essential. The must-have instruments include full skull base endoscopic instrument sets, endoscopic drills, shavers, and stereotactic neuronavigation with ability to fuse MRI and computed tomography images. Often this initial capital investment is more obtainable if a detailed business plan that includes the benefits of an endoscopic skull base practice is presented to the hospital before the development of the center. Other equipment that is very useful (but not necessarily immediately necessary) includes ultrasonic aspirators and non–heat-generating, oscillating, cutting, and tissue removal instruments. In addition, a fully integrated endoscopic OR suite (**Fig. 2**), which connects audio, video, and medical equipment in a more efficient way using booms, is certainly nice to have but not a necessity. Multiple monitors and panels throughout the suite facilitate surgeon-to-surgeon and surgeon-to-surgical team member interactions in an ergonomic setting. Observer education can also be enhanced through multiple wall-mounted monitors (**Fig. 3**). With the use of high-definition and enhanced video processing technology, crisp visualization of the endoscopic image

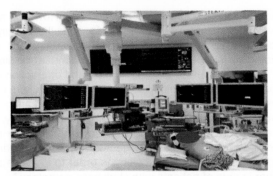

Fig. 2. Fully integrated endoscopic OR suite used for endoscopic skull base procedures at the Cleveland Clinic. Multiple monitors and panels throughout the suite facilitate surgeon-to-surgeon and surgeon-to-surgical team member interactions in an ergonomic setting. Wall-mounted high-definition monitors also enhance educational value to observers.

is further possible. Having a dedicated endoscopic OR suite with built-ins ensures all necessary equipment is always present and can greatly increase the efficiency of endoscopic skull base cases.

Perhaps one of the most meaningful decisions that impacts the long-term relationship of the otolaryngologist and the neurosurgeon is how to approach billing and reimbursement. The authors think that the best manner in which value and respect for the tandem is exemplified is in the equitable sharing of the professional reimbursement for procedures performed together. Admittedly, splitting the professional component of the fees is more readily accomplished in a salaried (nonincentivized) model such as the one in place at the Cleveland Clinic. However, a nonequal split or a case-by-

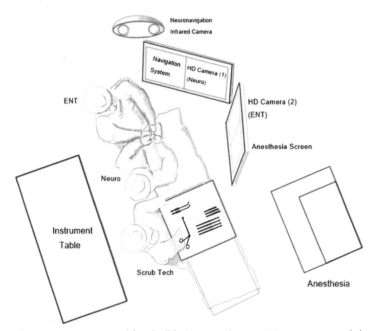

Fig. 3. Endoscopic OR setup used for skull base procedures. ENT, ears, nose, and throat; HD, high definition. (*Courtesy of* Ghaith Habboub, Cleveland, OH.)

case split inevitably forces a clear but artificial delineation of surgical roles. By not splitting the fees equitably, there is a risk that one party will not be as invested and possibly even consider alternative ways to spend their valuable time generating more revenue. This result, of course, would be a major detractor for the program and could fundamentally undermine the team concept. To prevent this distraction, the authors share the professional component of their charges evenly (50/50) and use the 2-surgeon modifier for all of their codes, when permissible. Other tips that may be helpful include the *coordinated* submission of charges to the insurance company from both departments to avoid unnecessary denials, delays, or circumstances in which one bill is paid and the other is not. Furthermore, the charges are sent out on the same day, with the same codes and the same supporting paperwork. Additionally, close follow-up throughout the complete billing process is imperative and should fall under the auspices of both departments.

WHEN

Logistical coordination and sharing of resources is essential to provide a seamless and efficient experience for patients with skull base pathologies. Coordination of operative days and sharing of OR block time between the otolaryngologist and neurosurgeon removes the uncertainty of surgical scheduling and allows for a higher volume of work to be performed more efficiently by staggering cases.

Other essential aspects that should be in place include having joint clinic days with referring specialists (eg, joint clinics between neurosurgery, otolaryngology, and endocrinology). This practice allows flexibility to add new patients in a same-day or timely manner, which is of special importance in settings where patients come from great distances for consultation. Priority is given to these patients so that they are not burdened by unnecessary scheduling obstacles and delayed treatment and to enhance the overall patient experience throughout the continuum of care.

Lastly, clinical care pathways are vital for successful implementation of skull base programs. They have become increasingly popular over the past few decades. The aim of these pathways is to enhance the quality of patient care by the implementation of protocols designed to easily guide patients through each stage of their care. Clinical care pathways are not only designed for increased patient safety and patient satisfaction but also allow for optimization of resources and a broader improvement of clinical outcomes. The authors have used these care paths to create a systematic approach to obtain preoperative medical clearance, preoperative imaging studies for neuronavigation, joint preoperative and education discussions (so as not to confuse patients by giving mixed opinions and expectations), and pre-established follow-up plans that include scheduling all postoperative visits preoperatively. Ultimately, appropriate planning and coordination of care makes this complex process translate into a streamlined patient experience, resulting in better care for individual patients and more efficient care delivery for the health system.[10]

HOW

Before establishing an endoscopic skull base program, it is imperative to obtain appropriate advanced training and exposure to contemporary endoscopic techniques. Although the pioneers of endoscopic skull base surgery had to break known barriers of surgery and explore unknown territories, it is no longer necessary or reasonable for current surgeons to repeat the mistakes of ignorance due to inadequate training. One option to gain fundamental exposure to endoscopic skull base surgery is to participate in an endoscopic skull base course that integrates cadaveric dissection. Many of these courses cover cross-disciplinary concepts in anatomy and surgical technique as well as encourage joint otolaryngology/neurosurgery team participation. They also allow experience with dealing with certain scenarios that may be unfamiliar to the surgeons (eg, dealing with emergencies such as pituitary apoplexy for the otolaryngologist or the workup and management of sinonasal pathology for the neurosurgeon). Participating as a team in one of the skull base courses is an excellent opportunity for the partners to work together in a safe environment and affords the opportunity to develop the joint vision and a shared operative philosophy. For more formal and extensive training, there are numerous clinical fellowships that incorporate endoscopic skull base surgery into their curriculum. These fellowships are available through the American Rhinologic Society[11] and the North American Skull Base Society.[12]

When starting to do endoscopic skull base surgery, it is wise to progress in a stepwise manner, starting with less complicated cases initially and gradually progressing to more difficult cases. This manner allows the team to learn to work together and focus on foundational elements, such as OR set up, where to stand, how to move instruments within the nose in concert, and so forth, rather than being overly distracted by the complexity of the procedure itself. Snyderman and colleagues[13] have categorized cases based on the level of difficulty and proposed a helpful stepwise approach to acquire the necessary skills to perform complex endoscopic skull base procedures.

WHY

There are clear advantages of using the endoscopic approach to the skull base. Primary reasons include improved patient care and patient experience. In addition to enhanced visualization through illumination and angled views, endoscopic approaches have been shown to positively impact outcomes in a variety of pathologies.[14–19] The team approach to skull base surgery allows each discipline to complement each other. A key example of the interplay between surgeons includes the endoscopic neurosurgeon offering expertise in the tumor removal, while the otolaryngologist creatively reconstructs the complex skull base defects while minimizing negative impact on nasal physiology.

A robust minimally invasive cranial base and pituitary surgery program can also greatly enhance academic training programs. Performing 2-surgeon tandem endoscopic cranial base and pituitary surgery provides a special environment for neurosurgery and otolaryngology trainees and is a unique opportunity for growth both intellectually and technically (**Fig. 4**). Each specialty contributes an otherwise foreign dimension of knowledge and perspective that would not have been learned had these procedures been completed in a separate traditional manner. The authors' trainees have greatly benefitted from the cross-pollination of ideas between disciplines. Attending lectures and performing cadaver dissection courses together are also strongly encouraged. Examples of this intermingling include otolaryngology residents and fellows getting experience with the tumor resection and neurosurgery trainees learning the fundamentals of endoscopic surgery in the sinus cavities and how to raise nasoseptal flaps. Another novel skill set that trainees develop when operating in this manner is the unique ability to operate bimanually in the nose. Bimanual manipulation allows for greater control and manipulation of tissue. Bimanual endoscopic surgery skills traditionally have not been a skill set that is garnered during otolaryngology residency training or even rhinology fellowships. However, the authors have gained an appreciation for the utilization of this technique and now use the 2-surgeon bimanual approach for a variety of operations, even when they are not working with their neurosurgeon, and have recently published on the advantages of this approach for non–skull base procedures including endoscopic orbital surgery.[20]

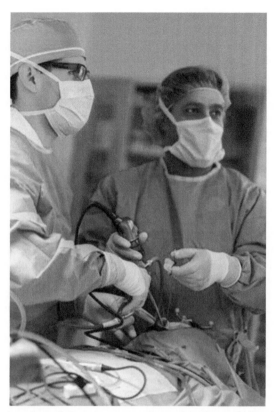

Fig. 4. Intraoperative view of the surgeon tandem using the multi-handed technique for endoscopic skull base surgery.

Expanding scientific publications, increasing patient word of mouth via electronic social outlets, and organized marketing campaigns from several large centers continue to highlight the advantages of endoscopic over traditional approaches to the skull base. The reputational and financial advantages of performing these complex operations have made it onto the radar screens of departmental and institutional leaders alike. The endoscopic approach to the cranial base will continue to proliferate and change the way we treat many patients in the years to come.

SUMMARY

Endoscopic skull base programs are valuable assets in the management of patients with complex neurologic and sinonasal pathologies. Not only do they allow contributions from 2 disciplines but they can also result in a more streamlined approach to comprehensive patient care, improved patient satisfaction, and improved outcomes. As with most new endeavors that are beyond the traditional approach, there is a great deal of up-front effort and investment required. A collaborative environment and understanding of required resources are essential to the development of a successful program.

REFERENCES

1. Jho HD, Carrau RL. Endoscopic endonasal transsphenoidal surgery: experience with 50 patients. J Neurosurg 1997;87:44–51.

2. Jho HD, Carrau RL. Endoscopy assisted transsphenoidal surgery for pituitary adenoma. Technical note. Acta Neurochir 1996;138:1416–25.
3. Kassam A, Gardner P, Snyderman C, et al. Endoscopic, expanded endonasal approach to the jugular foramen. Oper Tech Neurosurg 2005;8:35–41.
4. Kassam AB, Gardner P, Snyderman C, et al. Expanded endonasal approach: fully endoscopic, completely transnasal approach to the middle third of the clivus, petrous bone, middle cranial fossa, and infratemporal fossa. Neurosurg Focus 2005;19(1):E6.
5. Hirsch O. Endonasal method of removal of hypophyseal tumors. With a report of two successful cases. JAMA 1910;5:772–4.
6. Halstead A. Remarks on the operative treatment of tumors of the hypophysis. With the report of two cases operated on by an oronasal method. Trans Am Surg Assoc 1910;28:73–93.
7. Henderson WR. The pituitary adenomata. A follow-up study of the surgical results in 338 cases (Dr. Harvey Cushing's series). Br J Surg 1939;26(104):811–921.
8. McLaughlin N, Carrau RL, Kelly DF, et al. Teamwork in skull base surgery: an avenue for improvement in patient care. Surg Neurol Int 2013;4:36.
9. McLaughlin N, Laws ER, Oyesiku NM, et al. Pituitary centers of excellence. Neurosurgery 2012;71:916–24.
10. Rajasekaran K, Revenaugh P, Benninger MS, et al. Development of a quality care plan to reduce otolaryngologic readmissions: early lessons from the Cleveland Clinic. Otolaryngol Head Neck Surg 2015. [Epub ahead of print].
11. Available at: http://www.american-rhinologic.org/program_listing. Accessed October 26, 2015.
12. Rajasekaran K, Revenaugh P, Benninger M, et al. Development of a Quality Care Plan to Reduce Otolaryngologic Readmissions: Early Lessons from the Cleveland Clinic. Otolaryngol Head Neck Surg 2015;153(4):629–35. Available at: http://www.nasbs.org/nasbs-skull-base-fellowship-registry. Accessed October 26, 2015.
13. Snyderman C, Kassam A, Carrau R, et al. Acquisition of surgical skills for endonasal skull base surgery: a training program. Laryngoscope 2007;117(4):699–705.
14. Clark AJ, Jahangiri A, Garcia RM, et al. Endoscopic surgery for tuberculum sellae meningiomas: a systematic review and meta-analysis. Neurosurg Rev 2013;36:349–59.
15. Komotar RJ, Starke RM, Raper DM, et al. Endoscopic endonasal compared with microscopic transsphenoidal and open transcranial resection of craniopharyngiomas. World Neurosurg 2012;77:329–41.
16. Komotar RJ, Starke RM, Raper DM, et al. Endoscopic endonasal compared with microscopic transsphenoidal and open transcranial resection of giant pituitary adenomas. Pituitary 2012;15:150–9.
17. Komotar RJ, Starke RM, Raper DM, et al. Endoscopic endonasal versus open transcranial resection of anterior midline skull base meningiomas. World Neurosurg 2012;77:713–24.
18. McLaughlin N, Eisenberg AA, Cohan P, et al. Value of endoscopy for maximizing tumor removal in endonasal transsphenoidal pituitary adenoma surgery. J Neurosurg 2013;118:613–20.
19. Eytan DF, Kshettry VR, Sindwani R, et al. Surgical outcomes after endoscopic management of cholesterol granulomas of the petrous apex: a systematic review. Neurosurg Focus 2014;37(4):E14.
20. Stokken J, Gumber D, Antisdel J, et al. Endoscopic surgery of the orbital apex: outcomes and emerging techniques. Laryngoscope, in press.

Skull Base Anatomy

Chirag R. Patel, MD[a,b], Juan C. Fernandez-Miranda, MD[b,c],
Wei-Hsin Wang, MD[c,d], Eric W. Wang, MD[a,b,*]

KEYWORDS

- Endoscopic endonasal • Skull base • Cranial base • Anatomy • Pituitary
- Cavernous • Sella

KEY POINTS

- The sphenoid bone is at the center of the skull base and understanding its anatomy from multiple perspectives is important to understanding endonasal approaches.
- Within the sphenoid sinus, the lateral opticocarotid recess is a key landmark for identifying the locations of the parasellar carotid artery and optic nerve.
- The tuberculum sella is the anterior and superior limit of the sella. Limited removal of the tuberculum during pituitary surgery helps avoid CSF leak, while complete removal allows for access to the suprasellar space.
- The major neurovascular structures of the cavernous sinus are located in the lateral compartment and lateral wall.
- The clivus can be divided into thirds. The upper third corresponds to the dorsum sella, the middle third is in the sphenoid sinus below the sella, and the lower third behind the nasopharynx.

INTRODUCTION

The nasal cavity has been used as a corridor to access the midline skull base since the turn of the twentieth century. The transsphenoidal route to the pituitary was initially explored in the 1890s because of the high mortality associated with early transcranial approaches. Although the transsphenoidal approach showed some

Disclosure Statement: The authors have nothing to disclose.
[a] Department of Otolaryngology, University of Pittsburgh Medical Center, 200 Lothrop Street, Suite 500, Pittsburgh, PA 15213, USA; [b] Center for Cranial Base Surgery, University of Pittsburgh Medical Center, 200 Lothrop Street, Suite 500, Pittsburgh, PA 15213, USA; [c] Surgical Neuro-anatomy Lab, Department of Neurological Surgery, University of Pittsburgh Medical Center, 200 Lothrop Street, PUH B-400, Pittsburgh, PA 15213, USA; [d] Department of Neurosurgery, Neurological Institute, Taipei Veterans General Hospital, National Yang-Ming University, Taipei, Taiwan
* Corresponding author. Department of Otolaryngology, University of Pittsburgh Medical Center, 200 Lothrop Street, Suite 500, Pittsburgh, PA 15213.
E-mail address: wangew@upmc.edu

promise, it fell largely out of favor as neurosurgeons became increasingly proficient with transcranial approaches. It was not until the 1960s when Gerard Guiot was able to publish excellent results with the transsphenoidal approach that it began to regain popularity. He was also the first to report trying to use an endoscope in transsphenoidal surgery, but he abandoned it because of poor visualization compared with the microscope.[1]

It was also in the 1960s that Harold Hopkins introduced his rod-lens system, greatly improving on the prior 100 years of endoscopy. Combined with cameras and evolving video technology, endoscopy took a big step forward in the medical field. Otolaryngologists began using the rod-lens in the nasal cavity and endoscopic sinus surgery was born. Simultaneously, neurosurgeons began using these new endoscopes as adjuncts to their microscopic resections. These two parallel developments finally came together in the 1990s when the first multidisciplinary endoscopic skull base teams were formed.[2]

Endoscopic endonasal surgery has now become an invaluable alternate means of accessing and treating pathology of the skull base. It offers a direct route for accessing the anterior, middle, and posterior cranial fossa. It has been shown to be safe and effective, but requires a detailed understanding of the intricate anatomy to be successful. This article reviews the anatomy of the midline skull base from the frontal sinus to the clivus, with special attention to the endonasal perspective.

SPHENOID BONE

The sphenoid bone sits at the center of the skull base, and knowing its anatomy is central to understanding endonasal approaches. The sphenoid bone has been described as resembling a bat with its wings outstretched (**Fig. 1**). It consists of a central body, which is cuboidal in shape and houses the sphenoid sinus at its center. The sella turcica is located superiorly and the upper clivus posteriorly. The lesser wings extend from the superolateral aspect of the body and the greater wings from the inferior aspect of the body. The superior orbital fissure is the space between the greater and lesser wings. The paired pterygoid processes and pterygoid plates project downward from the body on either side.

The lesser wings extend laterally to form part of the floor of the anterior cranial fossa. The inferior surfaces of the lesser wings form the posterior roof of the orbits. Medially the lesser wings join with the planum sphenoidale, which forms the roof of the sphenoid sinus. The planum articulates anteriorly with the cribriform plate. At the posteromedial ends of the lesser wings are the anterior clinoid processes and the optic canals. The optic canals are separated from the superomedial aspect of the superior orbital

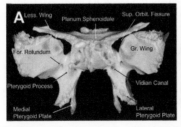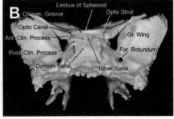

Fig. 1. (*A*) Sphenoid bone, anterior view. (*B*) Sphenoid bone, posterior view. Ant. Clin., anterior clinoid; Chiasm., chiasmatic; For., foramen; Gr., greater; Less., lesser; Post. Clin., posterior clinoid; Sup. Orbit., superior orbital; Tuber., tuberculum.

fissure by a piece of bone known as the optic strut. The optic strut extends from the body of the sphenoid to the base of the anterior clinoid. Between the two optic foramina is a shallow depression known as the chiasmatic groove or prechiasmatic sulcus. This groove is bounded by the planum sphenoidale anteriorly and tuberculum sella posteriorly.[3] At the junction of the prechiasmatic sulcus and planum sphenoidale is a bony ridge known as the limbus of the sphenoid.

When viewed from above, the center of the sphenoid body contains the sella turcica, a saddle shaped depression that houses the pituitary gland. It is bound anteriorly by the tuberculum sella and posteriorly by the dorsum sella. The dorsum sella also makes up the upper clivus. The posterior clinoid processes project from the superolateral aspects of the dorsum sella. On either side of the sella are the cavernous sinuses and the carotid arteries. The medial wall of the cavernous sinus marks the lateral boundary of the sella.[3,4]

In addition to the paired anterior and posterior clinoids, there is also a pair of middle clinoids. The middle clinoid is a variable length piece of bone that extends from the superolateral aspect of the sella toward the apex of the anterior clinoid. Its length can vary from being nonexistent to attaching to the anterior clinoid to form a complete osseous ring known as the caroticoclinoidal ring. The most common finding is a short segment of bone that does not extend all the way to the anterior clinoid. It is located at the inner bend of the anterior genu of the parasellar carotid as it loops around this middle clinoid. It is an important endonasal landmark because it marks the level of the roof of the cavernous sinus and the transition point between the cavernous and paraclinoidal segments of the internal carotid artery (ICA).[5]

The roof of the sella is formed by the diaphragma sella, a dural structure that extends from the tuberculum sella to the dorsum sella. It is continuous laterally with the roof of the cavernous sinus. In the center of the diaphragma is an opening known as the pituitary aperture, which transmits the pituitary stalk. This opening is variable in size and thickness. The arachnoid layer is located just above the diaphragma and so typically there is no cerebrospinal fluid (CSF) within the sella.[3,6]

SPHENOID SINUS

The sphenoid sinus varies considerably in size, shape, pneumatization, and septation. The degree of pneumatization varies with age, with most pneumatization occurring in adolescence. There are three types of pneumatization patterns in adults: conchal, presellar, and sellar. The conchal type has little to no pneumatization. The presellar type has some pneumatization but does not extend beyond the plane of the tuberculum sella. The sellar type is the most common and the cavity extends beyond the floor of the sella and often into the clivus creating a depression called the clival recess (**Fig. 2**A).

With greater pneumatization, the major sphenoid landmarks become more apparent (see **Fig. 2**). In the center of the sphenoid sinus is the sella turcica, which is a bulge into the sinus when viewed from below. Beneath the sella is the middle clivus and in most cases the clival recess. On either side of the clival recess is the bone that covers the vertical paraclival segment of ICA. As the carotid artery courses superiorly and enters the cavernous sinus, it turns and runs in a horizontal plane anteriorly before turning again and looping back on itself to go posteriorly. This loop occurs around the previously mentioned middle clinoid. This anterior genu of the carotid, which corresponds with the paraclinoidal segment, is the most superficial when viewed from the sphenoid sinus, and it often forms a prominence in the lateral sinus wall on either side of the sella.

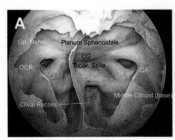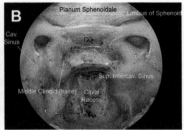

Fig. 2. (*A*) Sphenoid sinus. Note how the base of the middle clinoid sits at the inner aspect of the genu of the paraclinoidal segment of the carotid. (*B*) Sphenoid sinus with most of the bone removed. The tuberculum has been removed revealing the superior intercavernous sinus. Note the dural fold that corresponds to the bony limbus of the sphenoid, demarcating the transition from chiasmatic groove to planum sphenoidale. Cav., cavernous; CG, chiasmatic groove; OCR, opticocarotid recess; Op., optic; Sup. Intercav., superior intercavernous.

Above the prominence of the carotid runs the optic nerve prominence as it courses from the cisternal segment to the optic canal (see **Fig. 2**). Just lateral and between the carotid and optic nerve there is often a depression known as the opticocarotid recess (OCR). The OCR is the result of pneumatization of the previously described optic strut. With extensive pneumatization, the OCR can be quite prominent. In addition to helping identify the location of the carotid artery and optic nerve, it also demarcates the level at which the optic nerve enters the true optic canal and becomes most susceptible to injury. Also, there can be dehiscence of the bone overlying the carotid artery or the optic nerve and these should be noted before any surgery involving the sphenoid sinus.

PITUITARY GLAND

The human pituitary gland is composed of two embryologically, anatomically, and functionally distinct parts. There is an anterior lobe or adenohypophysis, and a smaller posterior lobe or neurohypophysis. The anterior lobe develops from an invagination of oral ectoderm known as Rathke's pouch. It is a glandular structure that is responsible for the production and release of growth hormone, prolactin, adrenocorticotropic hormone, thyroid-stimulating hormone, luteinizing hormone, and follicle-stimulating hormone.[7]

In contrast, the posterior lobe develops as a direct extension of neural ectoderm from the floor of the third ventricle. It is a projection of unmyelinated axons and specialized glial cells called pituicytes from the hypothalamus. It is not a glandular structure like the anterior gland, but rather stores and releases oxytocin and vasopressin, which is produced by hypothalamic cell bodies.[7] Grossly it is often distinguishable from the anterior gland by its lighter color.[3]

The anterior gland receives its blood supply from the superior hypophyseal arteries. They arise from the medial aspect of the supraclinoidal segment of the carotid artery approximately 5 mm distal to the ophthalmic artery (**Fig. 3**A). Each superior hypophyseal artery typically gives off three branches: one to the optic nerve (recurrent branch), one to the undersurface of the optic chiasm and upper infundibulum (anastomotic branch), and one to the lower infundibulum and diaphragm (descending branch). The branch to the upper infundibulum anastomoses with the branch from the contralateral superior hypophyseal artery to form a capillary network. A portal venous system drains the capillary plexus of the superior hypophyseal arteries, which delivers blood to the anterior gland.[7,8] This allows the delivery of hypothalamic prohormones to the

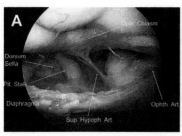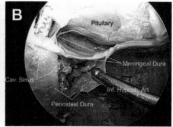

Fig. 3. (*A*) Roof of sella and suprasellar space with ophthalmic artery and superior hypophyseal artery shown. (*B*) Dural layers of the sella and cavernous sinus. The two layers of the sella separate laterally to form the cavernous sinus. The inferior hypophyseal artery is seen coming from the posterior aspect of the cavernous sinus. Inf. Hypoph. Art., inferior hypophyseal artery; Ophth. Art., ophthalmic artery; Pit., pituitary; Sup. Hypoph. Art., superior hypophyseal artery.

adenohypophysis. The posterior gland has been thought to receive most of its blood supply from the inferior hypophyseal arteries. The inferior hypophyseal artery is a branch of the meningohypophyseal trunk, which is the first branch of the internal carotid within the cavernous sinus (**Fig. 3**B). Recent evidence, however, has shown that sacrifice of both inferior hypophyseal arteries does not cause posterior pituitary dysfunction (ie, diabetes insipidus), suggesting alternative vascular supply by the superior hypophyseal arterial system.[9] Venous drainage from the anterior and posterior gland comes together and drains into the cavernous sinus.

Most of the pituitary gland is covered by two layers of dura: an outer periosteal layer and inner meningeal layer. These two layers separate laterally to form part of the cavernous sinus (see **Fig. 3**B). Anteriorly, the outer periosteal layer continues laterally to form the anterior sphenoidal wall of the cavernous sinus, and the inner meningeal layer stays attached to the gland and turns posteriorly toward the dorsum sella to form the medial wall of the cavernous sinus.[9] This medial wall also serves as the lateral wall of the sella. It is commonly compressed and occasionally even invaded by pituitary tumors. Also, the presence of two dural layers in the sellar region is the basis for the presence of intercavernous venous connections, which can exist anywhere along the anterior, posterior, or inferior aspects of the gland.

CAVERNOUS SINUS

The cavernous sinus is a venous lake that communicates with multiple venous tributaries and spaces: basilar plexus; superior and inferior petrosal sinuses; superior and inferior ophthalmic veins; veins of foramen rotundum, foramen spinosum, foramen ovale, and the foramen of Vesalius; deep middle cerebral vein; superficial sylvian vein; and the contralateral cavernous sinus via intercavernous connections. In addition to transmitting venous blood, it contains multiple neurovascular structures.[4]

The cavernous sinus is surrounded by five walls of dura. The anterior and medial walls as described previously; posterior wall which faces the posterior cranial fossa; the roof, which is continuous with the diaphragma sella; and the lateral wall. The lateral and medial walls come together inferiorly at the second division of the trigeminal nerve (V2) to mark the inferior limit of the cavernous sinus. The lateral wall of the cavernous sinus is a continuation of the outer periosteal dural layer of the middle fossa. It is tightly adherent to the inner meningeal layer of dura that covers the temporal lobe. Both dural layers come together at the level of the anterior petroclinoidal fold, which marks the transition from the lateral wall to the roof of the cavernous sinus. The meningeal layer goes on to form the outer layer of the roof of the cavernous sinus and diaphragma sella. Inferiorly, the periosteal layer of the middle fossa continues against the sphenoid bone to become the posterior wall of the cavernous sinus and floor of the sella.[4,9]

Within the cavernous sinus is the cavernous carotid artery and its branches (**Fig. 4**A). The cavernous carotid has three segments and two genua: posterior vertical segment, posterior genu, horizontal segment, anterior genu, and anterior vertical segment or paraclinoidal segment.[4,9] The cavernous carotid has two main branches (**Fig. 4**B). The meningohypophyseal trunk is the first branch of the cavernous carotid and comes off the posterior aspect of the posterior genu. It has three branches: the inferior hypophyseal artery, which supplies the posterior pituitary gland; the tentorial artery (artery of Bernasconi-Cassinari), which supplies the tentorium, oculomotor nerve, and trochlear nerve; and the dorsal meningeal artery, which supplies the upper clivus and abducens nerve.[3,4]

The second branch of the intracavernous carotid is the inferolateral trunk, or artery of the inferior cavernous sinus. It typically originates on the lateral or inferior surface of the middle third of the horizontal segment, approximately 5 to 8 mm distal to the meningohypophyseal trunk (see **Fig. 4**B). On rare occasions it has been described as originating from the meningohypophyseal trunk. It passes superior to the abducens nerve then turns downward between abducens and ophthalmic division of trigeminal nerve (V1) to supply the inferolateral wall and V1 and V2.[3,4]

The nerves of the cavernous sinus are the oculomotor, trochlear, V1, abducens nerve, and sympathetic plexus around the carotid. The abducens nerve and sympathetic plexus are the only of these that course entirely within the cavernous sinus. The abducens nerve leaves the pontomedullary junction and pierces the clival dura as it courses upward toward the cavernous sinus. It travels through Dorello's canal to enter the cavernous sinus through the posterior wall. It passes lateral to the cavernous carotid and goes through the lateral compartment medial to V1 to reach the superior orbital fissure.[3,4]

The remaining nerves run within the lateral wall of the cavernous sinus. The oculomotor nerve exits the midbrain and passes between the superior cerebellar artery and posterior cerebral artery as it travels anteriorly. It then enters the posterior roof of the cavernous sinus in an area called the oculomotor triangle. This triangle is defined by

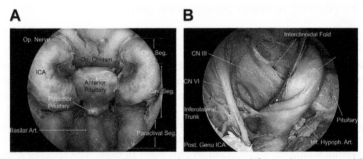

Fig. 4. (*A*) Sphenoid sinus with all bone and dura removed from planum to middle clivus. The different divisions of the carotid are seen. (*B*) Cavernous sinus exposed. The inferior hypophyseal artery is seen coming from the posterior aspect of the posterior genu as a branch of the meningohypophyseal trunk. The inferolateral trunk is seen coming off the middle of the horizontal segment. The oculomotor triangle and lateral wall of the cavernous sinus is seen. Art., artery; Cav. Seg., cavernous segment of ICA; Clin. Seg., clinoidal segment of ICA; CN, cranial nerve; Inf. Hypoph. Art., inferior hypophyseal artery; Paraclival Seg., paraclival segment of ICA; Post., posterior.

three dural folds: the previously mentioned anterior petroclinoidal fold, which extends from anterior clinoid to the petrous apex; the posterior petroclinoidal fold, which extends from posterior clinoid to the petrous apex; and the interclinoidal fold, which runs between the anterior and posterior clinoids. The oculomotor nerve runs parallel and just lateral to the interclinoidal fold.[3,4,9] A small cuff of arachnoid lined dura accompanies the oculomotor nerve as it enters the oculomotor triangle to create a variable sized CSF-filled space known as the oculomotor cistern. This cistern typically ends at the anterior roof of the cavernous sinus, also known as the clinoidal triangle. This is where the oculomotor nerve becomes incorporated into the lateral cavernous sinus wall, running under the anterior clinoid and lateral to the paraclinoidal ICA on its way to the superior orbital fissure.[10]

The trochlear nerve also enters the oculomotor triangle posterolateral to the oculomotor nerve at the junction of the anterior and posterior petroclinoidal folds. It travels in the lateral wall of the cavernous sinus below the oculomotor nerve toward the superior orbital fissure. The ophthalmic nerve (V1) travels inferior to the trochlear nerve in the lateral cavernous sinus wall and also enters the superior orbital fissure. These neural relationships divide the lateral cavernous sinus wall into two triangles: the supratrochlear triangle between the oculomotor and trochlear nerves; and the infratrochlear triangle, or Parkinson triangle, between the trochlear and trigeminal nerves.[4]

The carotid artery divides the cavernous sinus into multiple (venous) compartments: superior, inferior, posterior, and lateral. These compartments can be selectively occupied by invasive adenomas. The superior compartment (**Fig. 5**A) is located between the horizontal cavernous segment of the ICA and the inner aspect of the roof of the cavernous sinus. There are three distinguishable structures in this compartment: the undersurface of the paraclinoidal ICA medially and anteriorly, the dura of the oculomotor triangle that covers the inferior aspect of oculomotor nerve laterally and posteriorly, and the interclinoidal ligament.

The inferior compartment (**Fig. 5**B) lies below the horizontal cavernous carotid and anterior to the posterior vertical carotid. It contains the abducens nerve as it travels just lateral and below the horizontal cavernous carotid. It also contains the sympathetic plexus that sits around the carotid just medial to the abducens nerve. The anterior wall of this compartment corresponds to the anterior or sphenoidal wall of the cavernous sinus.

The posterior compartment (**Fig. 5**C) is located behind the posterior vertical ICA and posterior genu. The abducens nerve enters the cavernous sinus at the inferior aspect of this compartment after passing under the petrosphenoidal Gruber's ligament and runs behind the posterior vertical carotid. Finally, the lateral compartment (see **Figs. 4**B and **5**B) is located lateral to the horizontal carotid and anterior genu. All of the cranial nerves are located in this compartment as they travel toward the superior orbital fissure.

SUPRASELLAR SPACE

The suprasellar space extends from the diaphragma inferiorly to the floor of the third ventricle superiorly. Access to the suprasellar space is obtained by removing the tuberculum sella, prechiasmatic sulcus, and posterior planum sphenoidale. The suprasellar space is divided into the infrachiasmatic, suprachiasmatic, and retrochiasmatic areas.

Within the infrachiasmatic space is found the inferior surface of the optic chiasm and the infundibulum in the midline (see **Fig. 3**A; **Fig. 6**A). The infundibulum is covered by the suprasellar cistern arachnoid anteriorly and by the membrane of Lillequist

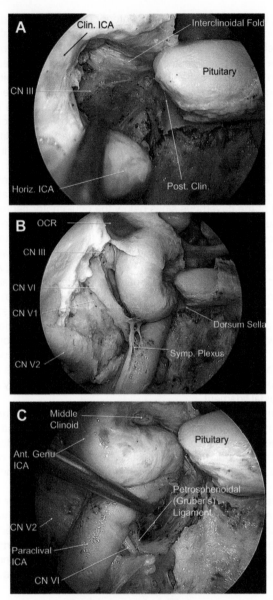

Fig. 5. (*A*) Cavernous sinus, superior compartment. (*B*) Cavernous sinus, inferior and lateral compartments. (*C*) Cavernous sinus, posterior compartment. Ant., anterior; Clin. ICA, clinoidal segment of ICA; Horiz., horizontal; Lam. Pap., lamina papyracea; Symp., sympathetic.

posteriorly. The optic nerves course anterolaterally from the chiasm to enter the optic canal. The ophthalmic artery is the first branch of the supraclinoidal carotid above the distal dural ring. It arises from the ventral surface of the carotid to enter the optic canal where it travels inferior to the optic nerve. The superior hypophyseal artery arises just distal to the ophthalmic artery on the medial aspect of the supraclinoidal carotid. The same arachnoid membrane that covers the infundibulum anteriorly also surrounds the

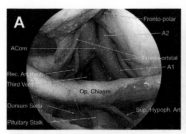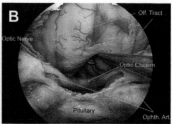

Fig. 6. (*A*) Infrachiasmatic and suprachiasmatic suprasellar spaces. (*B*) Suprachiasmatic suprasellar space. A1, first (horizontal) segment of anterior cerebral artery; A2, second (vertical) segment of anterior cerebral artery; ACom, anterior communicating artery; Olf., olfactory; Rec. Art. Heub., recurrent artery of Heubner; Vent., ventricle.

superior hypophyseal artery branches. Tuberculum sellae meningiomas that extend into this area displaces the infundibulum and superior hypophyseal arteries posteriorly.

The suprachiasmatic space extends above the optic chiasm (see **Fig. 6**). The posterior aspect of each olfactory tract is found here as they divide to become the olfactory striae just above each optic nerve. The A1 segment of the anterior cerebral artery runs from the carotid bifurcation to the midline just above the optic chiasm. It anastomoses to its counterpart here via the anterior communicating artery. From here, the A2 segments arise and enter the interhemispheric fissure. There are two important arterial branches in the suprachiasmatic space. One is the recurrent artery of Heubner, which travels from the midline to the anterior perforated substance. The other is the frontoorbital artery, which is the first cortical branch of the A2 segment and is often involved with tumors in this area. Planum meningiomas typically occupy this anatomic region and displace the optic chiasm and associated vascular structures posteriorly and/or inferiorly.

The retrochiasmatic, or retroinfundibular, space extends from the infundibulum anteroinferiorly to the posterior perforated substance and cerebral peduncles posteriorly. It is bounded by the floor of the third ventricle superiorly. The Lillequist membrane provides access to the interpeduncular cistern where the basilar apex is visible posteriorly. The posterior communicating arteries run in the lateral recess of the interpeduncular cistern along with the oculomotor nerves, which is seen traveling between the superior cerebellar artery and posterior cerebral artery. Craniopharyngiomas often occupy this anatomic space.[11]

ANTERIOR CRANIAL BASE

The anterior two-thirds of the anterior cranial base is composed of the ethmoid and frontal bones, and the posterior one-third is formed by the planum sphenoidale (**Fig. 7A**). The ethmoid bone consists of the cribriform plate and crista galli in the midline; the ethmoid roofs (fovea ethmoidalis) superiorly; and the lamina papyracea laterally, which separates the ethmoid sinuses from the orbit. The perpendicular plate of the ethmoid joins the vomer to become the bony septum.[12]

Once the ethmoid roof is completely exposed, one should be able to see from the planum sphenoidale to the frontal sinus (**Fig. 7B**). Two major arteries can be seen coursing across the ethmoid roof. The posterior ethmoid artery is found at the junction of the planum sphenoidale and the cribriform plate. The anterior ethmoid artery is found at the posterior aspect of the frontal recess, posterior to any supraorbital ethmoid air cell.

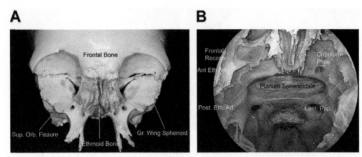

Fig. 7. (*A*) Bones of the anterior skull base. (*B*) Anterior skull base exposed from frontal sinus to sella. Ant. Eth. Art., anterior ethmoid artery; Gr., greater; Lam. Pap., lamina papyracea; Post. Eth. Art., posterior ethmoid artery; Sup. Orb., superior orbital.

The posterior ethmoid artery is typically within bone and runs almost directly from lateral to medial. The anterior ethmoid artery is more variable and is sometimes found in a bony mesentery because of pneumatization of the ethmoid roof around it. It also tends to run obliquely across the skull base from posterolateral to anteromedial. It is important to identify these vessels and avoid transecting them too close to the orbit to avoid having them retract into the orbit resulting in a retrobulbar hemorrhage.

The cribriform plate transmits the olfactory filae through small bony channels. These filae have dural invaginations that follow them into the cribriform, which makes this area very susceptible to iatrogenic and spontaneous CSF leaks. The bone of the ethmoid roof also tends to be quite thin and is a common location for iatrogenic CSF leaks.

Once the dura of the anterior cranial base has been opened, the olfactory bulbs and olfactory tracts are seen. The fronto-orbital branches of the anterior cerebral arteries should be visible medially. They provide vascular supply to the olfactory tracts and cortical surface. Superiorly the gyri recti are found medially and the orbital gyri laterally. The frontopolar arteries run within the interhemispheric fissure. The falx cerebri is located in this fissure and attaches to the crista galli, separating the left and right hemispheres. The height of the falx decreases posteriorly, which is important to note because the falx must be divided to remove the anterior skull base dura in a craniofacial resection procedure.

CLIVUS

The clivus can be divided into thirds (**Fig. 8**A). The upper third or "sellar" clivus is made up of the dorsum sella and posterior clinoids down to approximately the level of the floor of the sella. Dorello's canal is located at the transition point between upper and middle clivus, just a few millimeters below the floor of the sella. The middle third or "sphenoidal" clivus extends from the floor of the sella to the choana. The lower third or "nasopharyngeal" clivus extends from there down to foramen magnum and corresponds to the nasopharynx. Although the upper two-thirds of the clivus is considered part of the sphenoid bone, the lower third is considered part of the occipital bone.

The middle clivus is the tallest of the three segments. It is bounded laterally by the vertical paraclival carotid arteries, petroclival fissure, and foramen lacerum. Foramen lacerum and the choana are at approximately the same level and so foramen lacerum also serves as a landmark to define the transition between middle and lower clivus. A middle transclival approach provides access to the prepontine cistern (**Fig. 8**B). Here is found the basilar trunk, anterior inferior cerebellar artery, abducens nerve, and the ventral surface of the pons. Exposing and gently lateralizing the paraclival carotid

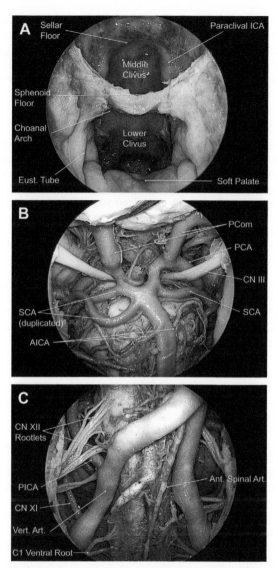

Fig. 8. (*A*) Divisions of the clivus. (*B*) Ventral pons after middle clivus removed and dura opened. (*C*) Ventral medulla after lower clivus removed and dura opened. AICA, anterior inferior cerebellar artery; Ant. Spinal Art., anterior spinal artery; Eust., Eustachian; PCA, posterior cerebral artery; PCom, posterior communicating artery; PICA, posterior inferior cerebellar artery; SCA, superior cerebellar artery; Vert. Art, vertebral artery.

can allow access to the petrous apex, free edge of the tentorium, trochlear nerve, and posterior root of the trigeminal nerve. The facial nerve, vestibulocochlear nerve, and internal acoustic canal are not accessible from an endonasal approach unless the paraclival carotid is sacrificed.

The inferior clivus is covered by the pharyngobasilar fascia, longus capitis muscles, and rectus capitis muscles. Once these are detached, one can gain exposure of the foramen magnum, anterior ring of C1, occipital condyles, atlanto-occipital joint, the apical ligament, and the tectorial membrane. An inferior transclival approach provides access to the premedullary cistern and its contents: vertebral arteries, vertebrobasilar junction, posterior inferior cerebellar artery, anterior spinal arteries, hypoglossal canal and nerves, lower cranial nerves, and ventral medulla (**Fig. 8**C). Laterally, access to the jugular foramen is limited by the Eustachian tubes, and requires Eustachian tube transection and/or mobilization to reach.[13]

SUMMARY

Technologic advances have greatly improved the ability to access the ventral skull base. The endonasal route has been expanded to allow access to the anterior, middle, and posterior cranial fossas. Understanding of the complex anatomy of the skull base has also greatly expanded. A detailed understanding of the various anatomic relationships provides one with the ability to determine the safest and most effective approach to lesions of the ventral skull base. It allows one to minimize morbidity, maximize patient safety, and continue advancing endoscopic endonasal surgery.

REFERENCES

1. Liu JK, Das K, Weiss MH, et al. The history and evolution of transsphenoidal surgery. J Neurosurg 2001;95:1083–96.
2. Doglietto F, Prevedello DM, Jane JA Jr, et al. Brief history of endoscopic transsphenoidal surgery–from Philipp Bozzini to the First World Congress of Endoscopic Skull Base Surgery. Neurosurg Focus 2005;19:E3.
3. Rhoton AL Jr. Anatomy of the pituitary gland and sellar region. In: Thapar K, Kovacs K, Scheithauer B, Lloyd RV, editors. Diagnosis and management of pituitary tumors. Totowa (NJ): Humana Press, Inc; 2001. p. 13–40.
4. Yasuda A, Campero A, Martins C, et al. Microsurgical anatomy and approaches to the cavernous sinus. Neurosurgery 2005;56:4–27 [discussion: 4–27].
5. Fernandez-Miranda JC, Tormenti M, Latorre F, et al. Endoscopic endonasal middle clinoidectomy: anatomic, radiological, and technical note. Neurosurgery 2012;71:ons233–9 [discussion: ons39].
6. Campero A, Martins C, Yasuda A, et al. Microsurgical anatomy of the diaphragma sellae and its role in directing the pattern of growth of pituitary adenomas. Neurosurgery 2008;62:717–23 [discussion: 17–23].
7. Lechan RM, Toni R. Functional anatomy of the hypothalamus and pituitary. Section 3b. In: De Groot LJ, Beck-Peccoz P, Chrousos G, et al, editors. Pituitary disease and endocrinology. South Dartmouth (MA): Endotext; 2000. Available at: www.endotext.org.
8. Krisht AF, Barrow DL, Barnett DW, et al. The microsurgical anatomy of the superior hypophyseal artery. Neurosurgery 1994;35:899–903 [discussion: 03].
9. Fernandez-Miranda JC, Gardner PA, Rastelli MM Jr, et al. Endoscopic endonasal transcavernous posterior clinoidectomy with interdural pituitary transposition. J Neurosurg 2014;121:91–9.
10. Everton KL, Rassner UA, Osborn AG, et al. The oculomotor cistern: anatomy and high-resolution imaging. AJNR Am J Neuroradiol 2008;29:1344–8.
11. Fernandez-Miranda JC, Gardner PA, Snyderman CH, et al. Craniopharyngioma: a pathologic, clinical, and surgical review. Head Neck 2012;34:1036–44.
12. Rhoton AL Jr. The anterior and middle cranial base. Neurosurgery 2002;51: S273–302.
13. Fernandez-Miranda JC, Gardner PA, Snyderman CH, et al. Clival chordomas: a pathological, surgical, and radiotherapeutic review. Head Neck 2014;36:892–906.

Anatomy, Physiology, and Laboratory Evaluation of the Pituitary Gland

Gregory K. Hong, MD, PhD[a], Spencer C. Payne, MD[b],
John A. Jane Jr, MD[c],*

KEYWORDS

- Pituitary diseases • Pituitary function tests • Pituitary gland • Pituitary hormones
- Pituitary neoplasms • Hypopituitarism

KEY POINTS

- Benign pituitary tumors are the most common cause of clinically relevant pituitary disease.
- The most significant anatomic consequence of an enlarging pituitary tumor is compression of the optic chiasm resulting in visual field loss.
- Evaluation of incidentally found pituitary tumors should include assessment for oversecretion of prolactin and growth hormone; assessment for Cushing disease should be undertaken if the clinical presentation is suspicious.
- First-line treatment of prolactinoma is medical therapy, not surgical resection.
- Perioperative assessment for adrenal insufficiency and hypothyroidism should be performed on all patients with a pituitary tumor as deficiencies of these hormones can lead to perioperative complications in the short term and can result in death in cases of long-term deficiency.

INTRODUCTION

The pituitary gland functions as a master regulator of numerous physiologic processes via its control of downstream endocrine glands. The pituitary controls the adrenals, gonads, and thyroid gland via secretion of specific regulating hormones into the systemic circulation. Growth and water balance also represent key physiologic processes directly influenced by the release of pituitary hormones. Pathology of the pituitary

Disclosures: The authors have nothing to disclose.
[a] Division of Endocrinology, Department of Medicine, University of Virginia Health System, PO Box 801406, Charlottesville, VA 22908, USA; [b] Department of Otolaryngology - Head & Neck Surgery, University of Virginia Health System, PO Box 800713, Charlottesville, VA 22908, USA; [c] Department of Neurosurgery, University of Virginia Health System, PO Box 800212, Charlottesville, VA 22908, USA
* Corresponding author.
E-mail address: johnajanejr@virginia.edu

Otolaryngol Clin N Am 49 (2016) 21–32
http://dx.doi.org/10.1016/j.otc.2015.09.002
0030-6665/16/$ – see front matter © 2016 Elsevier Inc. All rights reserved.

oto.theclinics.com

gland is primarily caused by benign pituitary tumors (adenomas)[1] that can result in hormonal hypersecretion, impairment of normal pituitary function, or mass effect on surrounding structures. Other sellar lesions, such as cysts or nonadenomatous tumors, can also cause mass effect or impairment of pituitary function.[2] Pituitary diseases cause varied clinical presentations which manifest across all medical disciplines; a basic understanding of pituitary anatomy, physiology, and the process for evaluating pituitary dysfunction is critical for any skull base surgeon.

This article reviews relevant anatomic relationships between the pituitary gland and surrounding structures while also examining the regulation and downstream action of pituitary hormones. Dysfunction of the pituitary gland which typically results from benign pituitary tumors and the clinical manifestations of these tumors, ranging from mass effects on surrounding structures to hormonal hypersecretion or hyposecretion, is reviewed. The biochemical evaluation of suspected pituitary function abnormalities is then presented and suggested testing strategies are outlined for various disease states.

BASIC ANATOMY

The pituitary gland lies in the sella turcica at the base of the skull and consists of 2 lobes (anterior and posterior) which arise from different embryologic origins. The anterior lobe originates from the oropharynx (Rathke's pouch) and grows upward during development where it meets tissue of neural origin growing inferiorly; this neural tissue forms the posterior lobe.[3] On completion of development, the posterior lobe contains nerve endings of neurons originating in the hypothalamus. The pituitary stalk connects the hypothalamus to the pituitary gland and serves to transmit the axons of the hypothalamus to the posterior lobe; it also transmits regulatory hormones from the hypothalamus to the anterior lobe via a portal system. The anterior lobe is larger than the posterior lobe and represents approximately two-thirds of total pituitary volume.

Pituitary tumors may cause symptoms as a result of a mass effect on surrounding structures,[4] hence an understanding of clinically relevant surrounding structures is paramount. Dura surrounds the pituitary gland and continues superiorly to form a roof over the sella (diaphragma sella). The cavernous sinuses contain cranial nerves (CN) 3, 4, 6, and the first and second branches of the fifth cranial nerve (V1 and V2). The optic chiasm rests approximately 5 to 10 mm above the diaphragma sella. Enlargement of the gland caused by inflammation, infiltration, or tumor growth can result in compression of these structures leading to bitemporal hemianopsia (from compression of the optic chiasm), extraocular muscle dysfunction (from palsies of CN 3,4, or 6), or ipsilateral facial pain (from involvement of the V1 and V2 branches).[5] Pituitary adenomas are classified based on their functional status (nonfunctioning vs hormonally active) and size; tumors up to 1 cm in diameter are microadenomas, whereas tumors greater than 1 cm are macroadenomas.

PHYSIOLOGY

The anterior pituitary gland consists of 5 separate cell types each of which secrete different hormones. Each cell type originates from a common progenitor cell in response to expression of specific transcription factors; deficiencies in these transcription factors result in genetic syndromes of hypopituitarism caused by a lack of particular anterior pituitary cell types.[6] Secretion of hormones from the anterior pituitary is a tightly regulated process influenced by physiologic stimuli and feedback control from downstream effector organs. In general, releasing hormones from the hypothalamus travel to the pituitary gland via the portal hypophysial circulation; these releasing hormones trigger the release of anterior pituitary hormones which then act on their target organ to exert biologic effects (eg, lactation in the breast in response to prolactin) or to induce hormone secretion from the target organ (eg, secretion of cortisol from the adrenal gland in response to adrenocorticotropic hormone, ACTH). The physiologic functions of the various endocrine axes controlled by the anterior pituitary are listed in **Table 1**. It should be noted that growth hormone (GH) can also act directly on target tissues to regulate metabolism and body composition independent of its effects on increasing insulin-like growth factor 1 (IGF-1) secretion from the liver.[7]

Negative regulation of most anterior pituitary hormones occurs via feedback of target organ hormones on the hypothalamus and/or the anterior pituitary; an illustrative overview is provided in **Fig. 1**. Negative control of thyroid hormone (free T4, FT4), cortisol, GH, and the reproductive hormones is achieved via this paradigm. It should be noted that negative regulation of GH is also mediated by somatostatin, a hormone which increases in response to GH and IGF-1. This physiology has been exploited through the use of synthetic somatostatin analogues to treat GH-producing tumors.[8]

Regulation of prolactin differs from other anterior pituitary hormones in that prolactin secretion is tonically inhibited by dopamine originating from hypothalamic neurons. Physiologic triggers of prolactin secretion (sleep, stress, suckling, pregnancy) decrease hypothalamic secretion of dopamine, thereby allowing lactotrophs to secrete prolactin. Pharmacologic blockade of lactotroph dopamine receptors (eg, by antipsychotics) also leads to increased prolactin secretion.

OVERVIEW OF PITUITARY DYSFUNCTION

Abnormalities of pituitary function can occur as a result of inappropriate/unregulated hormonal secretion or deficient hormonal secretion. Hormonal hypersecretion often results in physical and biochemical findings characteristic of a particular hypersecretion syndrome (eg, Cushing's disease, acromegaly). Hypopituitarism can present along a clinical spectrum that depends on the degree of deficiency of the hormone in question and whether this deficiency occurs in isolation or in combination with other pituitary hormones (panhypopituitarism).[9]

Table 1
Function of anterior pituitary hormones

Hormone	Target	Effects on Target	Downstream Effects
ACTH	Adrenal gland	Induction of cortisol secretion	Metabolism regulation; resistance to physiologic stress; maintenance of vascular tone
GH	Liver, skeleton, soft tissues	IGF-1 secretion (from liver); growth and regulation of nutrient metabolism	IGF-1 is primary mediator of growth
FSH and LH	Testes/ovaries	Secretion of testosterone or estrogen/progesterone	Maintenance of fertility, lean body mass, and bone density
PRL	Breast	Lactation	—
TSH	Thyroid gland	Induction of thyroid hormone (T4) secretion	Metabolism regulation

Abbreviations: ACTH, adrenocorticotropic hormone; FSH, follicle-stimulating hormone; GH, growth hormone; IGF-1, insulin-like growth factor 1; LH, luteinizing hormone; PRL, prolactin; TSH, thyrotropin-stimulating hormone.

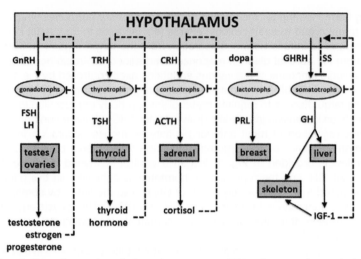

Fig. 1. Regulation of anterior pituitary hormones. ACTH, adrenocorticotropic hormone; CRH, corticotropin-releasing hormone; DOPA, dopamine; FSH, follicle-stimulating hormone; GH, growth hormone; GHRH, growth hormone–releasing hormone; GnRH, gonadotropin-releasing hormone; IGF-1, insulin-like growth factor 1; LH, luteinizing hormone; PRL, prolactin; SS, somatostatin; TRH, thyrotropin-releasing hormone; TSH, thyrotropin-stimulating hormone.

Several pituitary hypersecretion syndromes cause significant morbidity and shorten lifespan[10,11]; hence early diagnosis and appropriate management are critical. The various hypersecretion syndromes are summarized in **Table 2**. Of note, functional gonadotropin tumors (resulting in hypergonadism) are not discussed in this article as they are exceedingly rare.[12] Prolactinoma represents the most common hypersecretion

Table 2
Pituitary hypersecretion syndromes

Condition	Presentation	Important Considerations
Prolactinoma	Galactorrhea, hypogonadism	Medication history critical; surgery reserved for patients who fail medical therapy
Acromegaly ($\uparrow$GH)	Soft tissue overgrowth, hyperhidrosis, HTN, DM2	IGF-1 is preferred diagnostic test
Cushing disease ($\uparrow$ACTH)	Centripetal obesity, pigmented striae, insomnia, mood lability, skin thinning, proximal muscle weakness, HTN, DM2, hypogonadism	Presentation can be subtle and diagnosis challenging
TSH secreting adenoma (TSH-oma)	Weight loss, heat intolerance, hyperdefecation	Diagnosis suggested by hyperthyroid symptoms with $\uparrow$FT4 and $\uparrow$ (or inappropriately normal) TSH

Abbreviations: ACTH, adrenocorticotropic hormone; DM2, diabetes mellitus type 2; FT4, free T4; GH, growth hormone; HTN, hypertension; IGF-1, insulin-like growth factor 1; TSH, thyrotropin-stimulating hormone.

syndrome followed by acromegaly, Cushing's disease, and central hyperthyroidism caused by a thyrotropin-stimulating hormone (TSH) producing adenoma ("TSH-oma"), respectively.[13] In general, the preferred initial management of hypersecreting pituitary tumors is surgical removal,[14] with the exception of prolactinoma which can be treated medically in most cases.[15] Hence, it is critical for the skull base surgeon to exclude prolactinoma before resecting a pituitary tumor.

In all cases of suspected pituitary dysfunction (either hypopituitarism or hypersecretion syndromes) biochemical testing represents the initial diagnostic step. Once underproduction or inappropriate overproduction of pituitary hormones is confirmed then MRI of the sella (if not already done) should be performed to assess for a pituitary adenoma (the most common cause of pituitary dysfunction). Dedicated pituitary protocol MRI with 1.5-mm cuts provide clear definition of hypothalamic/pituitary anatomy; the addition of contrast is recommended and enhances detection of small pituitary tumors.[16]

DIAGNOSIS OF COMMON HYPERSECRETION SYNDROMES
Acromegaly

Acromegaly (GH excess) results in significant morbidity and increases mortality[10]; however, the diagnosis is often delayed by years due to insidious onset.[17] Assessment for GH oversecretion should be considered in patients with suggestive clinical features and is mandatory in any patient with a pituitary adenoma.[14] Measurement of IGF-1, a growth factor produced in the liver in response to GH stimulation, is the recommended screening test for GH oversecretion.[18] IGF-1 functions as an integrated measure of GH secretion over time and a normal IGF-1 level essentially excludes the diagnosis of acromegaly. Whereas measured serum GH levels are often increased in acromegaly, the pulsatile nature of GH secretion makes a random GH an unreliable means of diagnosing acromegaly.[19]

Once an increase in IGF-1 is demonstrated the diagnosis should then be confirmed with dynamic testing involving oral glucose loading (oral glucose tolerance test), typically done under the supervision of an endocrinologist. This test takes advantage of the ability of hyperglycemia to suppress GH secretion in normal individuals; lack of GH suppression is characteristic of acromegaly.[20]

Cushing's Disease

The proper diagnosis of Cushing's syndrome (hypercortisolism) can be a challenging endeavor requiring repeated assessment of endocrine function. Most cases of Cushing syndrome are caused by excess ACTH secretion from a pituitary adenoma (Cushing disease)[11]; the primary issue likely to be encountered by skull base surgeons surrounds the question of whether a patient with a known pituitary adenoma (usually incidentally found) could have Cushing's disease. This is a critical distinction to make as management of Cushing's disease includes surgical resection; whereas, there may be no acute indication for surgery with a small nonfunctional adenoma.

In general, only patients with multiple and progressive clinical features of hypercortisolism (previously described in **Table 2**) should be considered for biochemical screening.[21] Before undertaking a biochemical evaluation, a thorough history is essential as exogenous glucocorticoid use represents the most common cause of clinical hypercortisolism ("iatrogenic Cushing's").[22] Endogenous hypercortisolism from Cushing's disease is characterized by loss of appropriate feedback control leading to increased cortisol, loss of normal diurnal rhythm of cortisol secretion, and reduced ability of steroids (endogenous or exogenous) to inhibit ACTH secretion.

These characteristics can be assessed using 3 biochemical tests: (1) 24-hour urinary free cortisol (UFC) excretion (assesses total cortisol production), (2) late night salivary cortisol collection (assesses whether diurnal rhythm is present), and (3) 1 mg dexamethasone suppression test (assesses whether exogenous steroid can appropriately suppress ACTH/cortisol production). In general, at least 2 tests must be unequivocally abnormal (eg, 24 h UFC >3× upper limit of normal) to establish the diagnosis of Cushing's syndrome.[21] Diagnosis of Cushing's syndrome via these tests typically occurs in conjunction with an endocrinologist; a referral to an endocrinologist should be considered for any patients with a history of, or physical features suggestive of, hypercortisolism.

Conclusively establishing the diagnosis of Cushing's disease can be a challenging endeavor and a full discussion is beyond the scope of this article. Briefly, patients with unequivocally positive screening tests should have ACTH measured (to confirm the pituitary origin of hypercortisolism) followed by MRI of the pituitary. In cases where MRI is equivocal, then several options to localize ACTH overproduction to the pituitary exist, including high-dose dexamethasone suppression tests or sampling of ACTH levels in the inferior petrosal sinus.[23] While invasive, inferior petrosal sinus sampling has a sensitivity and specificity of greater than 90% and is the preferred option at pituitary centers where technical expertise and experience exists.

Prolactinoma

Diagnosis of prolactinoma is straightforward when prolactin is markedly increased (eg, >500 µg/L) with a visible pituitary adenoma on MRI. In general, prolactin levels parallel tumor size; most prolactinomas greater than 1 cm have prolactin concentrations greater than 250 µg/L.[24] Hyperprolactinemia in the absence of a pituitary tumor should prompt assessment for other causes of hyperprolactinemia (listed in **Table 3**). Drug-induced hyperprolactinemia is relatively common; increases are typically less than 200 µg/L, although certain atypical antipsychotics such as risperidone can rarely cause increases to greater than 200 µg/L.[25]

Hyperprolactinemia can also occur with any large sellar lesion as a result of compression of the pituitary stalk and subsequent interference with dopamine inhibitory signaling from the hypothalamus. This so-called "stalk effect" usually results in modest hyperprolactinemia (levels typically <100 µg/L).[26] Some prolactin immunoassays can result in falsely lowered prolactin values via a well-known phenomenon ("hook effect"); hence, many recommend diluting serum samples followed by reassessment of prolactin in cases of macroadenomas with mild increases in prolactin.[27]

Table 3	
Common nontumoral causes of hyperprolactinemia	
Physiologic	Pregnancy
	Stress
	Lactation/nipple stimulation
	Primary hypothyroidism
Pharmacologic	Antipsychotics (1st and 2nd generation)
	Antidepressants (TCA, SSRI)
	Anti-emetics (metoclopramide, prochlorperazine)
	Opioids, verapamil
Miscellaneous	Chest wall trauma/irritation (zoster, surgery)
	Renal failure (PRL renally cleared)

Abbreviations: SSRI, selective serotonin reuptake inhibitor; TCA, tricyclic antidepressant.

Dilution corrects for the hook effect and functional prolactin secreting tumors will have an increased prolactin after dilution.

Hypopituitarism

Hypopituitarism of the anterior lobe of the pituitary is a common finding with pituitary macroadenomas and other large sellar lesions, presumably from the mass effect of the tumor on the normal anterior pituitary.[4] Loss of GH secretion occurs first followed by gonadotropins, ACTH, and then TSH.[9] Hypopituitarism is less commonly seen with microadenomas, although hypogonadism often occurs in Cushing's disease and pro-lactinoma because of the suppressive effect of cortisol and prolactin on gonadotropin secretion. Sustained deficiency (eg, over months) of ACTH or TSH can result in significant morbidity. An acute stress (eg, anesthesia induction) in a patient with profound ACTH or TSH deficiency can be potentially fatal. Prolactin deficiency is uncommon and of minimal clinical consequence with the exception of the lactating female. Gonadotropins and GH are also not essential for life, although deficiencies of these hormones can lead to clinical syndromes. An overview of the syndromes resulting from deficiencies in anterior pituitary hormones is presented in **Table 4**.

Biochemical assessment for hypopituitarism is relatively straightforward, with the exception of GH and ACTH deficiency. Prolactin, thyroid hormone, and gonadotropin deficiency are easily demonstrated via simple biochemical testing (eg, low TSH and low free T4 in the case of central hypothyroidism). GH deficiency in adults can be a complex diagnosis to make; given that GH deficiency has minimal immediate consequences relevant to the skull base surgeon it will not be discussed in detail here. Briefly, a low IGF-1 level with multiple additional anterior pituitary hormone deficiencies typically indicates GH deficiency. In equivocal cases dynamic testing using insulin to provoke hypoglycemia (a potent GH stimulus) is required for a formal diagnosis.[28]

Assessment of ACTH sufficiency relies on demonstrating subnormal levels of the downstream adrenal hormone cortisol. Subnormal ACTH (and consequently cortisol) levels can occur as a result of hypothalamic/pituitary pathology; however, treatment with exogenous glucocorticoids represents the most common cause of low ACTH/cortisol levels because of suppression of ACTH secretion from exogenous

Table 4
Hypopituitary syndromes

Condition	Presentation	Important Considerations
GH deficiency	Fatigue, loss of lean body mass	Formal diagnosis can be complex and often requires dynamic testing
Secondary hypogonadism	Oligomenorrhea (female); low libido and erectile dysfunction (male)	Nontumoral causes include opioids, glucocorticoids, severe stress/illness, malnutrition
Secondary (central) hypothyroidism	Fatigue, weight gain, cold intolerance, constipation	Important to document decreased FT4 and decreased (or inappropriately normal) TSH
Secondary (central) adrenal insufficiency	Weight loss, heat intolerance, hyperdefecation	Recent/current treatment with glucocorticoids can also result in similar laboratory findings (↓ACTH, ↓Cortisol)

Abbreviations: ACTH, adrenocorticotropic hormone; FT4, free T4; GH, growth hormone; TSH, thyrotropin-stimulating hormone.

glucocorticoids. Secretion of ACTH and cortisol peaks in the morning (between 6:00 and 8:00 AM); cortisol levels are typically between 10 and 20 μg/dL at this time. A quick assessment of the hypothalamic–pituitary–adrenal (HPA) axis can be made with an 8:00 AM ACTH and cortisol measurement. An unequivocally low cortisol (eg, <3 μg/dL) indicates adrenal insufficiency[29]; concurrent demonstration of a low ACTH indicates that it is caused by hypothalamic/pituitary pathology. Conversely, a morning cortisol value greater than 17 μg/dL indicates normal adrenal function.[30] In most cases the morning cortisol is between these values; many clinicians use a morning cortisol value of greater than 10 μg/dL as rough criteria for indicating adequate adrenal function in a patient without suspicious symptoms. Although some studies report 100% sensitivity at this cutoff value,[29] others note a sensitivity of only 62% for diagnosing adrenal insufficiency at this value.[30] In equivocal cases with suggestive clinical symptoms, further dynamic testing should be pursued. One can assess cortisol following administration of 250 μg cosyntropin (synthetic ACTH); normal individuals increase cortisol to greater than 18 μg/dL within 60 minutes. The validity of this test relies on the development of adrenal atrophy over time because of chronically low levels of ACTH. Hence, individuals with recent (ie, within 4–6 weeks) damage to their hypothalamus/pituitary may still be able to respond to cosyntropin with a normal cortisol despite having ACTH deficiency.

Diabetes Insipidus

Central diabetes insipidus (DI) represents the primary disease process that results from posterior pituitary insufficiency. Compromise of the pituitary stalk from infiltrative disease (eg, sarcoidosis) or pituitary surgery can result in DI by damaging neurons responsible for secreting vasopressin/antidiuretic hormone (ADH) from the posterior pituitary.[31,32] Although less common with pituitary adenomas, DI can be a presenting feature of other nonadenomatous sellar tumors, such as craniopharyngioma or metastatic disease. ADH deficiency results in impaired urinary concentrating ability, and patients present with massive polyuria (>3 L/d), frequent urination (often every hour), and persistent thirst. Craving for ice-cold liquids is often a characteristic feature. Patients with an intact thirst center can maintain their hydration status via constant intake of fluid; if access to water is restricted then dehydration and hypernatremia quickly ensue. Whereas the diagnosis is formally made with a water deprivation test,[33] in many cases this is not necessary and empiric therapy with ADH analogues such as desmopressin (DDAVP) can be initiated in suggestive clinical settings (eg, persistent polyuria with dilute urine and extreme thirst following surgery on a large craniopharyngioma). Patients with DI are instructed to only drink when thirsty to avoid iatrogenic hyponatremia while on desmopressin.

EVALUATION OF PITUITARY INCIDENTALOMAS

Incidentally found lesions of the pituitary gland ("pituitary incidentaloma") are a common entity given the sheer numbers of MRI studies of the brain currently performed. Studies suggest a prevalence of at least 10% in the general population[34]; the majority (>90%) of these lesions are pituitary adenomas, usually nonfunctioning. Published guidelines recommend evaluation of all pituitary incidentalomas for hormonal dysfunction as well as for growth over time.[14]

Evaluation for hormonal dysfunction first occurs via a directed history and physical examination to ascertain whether the patient has characteristic symptoms/features consistent with hormonal hypersecretion or hypopituitarism. An overview of the initial objective evaluation of a pituitary incidentaloma is presented in **Table 5**. All patients

Table 5
Basic evaluation of pituitary incidentaloma

Test	Comments
Prolactin	>250 µg/dL is consistent with prolactinoma Macroadenoma stalk effect is usually <100 µg/dL (also repeat with diluted sample to rule out hook effect) Must interpret values in context of current medications
IGF-1	Any increase requires further endocrine evaluation (oral glucose tolerance test) for acromegaly
FT4	Ensures that patient is not profoundly hypothyroid before surgery
Cortisol (AM)	Ensures patient is not profoundly adrenally insufficient before surgery (see text for limitations of this test) Must perform thorough history; consider further testing (cosyntropin stimulation) if symptoms of adrenal insufficiency present

In addition to tests listed in the table, consider screening for hypercortisolism if the patient has clinical signs/symptoms of Cushing's disease. Formal visual field assessment should occur if an incidentaloma abuts the optic chiasm.

should be tested for oversecretion of prolactin and GH (via IGF-1); additional testing for Cushing's disease should be pursued in the presence of suggestive historical or physical examination features. Biochemical assessment should also always include evaluation of thyroid hormone status (FT4) and morning cortisol; further testing for adrenal insufficiency should be pursued when morning cortisol is equivocal and the patient has suggestive symptoms.

The decision to pursue surgical resection for an incidentaloma depends on the functional status and anatomic effect of the tumor. Hormonally active tumors (with the exception of prolactinoma) should be surgically resected. A nonfunctional lesion that compromises vision or results in cranial nerve palsy as a result of compression should also be surgically resected. Patients with lesions abutting or compressing the optic chiasm should have a formal visual field assessment as visual impairments may not be subjectively noticed by the patient or detected on confrontation testing. Most consider clinically significant growth over time as a relative indication for surgery. Although there is evidence that some tumor-induced hormone deficiencies may reverse following resection of a nonfunctioning tumor,[35] we typically do not use this as an indication for surgery in the absence of other indications. We are also cautious to use headache as an indication for surgery, particularly with microincidentalomas, given the lack of correlation with tumor size[36] and equivocal data regarding headache improvement after resection.[37] In general, we prefer a dedicated trial of medical therapy directed by a headache neurologist for at least 6 to 12 months before proceeding with resection solely for the purpose of headache relief. If surgery is not pursued, repeat biochemical assessment for hypopituitarism usually occurs on a yearly basis for incidentalomas 1 cm or greater. Longitudinal imaging surveillance is also recommended, although controversy exists over the optimal frequency and duration.[14]

PERIOPERATIVE EVALUATION OF PITUITARY FUNCTION

Assessment of pituitary function is a critical component of the perioperative management of a surgical patient with a sellar lesion. A thorough preoperative evaluation of pituitary function, performed using basic biochemical tests discussed in the preceding sections, ensures that the sellar lesion in question cannot be treated medically (eg, a prolactinoma) and that the patient does not have hypopituitary conditions (central hypothyroidism or adrenal insufficiency) which could pose a threat during anesthesia induction or the physiologic stress of surgery.

In the immediate postoperative period (48–72 h) careful monitoring for newly acquired DI (via strict recording of intake/output and serial measurements of urine specific gravity and serum sodium) and adrenal insufficiency (via early morning cortisol) should occur. Our general clinical practice involves initiating glucocorticoid replacement in patients with a morning cortisol of less than 10 µg/dL on either postoperative day 1 or 2, recognizing the limitations of such testing as outlined in the preceding sections. These patients are then evaluated formally for persistent HPA axis dysfunction at their postoperative visit, usually 2 to 3 months after their surgery. Transient hyponatremia, likely mediated by inappropriate ADH secretion, is a well-known complication of pituitary surgery which typically occurs 7 to 10 days postoperatively[38]; we suggest all patients have a sodium check approximately 1 week following discharge.

SUMMARY

The pituitary gland is an important regulator of multiple physiologic processes in the body. Tumors of the pituitary gland cause problems via mass effect, hypersecretion, or impairment of normal pituitary function. Relevant mass effect symptoms usually result from cranial nerve compression (optic chiasm; CN 3,4,6). A directed hormonal evaluation is a key step as hypersecreting tumors require surgical resection for cure; the exception being prolactinoma which usually responds to medical therapy. Evaluation of pituitary function perioperatively is critical to avoid morbidity from hypopituitarism. A thorough understanding of pituitary anatomy, physiology, and biochemical testing will allow the skull base surgeon to determine appropriate candidates for surgery and identify patients at high risk for perioperative complications from hypopituitarism.

REFERENCES

1. Bates AS, Van't Hoff W, Jones PJ, et al. The effect of hypopituitarism on life expectancy. J Clin Endocrinol Metab 1996;81(3):1169–72.
2. Freda PU, Post KD. Differential diagnosis of sellar masses. Endocrinol Metab Clin North Am 1999;28(1):81–117, vi.
3. Treier M, Rosenfeld MG. The hypothalamic-pituitary axis: co-development of two organs. Curr Opin Cell Biol 1996;8(6):833–43.
4. Feldkamp J, Santen R, Harms E, et al. Incidentally discovered pituitary lesions: high frequency of macroadenomas and hormone-secreting adenomas - results of a prospective study. Clin Endocrinol (Oxf) 1999;51(1):109–13.
5. Kim SH, Lee KC, Kim SH. Cranial nerve palsies accompanying pituitary tumour. J Clin Neurosci 2007;14(12):1158–62.
6. Pfaffle R, Klammt J. Pituitary transcription factors in the aetiology of combined pituitary hormone deficiency. Best Pract Res Clin Endocrinol Metab 2011;25(1): 43–60.
7. Butler AA, Le Roith D. Control of growth by the somatropic axis: growth hormone and the insulin-like growth factors have related and independent roles. Annu Rev Physiol 2001;63:141–64.
8. Gadelha MR, Kasuki L, Korbonits M. Novel pathway for somatostatin analogs in patients with acromegaly. Trends Endocrinol Metab 2013;24(5):238–46.
9. Vance ML. Hypopituitarism. N Engl J Med 1994;330(23):1651–62.

10. Swearingen B, Barker FG 2nd, Katznelson L, et al. Long-term mortality after trans-sphenoidal surgery and adjunctive therapy for acromegaly. J Clin Endocrinol Metab 1998;83(10):3419–26.

11. Ntali G, Asimakopoulou A, Siamatras T, et al. Mortality in Cushing's syndrome: systematic analysis of a large series with prolonged follow-up. Eur J Endocrinol 2013;169(5):715–23.

12. Ntali G, Capatina C, Grossman A, et al. Functioning gonadotroph adenomas. J Clin Endocrinol Metab 2014;99(12):4423–33.

13. Daly AF, Rixhon M, Adam C, et al. High prevalence of pituitary adenomas: a cross-sectional study in the province of Liege, Belgium. J Clin Endocrinol Metab 2006;91(12):4769–75.

14. Freda PU, Beckers AM, Katznelson L, et al. Pituitary incidentaloma: an endocrine society clinical practice guideline. J Clin Endocrinol Metab 2011;96(4):894–904.

15. Verhelst J, Abs R, Maiter D, et al. Cabergoline in the treatment of hyperprolacti-nemia: a study in 455 patients. J Clin Endocrinol Metab 1999;84(7):2518–22.

16. Hess CP, Dillon WP. Imaging the pituitary and parasellar region. Neurosurg Clin N Am 2012;23(4):529–42.

17. Rajasoorya C, Holdaway IM, Wrightson P, et al. Determinants of clinical outcome and survival in acromegaly. Clin Endocrinol (Oxf) 1994;41(1):95–102.

18. Katznelson L, Laws ER Jr, Melmed S, et al. Acromegaly: an endocrine society clinical practice guideline. J Clin Endocrinol Metab 2014;99(11):3933–51.

19. Dimaraki EV, Jaffe CA, DeMott-Friberg R, et al. Acromegaly with apparently normal GH secretion: implications for diagnosis and follow-up. J Clin Endocrinol Metab 2002;87(8):3537–42.

20. Giustina A, Chanson P, Bronstein MD, et al. A consensus on criteria for cure of acromegaly. J Clin Endocrinol Metab 2010;95(7):3141–8.

21. Nieman LK, Biller BM, Findling JW, et al. The diagnosis of Cushing's syndrome: an Endocrine Society Clinical Practice Guideline. J Clin Endocrinol Metab 2008;93(5):1526–40.

22. Hopkins RL, Leinung MC. Exogenous Cushing's syndrome and glucocorticoid withdrawal. Endocrinol Metab Clin North Am 2005;34(2):371–84.

23. Oldfield EH, Doppman JL, Nieman LK, et al. Petrosal sinus sampling with and without corticotropin-releasing hormone for the differential diagnosis of Cushing's syndrome. N Engl J Med 1991;325(13):897–905.

24. Klibanski A. Clinical practice. Prolactinomas. N Engl J Med 2010;362(13):1219–26.

25. Kearns AE, Goff DC, Hayden DL, et al. Risperidone-associated hyperprolactine-mia. Endocr Pract 2000;6(6):425–9.

26. Karavitaki N, Thanabalasingham G, Shore HC, et al. Do the limits of serum pro-lactin in disconnection hyperprolactinaemia need re-definition? A study of 226 patients with histologically verified non-functioning pituitary macroadenoma. Clin Endocrinol (Oxf) 2006;65(4):524–9.

27. Melmed S, Casanueva FF, Hoffman AR, et al. Diagnosis and treatment of hyper-prolactinemia: an Endocrine Society clinical practice guideline. J Clin Endocrinol Metab 2011;96(2):273–88.

28. Molitch ME, Clemmons DR, Malozowski S, et al. Evaluation and treatment of adult growth hormone deficiency: an Endocrine Society clinical practice guideline. J Clin Endocrinol Metab 2011;96(6):1587–609.

29. Schmidt IL, Lahner H, Mann K, et al. Diagnosis of adrenal insufficiency: evalua-tion of the corticotropin-releasing hormone test and Basal serum cortisol in com-parison to the insulin tolerance test in patients with hypothalamic-pituitary-adrenal disease. J Clin Endocrinol Metab 2003;88(9):4193–8.

30. Erturk E, Jaffe CA, Barkan AL. Evaluation of the integrity of the hypothalamic-pituitary-adrenal axis by insulin hypoglycemia test. J Clin Endocrinol Metab 1998;83(7):2350–4.
31. Nemergut EC, Zuo Z, Jane JA Jr, et al. Predictors of diabetes insipidus after transsphenoidal surgery: a review of 881 patients. J Neurosurg 2005;103(3):448–54.
32. Turcu AF, Erickson BJ, Lin E, et al. Pituitary stalk lesions: the Mayo Clinic experience. J Clin Endocrinol Metab 2013;98(5):1812–8.
33. Miller M, Dalakos T, Moses AM, et al. Recognition of partial defects in antidiuretic hormone secretion. Ann Intern Med 1970;73(5):721–9.
34. Hall WA, Luciano MG, Doppman JL, et al. Pituitary magnetic resonance imaging in normal human volunteers: occult adenomas in the general population. Ann Intern Med 1994;120(10):817–20.
35. Arafah BM. Reversible hypopituitarism in patients with large nonfunctioning pituitary adenomas. J Clin Endocrinol Metab 1986;62(6):1173–9.
36. Levy MJ, Jager HR, Powell M, et al. Pituitary volume and headache: size is not everything. Arch Neurol 2004;61(5):721–5.
37. Levy MJ, Matharu MS, Meeran K, et al. The clinical characteristics of headache in patients with pituitary tumours. Brain 2005;128(Pt 8):1921–30.
38. Olson BR, Gumowski J, Rubino D, et al. Pathophysiology of hyponatremia after transsphenoidal pituitary surgery. J Neurosurg 1997;87(4):499–507.

Imaging in Endoscopic Cranial Skull Base and Pituitary Surgery

Renato Hoffmann Nunes, MD[a,b,c], Ana Lorena Abello, MD[a,d],
Adam M. Zanation, MD[e,f], Deanna Sasaki-Adams, MD[e],
Benjamin Y. Huang, MD, MPH[a],*

KEYWORDS

- Endoscopic skull base surgery • CT • MRI • Nasoseptal flap • Skull base

KEY POINTS

- The feasibility of endoscopic endonasal approaches, the potential surgical risk, and tumor resectability depend on critical anatomic structures in the surgical corridors that can be assessed by preoperative imaging studies.
- Computed tomography scan yields the best overall evaluation of the bony architecture of the skull base.
- MRI is the best imaging modality to evaluate the soft tissues and to demonstrate the location of a lesion and its relationship to adjacent neurovascular structures.
- Neoplastic recurrences typically occur at the interface of the flap recipient bed and reconstructive tissue and appear as new or growing infiltrative enhancing tissue similar to the resected tumor.

INTRODUCTION

Although traditional open techniques still play an important role in skull base surgery, they continue to carry significant perioperative risks and morbidity with prolonged recovery times, in part because they require some degree of brain retraction and

Disclosures: The authors have nothing to disclose.
[a] Department of Radiology, University of North Carolina at Chapel Hill, 101 Manning Drive, CB#7510, Chapel Hill, NC 27599, USA; [b] Division of Neuroradiology, Fleury Medicina e Saúde, Santa Casa de Misericórdia de São Paulo, Rua Cincinato Braga, 282, Bela Vista, São Paulo, São Paulo 01333-910, Brazil; [c] Santa Casa de Misericórdia de São Paulo, Serviço de Diagnostico por Imagem, Rua Dr. Cesário Motta Junior 112, Vila Buarque, São Paulo, São Paulo 01221-020, Brazil; [d] Department of Radiology, Universidad del Valle, Calle 13#100-00 Cali, Valle del Cauca, Colombia; [e] Department of Neurosurgery, University of North Carolina at Chapel Hill, 170 Manning Drive, CB#7070, Chapel Hill, NC 27599, USA; [f] Department of Otolaryngology-Head and Neck Surgery, University of North Carolina at Chapel Hill, 170 Manning Drive, CB#7060, Chapel Hill, NC 27599, USA
* Corresponding author. Department of Radiology, University of North Carolina Chapel Hill, 101 Manning Drive, CB#7510, Chapel Hill, NC 27599-7510.
E-mail address: bhuang@med.unc.edu

Otolaryngol Clin N Am 49 (2016) 33–62
http://dx.doi.org/10.1016/j.otc.2015.09.003
0030-6665/16/$ – see front matter © 2016 Elsevier Inc. All rights reserved.

oto.theclinics.com

Abbreviations	
ASB	Anterior skull base
CN	Cranial nerve
CSB	Central skull base
CSF	Cerebrospinal fluid
CT	Computed tomography
CTA	Computed tomography angiography
DWI	Diffusion-weighted imaging
EEA	Endoscopic endonasal approaches
ESBR	Endoscopic skull base reconstructions
FDG-PET	F18-fluorodeoxyglucose positron emission tomography
FLAIR	Fluid-attenuated inversion recovery
ICA	Internal carotid artery
IOF	Inferior orbital fissure
ITAC	Intestinal type adenocarcinomas
MRA	Magnetic resonance angiography
MRI	Magnetic resonance imaging
NPL	Nasopalatine line
NSF	Nasoseptal flap
PPF	Pterygopalatine fossa
SOF	Superior orbital fissure
STIR	Short-tau inversion recovery
T1WI	T1-weighted image
T2WI	T2-weighted image

neurovascular manipulation to access the skull base. In an attempt to address some of the shortcomings of open skull base surgery, less invasive endoscopic endonasal approaches (EEAs) to the skull base have been developed and have become increasingly accepted and widely adopted.[1]

In recent years, EEAs have become standard for the treatment of a variety of sinonasal and central skull base diseases. Important factors leading to the popularization of these techniques include an improved understanding of the anatomy of the skull base anatomy; imaging advances that allow easy acquisition and reconstruction of high-resolution, multiplanar images of the skull base; and the rapid development of imaging-based operative navigation systems. In modern practice, the preoperative radiographic evaluation is not only useful for diagnosis but is also invaluable for surgical mapping to ensure safe and optimal surgical outcomes.[2] These techniques were initially developed for paranasal sinus surgery, but their indications have been gradually extended to include endoscopic resection of pituitary tumors, as well as lesions of the clivus, olfactory cleft, planum sphenoidale, petrous apex, and infratemporal fossa. The EEA provides access to almost all regions of the skull base situated anterior to the foramen magnum.[3]

Principles of endoscopic endonasal skull base surgery involve selecting a surgical corridor with an optimal visual field, thus minimizing the need for neurovascular manipulation. If these preconditions are met, the outcomes after an EEA compare favorably with conventional techniques, while providing the advantages of a lack of external incisions or scars, decreased trauma to soft tissue and bone, less disturbance of craniofacial growth in pediatric patients, fewer complications, reduced risk of neurologic damage, improved postoperative quality of life, decreased lengths of hospital stays, and faster recovery times.[4]

A major criticism of endoscopic techniques is that they do not allow en bloc resection of tumors. However, the tumors are also often fragmented in the course of open surgery, and the most important aspect is not en bloc resection, but complete resection of the tumor margins. Tumors of the skull base often demonstrate exophytic growth into paranasal sinuses from a smaller pedicle. However, the endonasal approach often allows resection without damaging adjacent healthy tissues, which is not the case with conventional open surgery, in which the skin, bone, and sometimes dura mater are opened to provide access to the tumor, with a risk of tumor seeding.[3]

The aims of this article were to review techniques for imaging the skull base, to depict the anatomy of the anterior and central skull base, to illustrate the most common cranial base pathologies that may be amenable to EEA, to briefly review the various endoscopic approaches in EEA and key presurgical anatomic considerations and contraindications to each of these, and to understand the expected postoperative imaging appearance of the common endoscopic skull base reconstructions (ESBR), recognizing the most frequent complications.

IMAGING TECHNIQUE

Given the diversity of pathologic findings of the skull base, a combination of imaging studies may be required to assess a particular lesion fully. Computed tomography (CT) and MRI often play complementary roles in evaluation of the skull base pathology, and both may be considered essential for an initial radiologic workup.[5]

High-resolution nonenhanced CT reconstructed with a bone algorithm yields the best overall evaluation of the bony architecture of the anterior and central skull base. Cortical margins, neuroforamina, trabecular bone, and tumoral or soft tissue calcifications can be evaluated with excellent detail.[5]

MRI is considered the best imaging study to evaluate the soft tissues of the skull base. MRI further details the location of a lesion and its relationship to adjacent neurovascular structures. In cases of a sinonasal tumor with skull base involvement, MRI distinguishes the neoplasm from inspissated secretion and defines the extranasal and intracranial extent of the tumor.[2] The presence of fat in the soft tissues and in the marrow spaces is extremely useful in defining normal anatomy and in identifying areas of potential pathology, particularly on spin-echo T1-weighted images (T1WI), on which fat demonstrates high signal intensity. Short-tau inversion recovery (STIR) or fat-suppressed T2-weighted images (T2WI) are used to suppress signal related to fat and maximize T2 signal related to infection, inflammation, fluid, or neoplasm. These sequences are commonly performed in the axial and/or coronal planes.[5]

Postcontrast gadolinium-enhanced images should be performed in at least 2 planes (usually the axial and coronal planes) and are essential for detecting disease of the suprahyoid soft tissues, the bone marrow, and the meninges, as well as perineural tumor spread. One or both of these enhanced sequences are typically performed with fat saturation. However, with fat-suppression techniques, susceptibility artifacts are common in the skull base because of field inhomogeneity and multiple air-bone–soft tissue interfaces.[5,6] **Table 1** outlines our MR protocol for imaging of the skull base. This protocol includes whole brain and dedicated skull base sequences and extends from the vertex to the hard palate.

Ultimately, imaging protocols may need to be individualized depending on the particular lesion or clinical question. Pituitary adenoma evaluation, for instance, often requires dynamic contrast-enhanced imaging, for detection of small lesions. Magnetic resonance angiography (MRA) or CT angiography (CTA) can be used to evaluate the vessels of the skull base and their relationships to resection targets. High-resolution heavily T2-weighted sequences are excellent at depicting cranial nerves (CNs) and vessels as they course through the basilar cisterns.[5]

Other modalities may occasionally be used to evaluate the skull base. F18-fluorodeoxyglucose positron emission tomography (FDG-PET) can be used in the

Table 1
MRI protocol for skull base evaluation

Sequence	Plane	Slice Thickness, mm	Coverage
Precontrast			
EPI DWI	Axial	5	Entire brain
Spin-echo T1W	Sagittal	4	Entire brain
Fat-suppressed TSE T2	Axial	5	Entire brain
FLAIR	Axial	5	Entire brain
Fat-suppressed TSE T2W	Axial	4	Paranasal sinuses and skull base
TSE T1W	Axial	4	Paranasal sinuses and skull base
3D T1 MPRAGE	Axial	1	Entire brain and skull base
Postcontrast			
Fat-suppressed SE T1W	Axial	4	Paranasal sinuses and skull base
Fat-suppressed SE T1W	Coronal	3	Tip of nose through brainstem
3D T1 MPRAGE	Axial with additional sagittal and coronal reconstructions	1	Entire brain and skull base
3D CISS	Axial	0.7	Paranasal sinuses and skull base

Abbreviations: 3D, 3 dimensional; CISS, constructive interference in steady state; DWI, diffusion-weighted image; EPI, echo planar imaging; FLAIR, Fluid-attenuated inversion recovery; MPRAGE, magnetization prepared rapid acquisition gradient recalled echo; T1W, T1-weighted; T2W, T2-weighted; TSE, turbo spin-echo.

posttreatment follow-up of skull base tumors to differentiate posttreatment changes from persistent or recurrent neoplasm. No routine role has been found in the primary evaluation of patients presenting with skull base lesions, however.[6] Conventional angiography may be necessary for preoperative embolization of highly vascular lesions to facilitate surgical resection and to reduce intraoperative hemorrhage.[5]

ANATOMY OF ANTERIOR SKULL BASE

The floor of the anterior cranial fossa, often referred to as the anterior skull base (ASB), is formed by the roof of the nasal cavity and ethmoid sinuses, the roof of the orbits on either side of the ethmoid roofs, and the lesser wings of the sphenoid bone posteriorly.[7]

The midline cribriform plate, which forms the roof of the nasal cavity, is traversed by multiple olfactory nerves that extend from the olfactory mucosa to the olfactory bulbs.[7] The cribriform plate is separated into right and left halves by the insertion of the nasal septum. On either side of the cribriform plate is the fovea ethmoidalis or ethmoid roof, which is formed by the medial extension of each orbital plate and is generally located more superiorly than the cribriform plate. A thin, usually vertically oriented bone plate (lateral lamella), connects the cribriform plate with each fovea ethmoidalis.[8] In adults, the olfactory fossae are variable depressions on either side of the crista galli, which contain the olfactory bulbs; each fossa is bounded inferiorly by the cribriform plate and laterally by the lateral lamella (**Fig. 1**). Because of the relative fragility of the

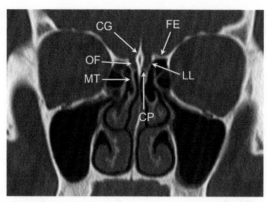

Fig. 1. Anatomy of the anterior skull base on coronal CT. CG, crista galli; CP, cribriform plate; FE, Fovea ethmoidalis; LL, lateral lamella; MT, middle turbinate insertion into the cribriform plate; OF, olfactory fossa.

bone of the cribriform plate and fovea ethmoidalis, they can be easily violated if care is not taken during EEA. The middle turbinate is delicately attached to the cribriform plate, so detachment of this structure at its insertion during EEA may tear the adjacent dura, resulting in cerebrospinal fluid (CSF) rhinorrhea.[7] Although the thin cribriform plate is easily crossed by tumors, the orbital plates of the frontal bone, which are made of thick compact bone, constitute a barrier to tumor growth into the anterior cranial fossa. Therefore, it is not surprising that most tumors violating the anterior skull base arise from the sinonasal region.[9]

The ethmoid cells are divided by the posterior attachment of the middle turbinate (the basal lamella) into an anterior group, which drains anteriorly into the ethmoid bulla and hiatus semilunaris, and a posterior group which drains into the sphenoethmoidal recess (**Fig. 2**). The basal lamella extends superiorly within the ethmoid complex to reach the fovea ethmoidalis. The anterior ethmoid cells comprise the anterior

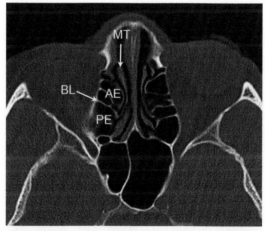

Fig. 2. The basal lamella on axial CT. The basal lamella (BL) represents the posterior attachment of the middle turbinate (MT) and divides the ethmoids into anterior ethmoid (AE) and posterior ethmoid (PE) cells.

two-thirds to three-quarters of the ethmoid complex. In the adult, the basal lamella is usually not a straight bony partition, but rather a curved structure almost inseparable from the other ethmoid septae, because it becomes remodeled by adjacent ethmoid cells as they develop. There is no basal lamella present along the anterior attachment of the middle turbinate. Instead, it is replaced by a medial lamella that attaches to the lateral cribriform plate.[10] The posterior ethmoid cells are important because of their variable relationship with the sphenoid sinus and their intimate association with the optic nerve at the orbital apex.[7]

The optic canal transmits the optic nerve and the ophthalmic artery. The anterior cranial base faces the frontal lobes with the gyri recti medially and the orbital gyri laterally, along with the branches of the anterior cerebral arteries medially and middle cerebral arteries laterally.[11]

Another important anatomic consideration is the medial orbital wall. Most of its surface is exceedingly thin (lamina papyracea). This is formed by a small portion of the frontal process of the maxilla, the lacrimal bone, the ethmoid bone, and the body of the sphenoid. Anteriorly is the lacrimal groove for the lacrimal sac. The groove communicates below with the nasal cavity through the nasolacrimal canal, which is approximately 1 cm long and contains the nasolacrimal duct, which drains into the inferior meatus of the nasal cavity. Also in the medial wall are 2 canals for the anterior and posterior ethmoidal nerves and vessels. These canals are situated at the level of the floor of the anterior cranial fossa, as their lower margins are formed by the upper margin of the ethmoid bone and their upper margins are formed by the under surface of the frontal bone. The anterior ethmoidal foramen is located at the frontal-ethmoidal suture and transmits the anterior ethmoidal vessels and nerve. The posterior ethmoidal foramen transmits the posterior ethmoidal vessels and nerve. These arteries often need to be identified and ligated/coagulated during procedures in the anterior cranial base (**Fig. 3**).[7,10,12]

Another important vessel to consider is the orbitofrontal branch of the anterior cerebral artery, due to its proximity to the anterior cranial base and the increased risk of injury to the vessel during procedures extending into the anterior cranial fossa

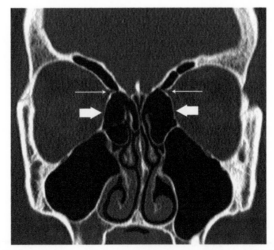

Fig. 3. Medial orbital wall on coronal CT. Anterior ethmoidal canals (*thin white arrows*), lamina papyracea (*thick white arrows*).

(**Fig. 4**).[11] Because of its small size, however, this vessel can be difficult to consistently visualize on noninvasive angiographic techniques like CTA and MRA.

ANATOMY OF THE CENTRAL SKULL BASE

The sphenoid bone is the foundation of the central skull base (CSB), which also contains the pituitary gland within the sella turcica and the parasellar cavernous sinuses. This bone and its foramina can be involved by primary pathologic processes of bone, extracranial disease that can extend intracranially, and intracranial disease that can extend extracranially.[10]

The shape of the sphenoid bone resembles that of a bird with wings outstretched. The central sphenoid body is a roughly cuboidal structure that houses the sphenoid sinuses, and the superior surface of the sphenoid body contributes to the floor of the anterior cranial fossa. Specifically, just posterior to the ethmoid bone, the ethmoid process of the sphenoid bone forms the flat region known as the planum sphenoidale, which represents the anterior portion of the roof of the sphenoid sinuses. The planum lies between the lesser sphenoid wings and separates the cribriform area anteriorly from the chiasmatic sulcus of the sella posteriorly (**Fig. 5**).[13] The greater wings of the sphenoid sweep laterally from the sphenoid body, reaching and contributing to the lateral surface of the calvarium. The lesser wings form the superior margin of the superior orbital fissure (SOF). The anterior clinoid processes define the posterior margins of each lesser wing. The pterygoid processes and their medial and lateral plates drop inferiorly from the junction of the body of sphenoid bone and the greater wing. The sphenoid bone is separated from the petrous apex of the temporal bone on either side by foramen lacerum.[13]

Many of the important neurovascular foramina of the skull base lay in this central compartment, including the intracranial opening of the SOF, which is traversed by CNs III, IV, VI, and V1 and the superior ophthalmic vein on their way from the cavernous sinus to the orbit; foramen rotundum, which gives passage to CN V2 between the cavernous sinus and the pterygopalatine fossa (PPF); the vidian canal, which contains the vidian nerve and artery extending from foramen lacerum to the

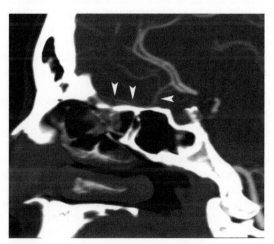

Fig. 4. Orbitofrontal branch of the anterior cerebral artery. Maximum intensity projection reconstruction from a CTA of the head demonstrating the course of the orbitofrontal artery (*arrowheads*) just above the anterior skull base.

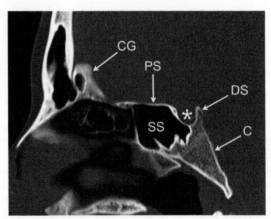

Fig. 5. Midsagittal CT demonstrating anatomy of the central skull base. C, clivus; CG, crista galli; DS, dorsum of the sella turcica; PS, planum sphenoidale, SS, sphenoidal sinus. Asterisk indicates the sella turcica.

high PPF; foramen ovale, which conveys V3 to the masticator space; and foramen spinosum, which is crossed by the middle meningeal artery (**Figs. 6–8**).[6,13]

The PPF is a primarily fat-filled space that tapers inferiorly into a common bony palatine canal that carries the palatine nerves. This canal ultimately divides into separate greater and lesser palatine canals, transmitting their respective nerves to the posterior hard palate. Superiorly, the PPF is contiguous with the inferior orbital fissure (IOF). The maxillary nerve continues from the PPF through the IOF, becoming the infraorbital nerve. Laterally, the PPF communicates with the infratemporal fossa through the pterygomaxillary fissure. Medially, the PPF is contiguous with the submucosa of the posterior nasal cavity through a gap or notch in the perpendicular plate of the palatine bone, referred to as the sphenopalatine foramen (see **Figs. 6** and **7; Fig. 9**).[5]

The body of the sphenoid bone also houses the sella turcica, which is located behind the planum sphenoidale and is bounded anteriorly by the tuberculum sellae and posteriorly by the dorsum sella. The posterior surface of the dorsum is continuous with the posterior surface of the body of the sphenoid and basiocciput, which collectively form the clivus. The sella turcica is covered superficially by a thin layer of dura, the diaphragma sellae, which stretches across the top of the sella and is perforated centrally by the pituitary stalk (see **Figs. 5–7**).[5,8,10,13]

The pituitary gland, also called the hypophysis, is a reddish-gray, bean-shaped gland with 2 distinct parts or "lobes," which differ in embryologic origin, structure, and function. These parts are the anterior pituitary (adenohypophysis) and the posterior pituitary (neurohypophysis). The overall height of the pituitary gland on coronal T1WI varies with both age and gender. In prepubescent children, a height of 6 mm or less is normal; in young girls of menstrual age, 9 mm is the upper limit of normal; and in pregnant women, the pituitary gland can measure 12 mm. The upper limit of normal in adult men and postmenopausal women is 8 mm. The neurohypophysis usually is of higher signal intensity on T1WI (the so-called posterior pituitary "bright spot") caused by the presence of neurosecretory granules. Of note, the neurohypophysis does not contain lipid and therefore does not suppress with fat-suppression techniques. The pituitary gland does not have a blood-brain barrier, so it normally enhances rapidly and intensely following contrast administration (**Fig. 10**).[14,15]

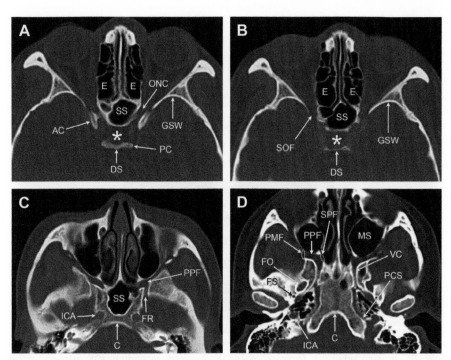

Fig. 6. (*A–D*) Axial CT images through the skull base, superior to inferior. AC, anterior clinoid; C, clivus; DS, dorsum sella; E, ethmoids; FO, foramen ovale; FR, foramen rotundum; FS, foramen spinosum; GSW, greater sphenoid wing; ICA, internal carotid artery canal; MS, maxillary sinus; ONC, optic nerve canal; PC, posterior clinoid; PCS, petroclival synchondrosis; PMF, pterygomaxillary fissure; PPF, pterygopalatine fossa; SOF, superior orbital fissure; SPF, sphenopalatine foramen; SS, sphenoidal sinus; VC, vidian canal. Asterisk indicates the sella turcica.

The cavernous sinuses are venous sinusoid structures situated between the layers of the dura, bordering the pituitary fossa and the lateral surfaces of the body of the sphenoid bone and forming much of the medial walls of the middle cranial fossae. Each cavernous sinus contains several nerves. The ophthalmic division of the trigeminal nerve (V1) passes from the Meckel cave into the cavernous sinus on the way to the SOF. The maxillary division of the trigeminal nerve (V2) has a shorter course within the cavernous sinus before entering the foramen rotundum. The third division of the trigeminal nerve (V3) exits almost directly from the Meckel cave through the foramen ovale and does not truly enter the cavernous sinus. The semilunar or gasserian ganglion, the convergence of the divisions of the trigeminal nerve, lies along the inferior lateral wall of the Meckel cave, which is a CSF-containing arachnoidal pouch protruding from the posterior cranial fossa and situated at the posterolateral aspect of the cavernous sinus. The oculomotor, trochlear, and abducens nerves traverse the entire anteroposterior length of the cavernous sinus before exiting the skull at the SOF.

The internal carotid arteries (ICAs) also traverse the cavernous sinuses. Each artery extends superiorly immediately after exiting the petrous carotid canal. This brings the artery into the cavernous sinus between the Meckel cave and the lateral wall of the sphenoid sinus. The artery then curves anteriorly before making a sharp bend upward to pass through the dura just below the optic nerve.[10] In some patients, the

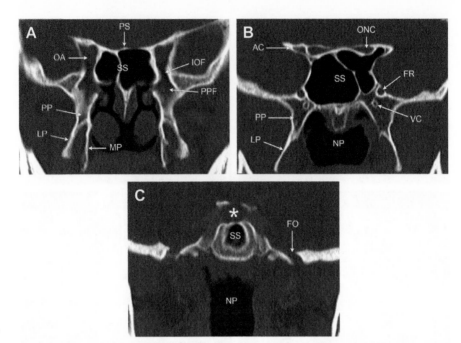

Fig. 7. (*A–C*) Coronal CT images through the CSB from anterior to posterior. AC, anterior clinoid; DS, dorsum sella; FO, foramen ovale; FR, foramen rotundum; IOF, inferior orbital
fissure; LP, lateral pterygoid plate; MP, medial pterygoid plate; NP, nasopharynx; OA, orbital
apex; ONC, optic nerve canal; PP, pterygoid process; PPF, pterygopalatine fossa; PS, planum
sphenoidale; SS, sphenoidal sinus; VC, vidian canal. Asterisk indicates the sella turcica.

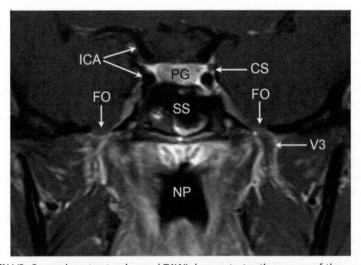

Fig. 8. CN V3. Coronal contrast-enhanced T1WI demonstrates the course of the mandibular
nerve (V3), which can be seen better on the left side passing through foramen ovale (FO).
CS, cavernous sinus; ICA, internal carotid artery; NP, nasopharynx; PG, pituitary gland; SS,
sphenoidal sinus.

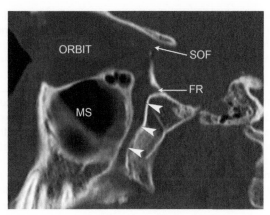

Fig. 9. Pterygopalatine fossa (*arrowheads*) on sagittal CT. FR, foramen rotundum; MS, maxillary sinus; SOF, superior orbital fissure.

intersphenoid septum may be deflected to one side and attach to the bony wall covering the carotid artery. In this situation, arterial injury may result if the septum is avulsed during surgery. In addition, the ICA may bulge into the sinus in some patients, making it more prone to injury during endoscopic sphenoid sinus surgery.

ANTERIOR SKULL BASE PATHOLOGY
Sinonasal Neoplasms

Most sinonasal neoplasms are epithelial in origin and include, in decreasing order of frequency, squamous cell carcinoma, intestinal-type adenocarcinoma, and minor salivary gland neoplasms. The remainder comprise neoplasms arising from the olfactory mucosa (esthesioneuroblastomas), nasal lymphoma, melanoma, and a variety of mesenchymal tumors including rhabdomyosarcoma, the most common in the pediatric age group. Regardless of histology, malignant neoplasms share aggressive imaging features usually presenting as enhancing ill-defined soft tissue masses spreading beyond the boundaries of the sinonasal cavities, eroding bone and often leading to

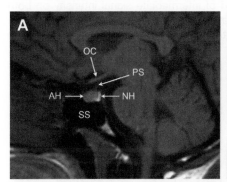
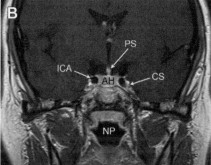

Fig. 10. Pituitary gland. (*A*) Sagittal precontrast T1WI demonstrates the posterior pituitary bright spot, which represents the neurohypophysis (NH) posterior to the adenohypophysis (AH). Note the relationship to the optic chiasm (OC) above and the sphenoid sinus (SS) below (PS, pituitary stalk). (*B*) Coronal postcontrast T1WI shows homogeneous enhancement of the adenohypophysis and pituitary stalk. Note the relationship of the pituitary gland to the ICA and cavernous sinus (CS) (NP, nasopharynx).

obstruction of sinus ostia and retention of secretions. Tumor spread is usually to the orbit, most commonly through the lamina papyracea, to the anterior cranial fossa through the cribriform plate, and to the PPF and retromaxillary fat through the posterior wall of the maxillary sinus or through the sphenopalatine foramen.[9]

Squamous Cell Cancer

Squamous cell carcinomas are the most common malignancies of the nose and paranasal sinuses, accounting for more than 70% of all malignancies. The maxillary antrum is the most frequent primary site, followed by the nasal cavity and ethmoid sinus. On imaging, these tumors are aggressive, often demonstrating bony destruction on CT. They show intermediate signal intensity on T2WI, reflecting high cellularity. They show intense homogeneous enhancement on postcontrast imaging, although usually to a lesser degree than normal sinonasal mucosa. This pattern helps to distinguish this entity from benign inflammatory processes, such as sinonasal polyposis, and from mucoceles, which do not erode bone and enhance peripherally. Because of the aggressive nature of squamous cell carcinomas, extension through the cribriform plate into the anterior cranial fossa is possible. Because of the presence of necrosis and hemorrhage, large tumors may be quite heterogeneous (**Fig. 11**).[9,16]

Adenocarcinoma

Adenocarcinomas comprise 10% of all sinonasal tumors and are subdivided into minor salivary gland tumors, intestinal type adenocarcinomas (ITAC), and neuroendocrine neoplasms.[9] Imaging features are usually nonspecific, and it is not possible to distinguish these tumors from squamous cell cancers based on imaging alone. Low-grade tumors show a less aggressive pattern of bone involvement, usually with remodeling and thinning rather than permeative destruction.[16]

Olfactory Neuroblastoma

Olfactory neuroblastomas, also known as esthesioneuroblastomas, comprise 3% of intracranial tumors and arise from the specialized olfactory epithelium. On CT scans, these lesions appear as solid, homogeneously enhancing superior nasal cavity masses with or without destruction of the adjacent bones, especially of the cribriform plate. Calcifications may occur in the tumor mass. Like other small-cell tumors, these tumors are slightly hyperdense on CT and of intermediate signal intensity on both T1WI and T2WI. In some of the larger tumors in which there is intracranial extension, the presence of small peripheral cysts at the interface with brain parenchyma, with

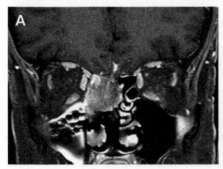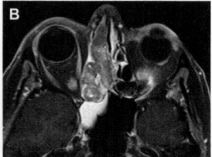

Fig. 11. Squamous cell carcinoma. (*A*, *B*) Coronal and axial postcontrast, fat-suppressed T1WI show a heterogeneously enhancing lesion in the superior nasal cavity, abutting the anterior skull base. The lesion does not invade the orbit or the anterior cranial fossa.

their broadest base at the tumor mass is reported as a specific (although insensitive) feature of this tumor (**Fig. 12**).[9,16]

Olfactory Groove and Planum Sphenoidale Meningiomas

This is the most common intracranial lesion affecting the anterior skull base from above. Meningiomas are best characterized on MRI. They are usually isointense to brain on both T1WI and T2WI, well circumscribed, and show intense and homogeneous gadolinium enhancement. Adjacent linear dural enhancement, referred to as a dural tail, is commonly seen. Meningiomas from the olfactory groove may extend through the cribriform plate into the ethmoid sinuses and nasal cavity. Associated bone changes include bone remodeling or bone sclerosis. Intratumoral calcifications are seldom seen (**Fig. 13**).[9,16] The associated hyperostosis of the skull base can require more detailed drilling before entering the intracranial cavity, which should be accounted for in planning the surgical approach.

CENTRAL SKULL BASE PATHOLOGY
Pituitary Adenoma

Adenomas are the most common pituitary tumors in adults. These lesions can be classified as microadenomas when smaller than 1 cm, or macroadenomas when larger

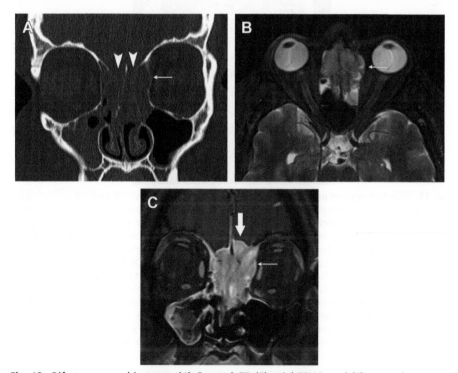

Fig. 12. Olfactory neuroblastoma. (*A*) Coronal CT, (*B*) axial T2WI, and (*C*) coronal postcontrast T1WI show a large, aggressive, enhancing mass arising in the nasal cavity at the skull base with extension into the anterior cranial fossa and dural invasion (*thick arrow on C*). There is osseous erosion of the cribriform plate (*arrowheads on A*). The left lamina papyracea is remodeled by the tumor and bowed laterally (*thin arrows on A–C*). Note on the T2WI the subtle hypointense line between the tumor and the orbital fat (*arrow on B*), indicating that the tumor has not violated the periorbita.

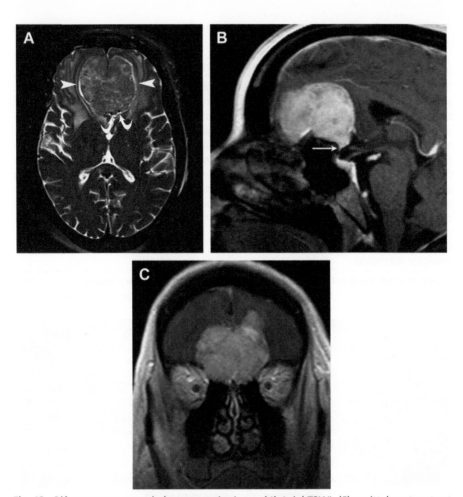

Fig. 13. Olfactory groove and planum meningioma. (*A*) Axial T2WI, (*B*) sagittal postcontrast T1WI, and (*C*) coronal postcontrast T1WI demonstrate a large intracranial mass sitting atop the anterior skull base and planum sphenoidale. The mass is heterogeneous on the T2WI, and there is a CSF cleft (*arrowheads* on *A*) apparent between the mass and the nearby brain parenchyma, indicating that the lesion is extra-axial in origin. Note also the relationship of the lesion to the anterior cerebral arteries (*curved arrows* on *A*). On the postcontrast images (*B, C*), the mass enhances homogeneously. A small tapered dural tail can be seen extending along the tuberculum sella (*arrow* in *B*), which is typical of meningiomas. On the coronal image (*C*), the tumor extends over the orbits, but does not extend over the far lateral aspects of either orbital roof, suggesting it may still be amenable to endoscopic resection; however, significant frontal lobe edema on (*A*) raises concern for possible subpial extension and indicates that this patient may not be an ideal candidate for an EEA.

than 1 cm.[8] Pituitary macroadenomas tend to fill and expand the sella and to extend superiorly into the suprasellar cistern through the diaphragm sella. Lateral growth may occur into the cavernous sinus, where the tumor may contact or even surround the cavernous carotid artery without narrowing its lumen, a distinctive feature of adenomas. Nonidentification of a normal pituitary gland suggests a tumor that is originating from the gland itself. Occasionally, macroadenomas show preferential inferior growth, destroy the sellar floor, and extend into the sphenoid body and sinus (invasive pituitary adenoma).[8,17] Macroadenomas are frequently of heterogeneous signal intensity, particularly on T2WI, with hyperintense areas reflecting cystic, necrotic, or hemorrhagic portions of the neoplasm. Similar to microadenomas, contrast enhancement of the tumors is usually not very prominent; the postcontrast images are primarily used to visualize the normal pituitary tissue, which demonstrates strong enhancement and may be seen displaced along the edges of the adenoma (**Fig. 14**). The frequent route of suprasellar spread in macroadenomas leads to a characteristic figure of 8 appearance because of tumor narrowing at the sellar diaphragm.[18]

Sellar Meningiomas

Meningiomas are the second most common tumor in the sellar region in adults.[19] Sellar meningiomas present as broad dural-based lesions, along the planum sphenoidale, filling in the sella. Usually the pituitary gland is compressed against the sellar floor, an important diagnostic clue. Other typical imaging features include increased pneumatization of the sphenoid sinus (pneumosinus dilatans) and hyperostosis of the planum sphenoidale with upward blistering, best appreciated on CT scans.[17] Meningiomas typically are similar to gray matter in CT density and in T1WI and T2WI signal intensity. They enhance homogeneously and brightly. Some diffuse calcification is not uncommon. Less commonly, they may have cystic areas, or even areas of fat. When meningiomas encase blood vessels, they tend to narrow the lumen more than other tumors, such as adenomas.[19]

Craniopharyngioma

Craniopharyngiomas are benign, slow-growing neoplasms of epithelial origin. They are the most common suprasellar lesion, and are most commonly entirely suprasellar in location. Approximately one-third, however, may extend into the sella, and occasionally they may be entirely intrasellar. They have a bimodal age distribution, with

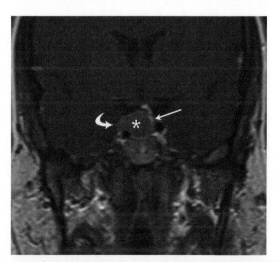

Fig. 14. Pituitary macroadenoma. Coronal postcontrast T1WI shows a mildly enhancing tumor (*asterisk*), located predominantly on the right aspect of the sella and displacing the pituitary stalk (*thin white arrow*) to the left. The lesions also extend lateral to the carotid artery into superolateral aspect of the cavernous sinus (*curved arrow*), which is an area to be avoided, given that the CNs III, IV, and VI pass through this region.

the first peak in incidence between 5 and 14 years of age, and the second peak in older adults aged 65 to 74 years. There are 2 histologic subtypes. The adamantinomatous subtype is seen mostly in children, whereas the squamous subtype occurs principally in older adults. This histologic variability in part accounts for the variability of imaging findings. The imaging hallmarks of craniopharyngioma are calcifications and cysts. Calcifications occur in approximately 80%, and may be nodular or curvilinear. Calcifications may be difficult to see on MRI, but are well depicted by CT. Cysts are present in almost all craniopharyngiomas. In children, the cystic parts tend to predominate, whereas in adults, solid parts are larger, and the cysts may be small or multiloculated. The cysts frequently contain highly proteinaceous fluid, which may be very bright on precontrast T1WI. The solid portions and cyst walls of all craniopharyngiomas enhance, usually heterogeneously (**Fig. 15**).[19] Three types of craniopharyngioma have been designated, based on its relationship to the infundibulum. A type I tumor grows anterior to the infundibulum and has a plane between it and the infundibulum, a type II tumor grows within the stalk, and a type III tumor is posterior to and often is surgically separable from the infundibulum. This last type may grow superiorly into the anterior third ventricle or posteriorly into the interpeduncular cistern. The relationship of the tumor to the stalk is important, because it has implications for the ability to preserve the pituitary stalk and determines the particular endonasal approach used to access the tumor.[20]

Chordoma

Chordomas are benign neoplasms thought to arise from remnants of the primitive notochord. They most commonly arise around the ends of the notochord, within the sacrum and clivus. Rarely, they may arise within the sella, in which case they are difficult to distinguish from pituitary macroadenomas. Although histologically benign, they can be quite aggressive, causing extensive bony destruction in the skull base. CT scan of patients with clival chordoma shows a bone-destroying mass, centered on the spheno-occipital synchondrosis. MRI shows a heterogeneous mass with internal septations, and heterogeneous enhancement (**Fig. 16**).[19]

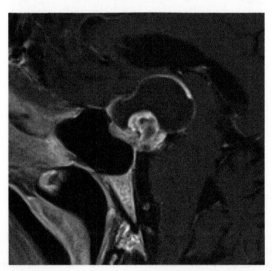

Fig. 15. Craniopharyngioma. Sagittal postcontrast T1WI shows a predominantly suprasellar cystic lesion with an enhancing nodule compatible with a craniopharyngioma.

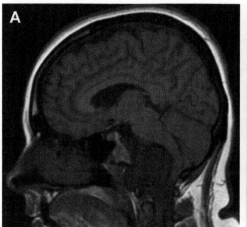
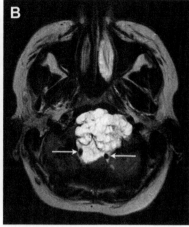

Fig. 16. Chordoma. (*A*) Sagittal T1WI demonstrate a hypointense mass centered in the clivus compressing the brainstem posteriorly. (*B*) On the axial T2WI, the lesion is very hyperintense and appears to encase the vertebral arteries (*arrows*), which would preclude complete resection.

PRESURGICAL CONSIDERATIONS IN ENDOSCOPIC ENDONASAL SURGERY

Effective EEA is now widely accepted for gross total resection of small and medium-sized tumors that are located in the midline or paramedian plane of the ventral skull base from the olfactory groove to the odontoid process of C2.[2] When planning the surgical approach, the surgeon decides on the target, the corridor, and an approach, minimizing the need for manipulating any vascular or neural components.[21] Preoperative imaging must be diligently reviewed to see where structures are compressed and altered from their original location.[22]

Determining the target is the first step. Based on its location, an approach and an entry point to the skull base, is selected to best access this target. Different types of approaches are used, including transfrontal, transcribriform, transclival, transsellar, and transtuberculum/transplanum (**Fig. 17**). After one is chosen, a corridor through which the selected approach will be achieved is chosen.[22]

Most of the corridors to the anterior skull base begin transnasally and then extend to include either transsphenoidal and/or transethmoidal corridors. Therefore, it is critical to understand the individual patient's sinonasal anatomy, especially of the ethmoid and sphenoid sinuses. Identifying anatomic variations, as well as the degree of the pneumatization of the sphenoid sinus and sellar morphology, allows a better preoperative evaluation and, consequently, a better surgical outcome.[22]

Limitations for Surgical Treatment

Some findings depicted on imaging are generally considered contraindications to surgical treatment with EEA alone for curative intent. These include regional metastases, direct invasion of the brain, orbits, or skin, and extensive systemic metastasis.[2]

Orbit invasion should be assessed by a combination of axial and coronal imaging demonstrating the normal orbital bony rim. Bony erosion and displacement of the periorbita are significant findings.[23] The normal periorbital lining is hypointense on both T1WI and T2WI on MRI and still can be clearly delineated when the adjacent sinus is filled with tumor or secretions. The low signal remains despite bony erosion, but infiltration of the periosteum results in loss of signal. When the thin and regular

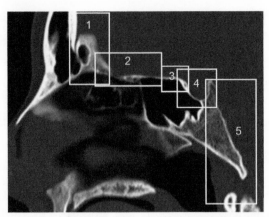

Fig. 17. Midline skull base approaches. Sagittal CT in the midsagittal plane shows the 5 anterior skull base entry points: (1) transfrontal, (2) transcribriform, (3) transtuberculum or transplanum, (4) transsellar, and (5) transclival.

hypointensity is still visible on T2 images between tumor and orbital fat, the periorbita is considered intact (see **Fig. 12**).[24] Other signs of orbital involvement include fat invasion, characterized by soft tissue stranding or infiltration within the extraconal fat that is contiguous with the primary tumor, and changes within the extraocular muscles, such as displacement, enlargement, or abnormal signal or attenuation. The orbital bone integrity must be assessed in addition to possible nasolacrimal system invasion.[25]

Dural invasion is a precursor to actual brain invasion and is consequently very important when considering the extent of resection. Dural involvement is best assessed with MRI. The normal dura is often not visible or, if seen, may be very subtle and show very thin enhancement following gadolinium contrast administration. Imaging assessment of this interface is critical in determining the extent of skull base invasion. A lesion is extracranial when the lesion abuts the fovea or cribriform plate without disrupting the bony integrity on CT or the cortical bone linear hypointensity on MRI. Any focal bony dehiscence or loss of hypointense MR signal suggests bone-periosteal invasion. Intracranial dural involvement is strongly suspected when there is dural enhancement with associated thickening (see **Fig. 12**). Nodular or pial enhancement both correlate strongly with dural invasion histologically, but thin linear dural enhancement also can be observed in other pathologies, including inflammatory, vascular, or infectious processes.[25,26]

Perineural tumor spread is frequently observed in paranasal carcinomas and should be assessed before treatment planning. CT is limited to indirect signs, including effacement of fat planes, enlargement of neuroforamina, or muscular atrophy due to nerve denervation. MRI can give direct visualization of perineural extension or spread, such as nerve enlargement and enhancement as well as indirect signs mentioned previously.[27] Replacement of normal CSF signal in the Meckel cave or convexity of the lateral aspects of the cavernous sinus also may suggest perineural disease (**Fig. 18**).[25]

Location is also remarkably important and can be easily assessed by imaging studies. Lesions situated posterior to the ICA or close to proximal branches of the circle of Willis or the CNs, lesions displaying vascular encasement or involvement of the pituitary stalk and/or of the hypothalamus, and lesions mostly located in the third ventricle increase the surgical difficulty and precipitate higher risks of complications. In such cases, the surgical aggressiveness is dictated by the resection goal and by the

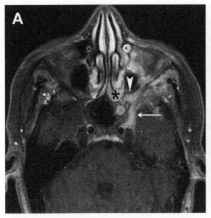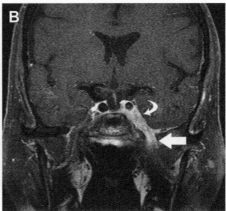

Fig. 18. Adenoid cystic carcinoma with perineural spread. (*A*) Axial postcontrast fat-sat T1WI reveals small enhancing left nasal cavity lesion (*asterisk*) with adjacent abnormal enhancement extending laterally into the left PPF (*arrowhead*) and posteriorly along CN V2 through foramen rotundum (*thin arrow*) and into the Meckel cave. (*B*) Coronal postcontrast fat-suppressed T1WI demonstrates abnormal enhancement and enlargement of the left cavernous sinus (*curved arrow*), indicating tumor invasion, as well as antegrade spread along CN V3 (*thick arrow*) through the foramen ovale.

pathology.[2] **Box 1** summarizes other relative contraindications to attempting curative surgical treatment with EEA.

Basic Anatomic Limits for EEA

Midline or paramedian plane ventral skull base lesions, located from the olfactory groove to the odontoid process of C2 are the best targets for EEA.[22] However, general anatomic limits must be considered for a purely endoscopic surgery.

Transcribriform

Lesions amenable to this approach (commonly sinonasal neoplasms, esthesioneuroblastoma, and meningioma) extend from the posterior frontal sinus and crista galli to

---

Box 1
Radiographic findings that indicate contraindications to endoscopic endonasal approaches

Brain invasion.

Orbital invasion.

Lateral skull base lesion.

Lesion in superolateral cavernous sinus.

Craniopharyngioma that is isolated to the third ventricle.

Lesion with major component extending over the orbital roof, optic canal, and lateral to foramen ovale.

Lesion arising from or extensively involving the frontal sinus.

Inability to reconstruct the skull base defect.

Adapted from Learned KO, Lee JYK, Adappa ND, et al. Radiologic evaluation for endoscopic endonasal skull base surgery candidates. Neurographics 2015;5(2):44.

the planum sphenoidale, across the roof of the ethmoid sinuses, and are flanked on either side by the lamina papyracea and orbits. Limitations for a purely endoscopic approach include periorbita invasion, which is also a contraindication to open surgical procedures, extension over the far lateral orbital roof, and frontal sinus involvement.[2,28–32] Frontal sinus extension disqualifies complete resection via a purely endonasal approach. Dural sinus invasion and lack of a cortical cuff between the lesion and the surrounding vessel are also related to a poor outcome. The A2 segments of the anterior cerebral arteries and the superior sagittal sinus are potential blind spots and should be assessed on preoperative imaging for vascular encasement. Subpial invasion of the gyrus recti and orbitofrontal gyri, usually characterized by the lack of a CSF plane between the tumor and the brain or brain edema, as well as leptomeningeal enhancement must be identified, as they are related to increased surgical risk and higher rates of incomplete resection (see **Fig. 13**).[2,25,31,32]

Transplanum

Lesions along the planum sphenoidale and tuberculum sella are usually resected via this approach. Moreover, it allows direct access to the lesions within the anterior suprasellar cistern and the anterior third ventricle. Consequently, meningiomas and craniopharyngiomas may be resected with this technique.[7] Special attention must be given to the optic canals and optic nerves, especially in cases of optic canal dehiscence. The relationship between the tumor and the surrounding structures must be assessed, with particular attention to the optic chiasmatic structures superiorly, laterally, and posteriorly, as well as the ICAs laterally, the anterior cerebral and communicating arteries superiorly, and the pituitary gland inferiorly (see **Fig. 14**).[28,33] The pituitary stalk and inferior frontal lobes should also be carefully evaluated. There are increased surgical difficulties with lesion extension into or lateral to the orbital apex or optic canals, extension behind vasculature or the infundibulum, and extension above the optic nerve. These are the potential locations in which to anticipate residual unresectable neoplasm on postoperative imaging evaluation.[34]

Transellar

This approach can be used when the lesion is located in the sella turcica, pituitary gland, parasellar region including cavernous sinus, and suprasellar cistern. The transellar EEA not only gives access to the sella and pituitary, but also provides access to lesions located in the suprasellar cistern and bilateral cavernous sinuses when combined with other approaches (transplanum, transclival). The common pathologies treated in this manner include pituitary adenoma and craniopharyngioma.[35–39] As is the case for the transplanum approach, neurovascular involvement and vascular encasement are considered relative contraindications for a purely EEA approach. It is also important to consider that extensive suprasellar neoplastic components may preclude a total resection via a purely endonasal route, because of the limitation of reach by instrumentation as well as the decrease in visibility of the deep-seated surgical field. A combined transnasal and transcranial approach may be the best surgical option in those cases. Proximity to and possible involvement of the optic chiasm and infundibulum by suprasellar craniopharyngiomas are important in determining the risk to pituitary gland function.[38] Craniopharyngiomas located either anterior or posterior to the pituitary stalk presenting with a clear plane separating it from these structures are the best candidates for a resection with least risk to pituitary function using either transellar or combined approaches. Lesions involving the stalk present the highest risk for panhypopituitarism. Isolated third ventricular craniopharyngiomas are generally not suited for EEA.[2]

Transclival

Lesions located along the midline clivus from the sella to the anterior foramen magnum may be accessed by EEA. Caudal exposure is limited by the nasal bones anteriorly and the hard palate posteriorly and the line connecting these 2 points, named the nasopalatine line (NPL), which extends to the spinal column above the level of the base of C2 and predicts the most inferior extent of surgical dissection (**Fig. 19**).[40] The EEA surgical corridor requires posterior septectomy, sphenoidectomy, and midline posterior nasopharyngectomy and clivectomy. The common pathologies addressed with this approach include clival lesions, such as chordomas and chondrosarcomas, and meningiomas. Attention should be given in the preoperative imaging assessment to the CNs, especially CN III and VI that can be better visualized on constructive interference in steady state or fast imaging using steady-state acquisition imaging, and to the vertebral and basilar arteries (see **Fig. 16**).[2,41] Clivectomy and dissection in transclival EEA are maintained in the midline between the petrous ICAs and lateral margins of the clivus to avoid inadvertent arterial or CN injury. Dehiscence of the carotid canal must be identified because it puts ICA at risk. Tumor involvement of the posterior clinoid, lateral dorsal clivus, and petrous apex along the courses of CN III and VI observed on preoperative imaging may be left untouched, and these locations should be carefully assessed on postoperative imaging for adjuvant treatment planning and follow-up.[2]

POSTOPERATIVE IMAGING OF ENDOSCOPIC ENDONASAL SURGERY

Effective closure of communications between the sinonasal cavity, aerodigestive tract, and the intracranial compartment can be addressed with a broad array of non-vascularized and vascularized tissues, including flaps and grafts that are selected based on the skull base surgical approach, as well as the location and size of the surgical defect.[34,42,43] Postsurgical evaluation requires a thorough understanding of the type and extent of surgical excision, packing material used, the preoperative

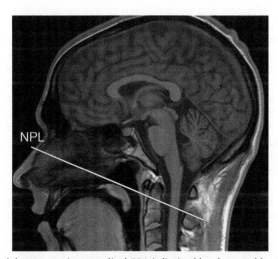

Fig. 19. NPL. Caudal exposure in transclival EEA is limited by the nasal bones anteriorly and the hard palate posteriorly and the line connecting these 2 points, the NPL, defines the most inferior boundary for surgical dissection. The NPL extends to the spinal column above the level of the base of C2.

appearance of the original tumor, and the expected evolution of the postoperative MRI findings.[34,44]

In general, the sole use of free grafts is suitable for reconstructions of small defects, but nonautologous biomaterials are avoided in oncologic patients in whom postoperative radiation is anticipated because of a high extrusion rate.[42] For most medium and large defects in skull base surgery, vascularized flaps in combination with nonvascularized grafts are required. The common vascularized flaps are free tissue transfers and pedicled regional or local flaps.[42] For even larger defects, fasciocutaneous, myocutaneous, and muscular free tissue transplants, as well as regional myocutaneous flaps are viable choices. Currently, ESBR commonly uses multilayer closure techniques using tissues that may include intracranial autologous fat graft, inlay subdural collagen matrix dural graft, inlay/onlay fascial graft, and onlay vascularized nasoseptal flaps (NSF), the latter of which are currently the workhorse in this type of surgery.[43]

Early Postoperative

Early postoperative imaging is critical following any tumor surgery, as inflammatory changes beyond 48 hours after surgery may produce abnormal contrast enhancement. In addition, time-sensitive degradation of blood and hemostatic synthetic materials begins during this period. These processes result in increased precontrast T1W signal that makes evaluation of contrast enhancement harder in the subacute stage.[44]

The postoperative appearance of endoscopic tumor resection is varied by the extent of sinonasal and skull base tumor involvement. Depending on the chosen approach and corridor, a combination of turbinectomy, ethmoidectomy, medial maxillectomy, septectomy, sphenoidectomy, and/or clivectomy may be seen.[45]

The sinonasal cavity typically contains postoperative debris and fluid, which can be heterogeneous on MRI, as well as nasal packing, nasal trumpets, or Foley catheter balloons to bolster the ESBR graft (**Figs. 20** and **21**).[2]

The tumor cavity in early postoperative imaging is occupied by postsurgical material and the beginnings of deoxyhemoglobin or oxyhemoglobin blood accumulation, which are hypointense and hyperintense on T2WI, respectively. Confounding factors like inflammatory changes and accumulation of methemoglobin containing bloodproducts (which are hyperintense on T1WI) have not yet begun.[44]

In the immediate postoperative period, the NSF, which is a mucoperichondrial-mucoperiosteal flap elevated off the nasal septum and anterior face of the sphenoid sinus with its vascular pedicle from the nasoseptal branch of the sphenopalatine artery,[45] is seen on MRI as a characteristic C-shaped, isointense structure underlying the surgical defect on the precontrast T1WI and T2WI that shows contrast enhancement on postgadolinium T1WI and a vascular pedicle (see **Figs. 20** and **21**).[2,44,46] It is important that the flap enhancement should not be mistaken for residual neoplasm, and its pattern does not predict CSF leak.[46,47]

The nasoseptal flap can desiccate and contract if its mucoperichondrial surface is not apposed to the denuded sinonasal cavity, with the highest risk for flap displacement or migration being along the superior margin of the surgical defect. However, it is important to recognize that MRI cannot differentiate the mucosal and mucoperichondrial surfaces and will show normal flap enhancement while missing this cause of failure.[2,44]

When multilayer grafts are used, the multilayer inlay and onlay graft material is seen as a linear hypointense, nonenhancing structure deep to the flap on precontrast and postcontrast T1WI and shows slight T2WI hyperintensity.[46]

Implanted muscles with fascia have characteristic striated muscle bundles, and variable MR signal intensity. They are usually seen as a round and T1WI hypointense

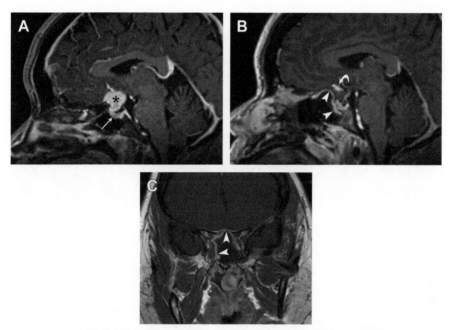

Fig. 20. Early postoperative changes after resection of planum sphenoidale meningioma with defect closure using a layered reconstruction with a pedicled nasoseptal flap. (*A*) Sagittal postcontrast T1WI demonstrates an enhancing midline lesion (*asterisk*) along the planum sphenoidale extending over the tuberculum sella that turned out to be a meningioma. Note the normal pituitary gland along the floor of the sella (*arrow*). (*B*) Sagittal and (*C*) coronal postcontrast T1WI acquired a few days after endoscopic resection and skull base repair. Given the depth of dissection, a layered reconstruction was performed using an abdominal dermal fat graft (*curved arrow*) with an overlay pedicled nasoseptal flap (*arrowheads*). The high signal intensity of the fat graft is due to the intrinsic short T1 of adipose tissue (not enhancement), whereas the increased signal intensity in the nasoseptal flap reflects enhancement of vascularized nasoseptal mucosal tissue. Synthetic collagen matrix was also used (intermediate signal material between the fat graft and nasoseptal flap in *B*).

structure, displaying slight peripheral enhancement. On T2WI, the denervated muscle commonly shows increased signal, whereas a line of low signal intensity represents the fascia.[48,49]

Identification of residual tumor at this early stage has a very high positive predictive value. The suggestive enhancement patterns are nodular or combined nodular and peripheral enhancement in the region of the resected tumor. Absence of enhancement or only thin, uniform, peripheral enhancement in the tumor region usually excludes tumor.[44,50]

Late Postoperative

On follow-up MRI, resolution of the postoperative debris and fluid superficial to the flap is depicted (see **Fig. 21**). The ESBR layers retract to the skull base with reduction in thickness but continued enhancement.[34,44] Gelfoam usually disappears in 3 to 6 months, but contrast-enhancing granulation tissue develops as the Gelfoam degrades, which could mimic recurrent tumor. On the other hand, fat packing usually disappears more slowly over 6 to 12 months and does not produce much contrast enhancement as it resolves.[44]

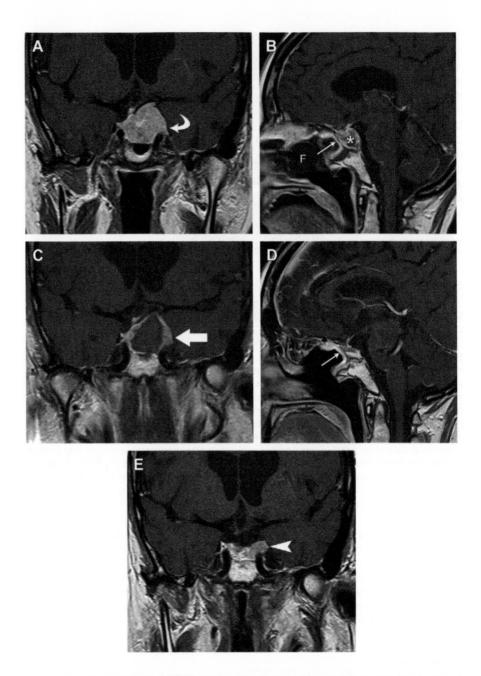

Even though retraction of NSF into the denuded skull base defect and the sinonasal cavity makes it less distinct, the flap maintains its basic configuration and location and should not be misinterpreted as an enhancing tumor (see **Fig. 21**).[34]

Myocutaneous flaps develop a variable MR signal intensity and enhancement as a result of multiple factors, including scar maturation, resorption of fat, muscle denervation, and, in some cases, sequelae of postoperative adjuvant radiation.[48,49] These robust flaps gradually loose tissue bulk as the muscle atrophies.[34]

Tumor recurrence typically has local mass effect and appears as infiltrative or nodular tissue that lacks the striated muscle architecture or fat composition of normal myocutaneous regional or free flaps. Even though differentiating tumor from surgical reconstruction material or granulation tissue is often difficult, some findings may aid the differentiation. First, on late follow-up scans, an NSF can be mistaken as tumor recurrence if one does not recognize that one was performed to close the skull base defect. Therefore, identifying its location in the early postoperative scan is quite important, allowing a more confident diagnosis. In addition, the location of neoplastic recurrence in skull base surgery is usually predictable, appearing as a new mass and/ or growing tissue at the interface of the flap recipient bed and the reconstructive tissue. Another important characteristic of tumor recurrence is that the signal intensity and/or enhancement of tumor are typically different from the abutting reconstructive layers and similar to the tumor on the pretreatment scan (see **Fig. 21**).[34]

In the postsurgical sella, it can be difficult in some situations to determine whether peripheral enhancement represents residual tumor, tumor capsule, or pituitary gland. Dynamic pituitary MRI can help to differentiate the normal enhancement of the residual pituitary gland from granulation tissue or tumoral enhancement, as the latter are typically milder and delayed.[50] Serial surveillance MRI helps in the differentiation among residual tumor, tumor capsule, or normal tissue, which in some cases may demonstrate tissue stabilization and conformation with a normal pituitary size and shape within the sella.[44]

Although it is not common, tumor may also deposit along the dura in distant sites from the operative cranial base.[48,51]

Complications

Diagnosis of CSF leak in the postoperative patient can be challenging due to the confounding factors of perioperative nasal irrigations, general inflammation, and the presence of nasal packing. A postoperative CSF leak can be confirmed with a beta-2 transferrin test. Subsequently, the goal is to identify where the leak is coming from to plan the repair. A thorough endoscopic examination of the nasal cavity may reveal the site of the leak. High-resolution CT scan is usually the first radiologic tool to investigate potential leakage sites in this clinical scenario.[22,52] Another noninvasive tool is the MR cisternography, which uses high-resolution, heavily T2-weighted sequences to show potential sites of CSF leaks, which may appear as areas of fluid-signal outside

◄───

Fig. 21. Incomplete resection of macroadenoma. (*A*) Coronal postcontrast T1WI demonstrates a sellar and suprasellar mass extending into the left cavernous sinus (*curved arrow*). The presence of tumor extending lateral to the carotid artery suggests that it may not be possible to achieve a complete resection. Postcontrast T1WI obtained 1 day (*B, C*) and 8 months (*D, E*) after minimally invasive endoscopic pituitary tumor resection and skull base repair. Immediate postoperative sagittal postcontrast T1WI (*B*) demonstrates a peripherally enhancing, fluid-filled resection cavity (*asterisk*) and defect closure with a pedicled nasoseptal flap (*thin arrow*). A Foley catheter balloon (labeled F in the figure) has been inflated in the nasal cavity to bolster the graft. Eight-month postoperative sagittal image (*D*) shows retraction of flap (*thin arrow*) and collapse of the resection cavity. Coronal image in the immediate postoperative period (*C*) demonstrates the fluid-filled resection cavity with enhancement on either side. The enhancing tissue on the right was thought to represent normal pituitary tissue (note the pituitary stalk displaced to the *right*), whereas the enhancing tissue on the left (*thick arrow*) was worrisome for residual tumor. This suspicion was confirmed on 8-month follow-up coronal image (*E*). Note how the residual tumor (*arrowhead*) enhances less avidly than the adjacent normal pituitary tissue.

of, but contiguous with, the cranial fossa. These studies are often used in correlation with the high-resolution CT scan, which will ideally show a bony defect in the same location. If a sizable defect is noted on CT, a follow-up MRI may be indicated to investigate for the possibility of a meningocele or encephalocele. If findings are inconclusive, CT cisternograms after intrathecal administration of iodinated contrast material (occasionally done in concert with nuclear cisternography), as well as MR cisternograms after intrathecal gadolinium injection, may identify the source of CSF leakage by demonstrating contrast-opacified CSF in the sinonasal cavities.[22,34,52,53]

Postoperative infections, including bacterial meningitis, are fairly uncommon, with an incidence of 1% to 2%. Risk factors for infection include male sex, complex

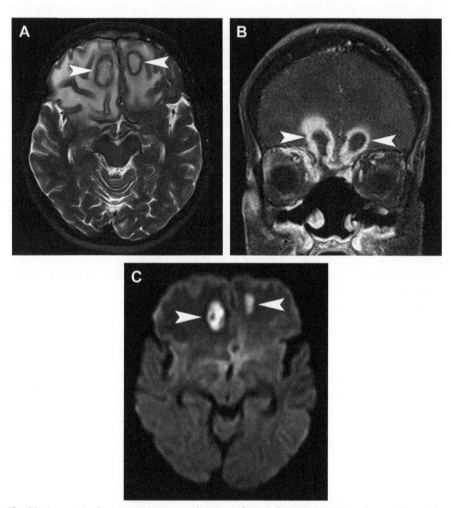

Fig. 22. Pyogenic abscess as a late complication of ESBR. (*A*) Axial T2WI performed 6 months after ESBR demonstrates extensive vasogenic edema in both frontal lobes surrounding discrete ovoid lesions (*arrowheads* in *A–C*), which are T2 hyperintense with hypointense rims. (*B*) A coronal postcontrast T1WI demonstrates the rims of these lesions to be thick, irregular, and enhancing. (*C*) Axial DWI demonstrates high signal intensity within the lesions centrally, indicating restricted diffusion and supporting the diagnosis of pyogenic abscess.

tumors, presence of an external ventricular drain or shunt, and postoperative CSF leak.[22] Meningitis usually presents on MRI as abnormal hyperintensities on fluid-attenuated inversion recovery (FLAIR) sequences in the subarachnoid space and leptomeningeal enhancement. Subdural empyemas are characterized on CT scan and MRI as peripherally enhancing extra-axial collections with signal intensities that differ from the CSF on MRI. They also characteristically display restricted diffusion on diffusion-weighted imaging (DWI). Cerebritis also can be easily identified as parenchymal areas of abnormal FLAIR signal, which can evolve into brain abscesses that appear as ring-enhancing brain lesions with restricted diffusion (**Fig. 22**).[54,55]

SUMMARY

The EEA allows management of both benign and malignant processes along the entire ventral skull base. The feasibility of endoscopic approaches, the potential surgical risk, and tumor resectability depend on tumor location and critical anatomic structures in the surgical corridors. The radiographic evaluation of skull base anatomy and its relationship with associated tumors remains critical for both preoperative planning and intraoperative guidance. A detailed understanding of the type and extent of surgical excision, packing materials and flaps used, original preoperative appearance of the lesion, and the expected chronologic postsurgical imaging appearance is essential for adequately evaluating the postoperative scan.

REFERENCES

1. Krischek B, Carvalho FG, Godoy BL, et al. From craniofacial resection to endonasal endoscopic removal of malignant tumors of the anterior skull base. World Neurosurg 2014;82(6 Suppl):S59–65.
2. Learned KO, Lee JYK, Adappa ND, et al. Radiologic evaluation for endoscopic endonasal skull base surgery candidates. Neurographics 2015;5(2):41–5.
3. Verillaud B, Bresson D, Sauvaget E, et al. Endoscopic endonasal skull base surgery. Eur Ann Otorhinolaryngol Head Neck Dis 2012;129(4):190–6.
4. Kasemsiri P, Carrau RL, Ditzel Filho LF, et al. Advantages and limitations of endoscopic endonasal approaches to the skull base. World Neurosurg 2014;82(6 Suppl):S12–21.
5. Chapman PR, Bag AK, Tubbs RS, et al. Practical anatomy of the central skull base region. Semin Ultrasound CT MR 2013;34(5):381–92.
6. Borges A. Imaging of the central skull base. Neuroimaging Clin N Am 2009;19(4):669–96.
7. Chong VF, Khoo JB, Fan YF. Imaging of the nasopharynx and skull base. Neuroimaging Clin N Am 2004;14(4):695–719.
8. Policeni BA, Smoker WR. Imaging of the skull base: anatomy and pathology. Radiol Clin North Am 2015;53(1):1–14.
9. Borges A. Skull base tumours part I: imaging technique, anatomy and anterior skull base tumours. Eur J Radiol 2008;66(3):338–47.
10. Som PM, Curtin HD. Head and neck imaging - 2 volume set expert consult- online and print. 5th edition. Philadelphia: Mosby Imprint Elsevier - Health Sciences Division; 2011. Available at: http://getitatduke.library.duke.edu/?sid=sersol&SS_jc=TC0000537456&title=Head%20and%20Neck%20Imaging%20-%202%20Volume%20Set%3A%20Expert%20Consult-%20Online%20and%20Print.
11. Rhoton AL Jr. The anterior and middle cranial base. Neurosurgery 2002;51(4 Suppl):S273–302.

12. Pinheiro-Neto CD, Fernandez-Miranda JC, Wang EW, et al. Anatomical correlates of endonasal surgery for sinonasal malignancies. Clin Anat 2012;25(1):129–34.

13. Laine FJ, Nadel L, Braun IF. CT and MR imaging of the central skull base. Part 1: techniques, embryologic development, and anatomy. Radiographics 1990;10(4):591–602.

14. Osborn AG. Osborn's brain: imaging, pathology, and anatomy. 1st edition. Salt Lake City (UT): Amirsys Pub; 2013.

15. Yousem DM, Grossman RI. Neuroradiology: the requisites. Requisites in radiology series. 3rd edition. Philadelphia: Mosby/Elsevier; 2010. Available at: http://VB3LK7EB4T.search.serialssolutions.com/?V=1.0&L=VB3LK7EB4T&S=JCs&C=TC0000450761&T=marc.

16. Parmar H, Gujar S, Shah G, et al. Imaging of the anterior skull base. Neuroimaging Clin N Am 2009;19(3):427–39.

17. Borges A. Skull base tumours Part II. Central skull base tumours and intrinsic tumours of the bony skull base. Eur J Radiol 2008;66(3):348–62.

18. Rumboldt Z. Pituitary adenomas. Top Magn Reson Imaging 2005;16(4):277–88.

19. Smith JK. Parasellar tumors: suprasellar and cavernous sinuses. Top Magn Reson Imaging 2005;16(4):307–15.

20. Gardner PA, Kassam AB, Rothfus WE, et al. Preoperative and intraoperative imaging for endoscopic endonasal approaches to the skull base. Otolaryngol Clin North Am 2008;41(1):215–30, vii.

21. Schwartz TH, Fraser JF, Brown S, et al. Endoscopic cranial base surgery: classification of operative approaches. Neurosurgery 2008;62(5):991–1002 [discussion: 1002–5].

22. Ivan ME, Jahangiri A, El-Sayed IH, et al. Minimally invasive approaches to the anterior skull base. Neurosurg Clin N Am 2013;24(1):19–37.

23. Eisen MD, Yousem DM, Loevner LA, et al. Preoperative imaging to predict orbital invasion by tumor. Head Neck 2000;22(5):456–62.

24. Kim HJ, Lee TH, Lee HS, et al. Periorbita: computed tomography and magnetic resonance imaging findings. Am J Rhinol 2006;20(4):371–4.

25. Singh N, Eskander A, Huang SH, et al. Imaging and resectability issues of sinonasal tumors. Expert Rev Anticancer Ther 2013;13(3):297–312.

26. Eisen MD, Yousem DM, Montone KT, et al. Use of preoperative MR to predict dural, perineural, and venous sinus invasion of skull base tumors. AJNR Am J Neuroradiol 1996;17(10):1937–45.

27. Chang PC, Fischbein NJ, McCalmont TH, et al. Perineural spread of malignant melanoma of the head and neck: clinical and imaging features. AJNR Am J Neuroradiol 2004;25(1):5–11.

28. Kassam A, Snyderman CH, Mintz A, et al. Expanded endonasal approach: the rostrocaudal axis. Part I. Crista galli to the sella turcica. Neurosurg Focus 2005;19(1):E3.

29. Kassam AB, Prevedello DM, Carrau RL, et al. Endoscopic endonasal skull base surgery: analysis of complications in the authors' initial 800 patients. J Neurosurg 2011;114(6):1544–68.

30. Harvey RJ, Winder M, Parmar P, et al. Endoscopic skull base surgery for sinonasal malignancy. Otolaryngol Clin North Am 2011;44(5):1081–140.

31. Snyderman CH, Pant H, Carrau RL, et al. What are the limits of endoscopic sinus surgery? The expanded endonasal approach to the skull base. Keio J Med 2009;58(3):152–60.

32. Lund VJ, Stammberger H, Nicolai P, et al. European position paper on endoscopic management of tumours of the nose, paranasal sinuses and skull base. Rhinol Suppl 2010;(22):1–143.

33. Gardner PA, Kassam AB, Thomas A, et al. Endoscopic endonasal resection of anterior cranial base meningiomas. Neurosurgery 2008;63(1):36–52 [discussion: 52–4].
34. Learned KO, Maralani PJ, Malloy K, et al. Skull base reconstruction: demystifying postoperative imaging evaluation. Neurographics 2015;5(2):56–63.
35. Komotar RJ, Starke RM, Raper DM, et al. Endoscopic skull base surgery: a comprehensive comparison with open transcranial approaches. Br J Neurosurg 2012;26(5):637–48.
36. Leng LZ, Greenfield JP, Souweidane MM, et al. Endoscopic, endonasal resection of craniopharyngiomas: analysis of outcome including extent of resection, cerebrospinal fluid leak, return to preoperative productivity, and body mass index. Neurosurgery 2012;70(1):110–23 [discussion: 123–4].
37. Stamm AC, Vellutini E, Balsalobre L. Craniopharyngioma. Otolaryngol Clin North Am 2011;44(4):937–52, viii.
38. Kassam AB, Gardner PA, Snyderman CH, et al. Expanded endonasal approach, a fully endoscopic transnasal approach for the resection of midline suprasellar craniopharyngiomas: a new classification based on the infundibulum. J Neurosurg 2008;108(4):715–28.
39. Ali ZS, Lang SS, Kamat AR, et al. Suprasellar pediatric craniopharyngioma resection via endonasal endoscopic approach. Childs Nerv Syst 2013;29(11):2065–70.
40. de Almeida JR, Zanation AM, Snyderman CH, et al. Defining the nasopalatine line: the limit for endonasal surgery of the spine. Laryngoscope 2009;119(2):239–44.
41. Xie T, Zhang XB, Yun H, et al. 3D-FIESTA MR images are useful in the evaluation of the endoscopic expanded endonasal approach for midline skull-base lesions. Acta Neurochir (Wien) 2011;153(1):12–8.
42. Schmalbach CE, Webb DE, Weitzel EK. Anterior skull base reconstruction: a review of current techniques. Curr Opin Otolaryngol Head Neck Surg 2010;18(4):238–43.
43. Harvey RJ, Parmar P, Sacks R, et al. Endoscopic skull base reconstruction of large dural defects: a systematic review of published evidence. Laryngoscope 2012;122(2):452–9.
44. Chaaban MR, Woodworth BA, Vattoth S, et al. Surgical approaches to central skull base and postsurgical imaging. Semin Ultrasound CT MR 2013;34(5):476–89.
45. Hadad G, Bassagasteguy L, Carrau RL, et al. A novel reconstructive technique after endoscopic expanded endonasal approaches: vascular pedicle nasoseptal flap. Laryngoscope 2006;116(10):1882–6.
46. Kang MD, Escott E, Thomas AJ, et al. The MR imaging appearance of the vascular pedicle nasoseptal flap. AJNR Am J Neuroradiol 2009;30(4):781–6.
47. Learned KO, Adappa ND, Loevner LA, et al. MR imaging evaluation of endoscopic cranial base reconstruction with pedicled nasoseptal flap following endoscopic endonasal skull base surgery. Eur J Radiol 2013;82(3):544–51.
48. Learned KO, Malloy KM, Loevner LA. Myocutaneous flaps and other vascularized grafts in head and neck reconstruction for cancer treatment. Magn Reson Imaging Clin N Am 2012;20(3):495–513.
49. Naidich MJ, Weissman JL. Reconstructive myofascial skull-base flaps: normal appearance on CT and MR imaging studies. AJR Am J Roentgenol 1996;167(3):611–4.
50. Dina TS, Feaster SH, Laws ER Jr, et al. MR of the pituitary gland postsurgery: serial MR studies following transsphenoidal resection. AJNR Am J Neuroradiol 1993;14(3):763–9.

51. Hudgins PA, Burson JG, Gussack GS, et al. CT and MR appearance of recurrent malignant head and neck neoplasms after resection and flap reconstruction. AJNR Am J Neuroradiol 1994;15(9):1689–94.
52. Carrau RL, Snyderman CH, Kassam AB. The management of cerebrospinal fluid leaks in patients at risk for high-pressure hydrocephalus. Laryngoscope 2005; 115(2):205–12.
53. Selcuk H, Albayram S, Ozer H, et al. Intrathecal gadolinium-enhanced MR cisternography in the evaluation of CSF leakage. AJNR Am J Neuroradiol 2010;31(1): 71–5.
54. Gasparetto EL, Cabral RF, da Cruz LC Jr, et al. Diffusion imaging in brain infections. Neuroimaging Clin N Am 2011;21(1):89–113, viii.
55. Maia AC Jr, Guedes BV, Lucas A Jr, et al. Diffusion MR imaging for monitoring treatment response. Neuroimaging Clin N Am 2011;21(1):153–78. viii-ix.

Sellar Lesions/Pathology

Damien Bresson, MD[a], Philippe Herman, MD[b], Marc Polivka, MD[c],
Sébastien Froelich, MD[d],*

KEYWORDS

- Sellar lesions • Pituitary tumors • Pituitary adenomas • Craniopharyngiomas
- Rathke's cleft cysts • Meningiomas

KEY POINTS

- Sellar conditions, dominated by pituitary adenomas, is extremely rich.
- Clinical symptoms are mainly visual and endocrine.
- Neuroimaging associated with careful clinical evaluation and adequate endocrinologic biochemical workup allows the diagnosis of most lesions preoperatively.
- Intrasellar aneurysm is rare but needs to be ruled out before any surgery to prevent dramatic bleeding.
- MRI and angio–computed tomography are needed for preoperative planning and intraoperative navigation.

INTRODUCTION

The sellar region is located in the central portion of the skull base, behind the posterior wall of the sphenoid sinus and between both cavernous sinuses. The pituitary gland formed by the adenohypophysis (anterior pituitary) and the neurohypophysis (posterior pituitary), lies in the sella turcica. Suprasellar growth is the main axis of extension of sellar tumors. The medial wall of the cavernous sinus that separates the pituitary fossa from the cavernous sinus is weak so that sellar tumors frequently infiltrate the cavernous sinus. Tumors of the pituitary gland and sellar region account for approximately 10% to 15% of all brain tumors and a large variety of neoplastic, inflammatory, vascular, or developmental lesions can be found in this region. Most tumors are pituitary adenomas (PAs) (9%) (**Table 1**).[1]

Disclosures: No conflict of interest.
[a] Neurosurgery Department, Assistance Publique-Hôpitaux de Paris, 2 rue Ambroise Paré, Paris 75010, France; [b] ENT Department, Lariboisière Hospital, Université Paris VII - Diderot, 2 rue Ambroise Paré, Paris 75010, France; [c] Department of Pathology, Lariboisiere Hospital, 2 rue Ambroise Paré, Paris 75010, France; [d] Neurosurgery Department, Assistance Publique-Hôpitaux de Paris, Université Paris VII - Diderot, 2 rue Ambroise Paré, Paris 75010, France
* Corresponding author.
E-mail address: sebastien.froelich@lrb.aphp.fr

oto.theclinics.com

Abbreviations

ACTH	Adrenocorticotropic hormone
CSF	Cerebrospinal fluid
CPs	Craniopharyngiomas
CT	Computed tomography
DI	Diabetes insipidious
GH	Growth hormone
ICA	Internal carotid artery
Ki-67 LI	Ki-67 labeling index
MRI	Magnetic resonance imaging
PAs	Pituitary adenomas
PRL	Prolactin
RCCs	Rathke's Cleft Cysts
TSH	Thyroid-stimulating hormone
vHL	von Hipple-Lindau disease
WHO	World Health Organization
WI	Weighted Imaging

Table 1
Classification of sellar and parasellar lesions

Neoplastic	Pituitary	Benign	Pituitary adenoma
		Malignant	Pituitary carcinoma
		Low-grade malignancy	Pituicytoma
	Nonpituitary tumors	Usually benign	Craniopharyngioma
			Meningioma
			Lipoma
			Schwannoma
			Gangliocytoma
			Hemangioblastoma
		Low-grade malignancy	Chordoma
			Chondrosarcoma/chondroma
			Langherans' cell histiocytosis
			Solitary fibrous tumors
			Plasmacytoma
		Malignant	Gliomas
			Germ cell tumor
			Primary Pituitary Lymphoma/ leukemia
			Pituitary metastasis
			Other (melanoma)
Nonneoplastic	Developmental lesions		RCC
			Epidermoid/dermoid cysts
			Arachnoid cyst
	Infectious, Inflammatory	Infectious	Pituitary abscess
			Pseudotumor tuberculosis
			Mycoses
		Immune	Hypophysitis
		Granulomatous	Sarcoidosis
			Wegener
	Vascular lesions		Aneurysms
			Carotido cavernous fistula
			Cavernous sinus thrombosis

However, other diagnoses should be excluded before surgery because the optimal therapeutic strategy may vary significantly from one lesion to another.

It is crucial, in a case of a sellar lesion, to perform first a complete diagnostic workup including endocrinologic, ophthalmologic, and neurologic assessments and neuroimaging studies.

In most cases, these studies will lead to a diagnosis of near certainty, preoperatively, but in some cases, a biopsy is still necessary to define the optimum treatment strategy before a more complex surgery that may not be required.

Most often, sellar and parasellar tumors require a multidisciplinary approach including endocrinologic care, surgery, radiation therapy, or primary medical treatment. For those lesions that have a high risk of recurrence, long-term follow-up, based mainly on regular ophthalmologic and endocrinologic examinations and MRI, is required. This article provides an overview of sellar diseases with emphasis on their most useful characteristics to clinical practice.

EMBRYOLOGY OF THE PITUITARY GLAND

The pituitary gland, located in the sella turcica is composed of 2 distinct parts, the adenohypophysis (anterior pituitary) and the neurohypophysis (posterior pituitary), which differ in terms of embryologic development, anatomy, and function. The 2 lobes have entirely separate embryonic origins, which later become structurally and functionally linked. The pituitary gland has both an ectodermic and neuroectodermic origin. A small sliver of tissue, the intermediate lobe, separates both lobes.

The pituitary differentiation, under the control of a complex cascade of signaling and transcription processes, occurs during the first trimester of gestation and finally results in the juxtaposition and interaction of the oral ectoderm forming Rathke's pouch, an upward invagination of the roof of the stomodaeum, and the neural ectoderm of the diencephalon, which bulges downward to form the infundibulum.[2]

Once in contact, both layers will proliferate. The cells of Rathke's pouch differentiate into the endocrine cells of the anterior pituitary. Rathke's pouch loses its connection with the roof of the primitive mouth and comes to lie anterior to the infundibulum and wrap around the pituitary stalk. It gives rise to pars distalis, pars tuberalis, and pars intermedia. The infundibulum gives rise to the pituitary stalk and the posthypophysis.

A network of blood vessels, the hypophyseal portal system, functionally links the anterior lobe to the hypothalamus and posterior lobe of the pituitary.

ANATOMICAL BOUNDARIES OF THE PITUITARY FOSSA

The anterior wall and the floor of pituitary fossa are formed by a bony wall that corresponds to the sellar prominence of the posterior wall of the sphenoid sinus. It is covered by a thin layer of periosteum. Superiorly, the anterior wall of the sella turcica continues with the tuberculum sellae. Laterally, the tuberculum sellae continues with the posterior edge of the optic strut. Above the tuberculum sellae is the chiasmatic sulcus. The chiasmatic sulcus is bounded posteriorly by the tuberculum sellae and anteriorly by the chiasmatic ridge, which forms the posterior border of the planum sphenoidale. The shape of the tuberculum sellae, chiasmatic sulcus, and optic strut is highly variable and correlates with the shape of the prominence and recess that are identified exocranially on the posterior wall of the sphenoid sinus.[3–5]

The ceiling of the pituitary fossa is formed by the diaphragma sellae that covers the pituitary gland. It has a central opening for the pituitary stalk. The diaphragma sellae is also highly variable in terms of thickness and size of the central opening. Those variations may also influence to some extent, the superior extension of sellar lesion, especially the macroadenomas (**Fig. 1**).

The medial wall of the cavernous sinus, which separates the cavernous sinuses from the pituitary fossa, has been the subject of numerous studies and controversies.[6,7] Some investigators state that there is no true medial wall and that it is only composed of a glandular capsule and of some connective tissue continuous with the supportive connective tissue of the cavernous sinus. This may account for the well-known extension of PAs and other sellar lesions in the posterior aspect of the cavernous sinus.[8] Histologic examination of this region supports those findings indicating that the pituitary gland and PAs are separated from the lateral sellar compartment, the so-called *cavernous sinus*, by a thin layer of loose connective tissue (**Fig. 2**).

The internal carotid artery (ICA) is in close contact with the pituitary gland. The position and the trajectory of the ICA along the lateral aspect of the pituitary gland are also highly variable and should be carefully evaluated on preoperative angiographic dedicated examinations.[9]

The posterior wall of the pituitary fossa is formed by the dorsum sellae. The posterior clinoid processes form the superolateral margin of the dorsum sellae.

SIGNS AND SYMPTOMS RELATED TO SELLAR LESIONS

The clinical symptomatology may be very rich and is primarily dependent on the hormones secretory active status (or nonsecretory) of the lesion, its effect on the hypothalamic-pituitary axis, its growth rate, and its upper extension toward the visual pathways and lateral extension toward the cavernous sinus.

Symptoms related to sellar regions are classified into 3 main categories: ophthalmologic, endocrine, and neurologic symptoms.

Sellar lesions may also be discovered on a routine computed tomography (CT) scan or MRI performed for another reason in a patient without any signs or symptoms of pituitary disease. The prevalence of these so-called pituitary incidentalomas estimated from autopsic series is 9.3% (range, 1.5%–26.7%).[10,11] Imaging series based on MRI, however, showed a prevalence of asymptomatic pituitary macroadenomas between 0.1% and 0.3%.[12,13]

Endocrine Symptoms

Endocrine symptoms are related to the hormone-secreting aspect of the primary lesion or the compression or invasion of the pituitary gland or pituitary stalk.

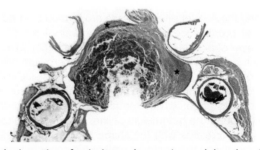

Fig. 1. Coronal histologic section of a pituitary adenoma in an adult cadaveric specimen (hematoxylin-eosin). The black stars indicate the normal pituitary gland. The red star indicates the pituitary stalk. The red arrows indicate the extension of the pituitary adenoma toward the right cavernous sinus without a true medial wall separating the adenoma and the cavernous sinus.

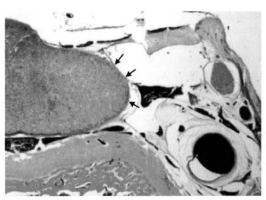

Fig. 2. Coronal histologic section of the sellar and left parasellar region of a newborn head (hematoxylin-eosin). The black arrows indicate the limit between the pituitary fossa and the cavernous sinus without clear dural medial wall.

Any of the different types of hormones produced by the hypophysis can be secreted in excess leading to a typical hypersecretory syndrome:

- Prolactin (PRL)-secreting adenoma produce the typical amenorrhea–galactorrhea syndrome in women and decreased libido, impotence, gynecomastia and hypogonadism in men. Osteoporosis concerns both sex.
- Growth hormone (GH)-secreting adenomas cause acromegaly (or gigantism before puberty).
- Adrenocorticotropic hormone (ACTH)-secreting adenomas are the main cause of Cushing's disease.
- Thyroid-stimulating hormone (TSH)-secreting adenomas are rare and lead to hyperthyroidism.
- Luteinizing hormone– and follicle-stimulating hormone–secreting adenomas are particular and account for most nonfunctioning PAs.[14] They are diagnosed by immunochemistry, and they rarely secrete active gonadotropin hormones that result in increased sex hormone levels. Anterior pituitary insufficiency caused by mass effect on the normal pituitary gland is much more frequent.[15]

Hypersecreting symptoms related to multiple hormones may explained either by a reversible transdifferentiation or a proliferation of more than one type of secreting cell.[16,17]

Nonfunctioning tumors (adenomas or nonpituitary tumors), on the other hand, usually present with symptoms related to mass effect. Pituitary insufficiency is frequent and a deficiency of at least one axis is present in 60% to 85% of nonfunctioning PAs.[18]

Mild hyperprolactinemia typically related to stalk disconnection is a common feature and usually not associated with clinically hyperprolactinema-related symptoms. Diabetes insipidus at the time of presentation is highly suggestive of nonpituitary lesion.[1]

Neurological Symptoms

Headache is a common symptom of sellar lesions with an incidence varying from 33% to 76%.[19,20] Headache characteristics are highly variable in terms of location and intensity. Headache can affect the frontal region but also the orbital, retro-orbital, and temporal regions. Bilateral headache is frequent. They are usually described as chronic, but acute headaches might occur in case of pituitary apoplexy, for example, Headache is supposed to be related to stretching and displacement of intracranial pain-sensitive structures located in blood vessels (internal carotid artery), cranial nerves (trigeminal nerve and ganglion), and dura mater (cavernous sinus lateral wall, medial wall and diaphragm sellae). Other mechanisms, such as inflammation and meningeal irritation, may also be involved.[21] Raised intracranial pressure, most often caused by obstructive hydrocephalus, may be another mechanism of headache. In such cases, papilledema owing to optic disc swelling caused by increased intracranial pressure is easily diagnosed with the help of ophthalmoscopy. Nausea and vomiting are also classical accompanying symptoms of increased intracranial pressure.

Other neurologic symptoms are less common and are usually related to large or giant lesions with intracranial extension far beyond the limit of the sella. Anosmia may be encountered for lesions compressing the olfactory tracts. Cognitive deficit may be explained by compression of the frontal lobes (frontal syndrome) or masse effect on the temporal lobes (memory impairment).

Upward extension toward the hypothalamus may also produce hypothalamic obesity caused by the disruption of the control of appetite.

Visual Symptoms

Visual loss is a common presenting symptom and related to the proximity of the optic nerve, chiasma, and optic tracts. A detailed neuro-ophthalmologic examination including ophthalmoscopy, visual acuity, and visual field testing (automatic static or Goldman perimetry) is needed.[22] Lesions compressing the cisternal portion of the optic nerve and chiasma can produce a variety of visual field defects including central visual field loss or peripheral visual field loss. Visual acuity is decreased in the case of central visual field loss. The most typical presentation is bitemporal hemianopia. However, junctional scotoma, quadranopsia, or unilateral temporal scotoma may be seen depending on the site and extent of the compression.[23]

Visual loss is usually progressive for slow-growing lesions leading to insidious visual loss and to delayed diagnosis. Rare acute visual loss can occur in the case of acute optic nerve compression, such as of pituitary apoplexy, for example.

Diplopia may occur in the case of abducens nerve palsy related to increased intracranial pressure. Other causes of diplopia are direct compression of the cranial nerves VI, IV, or III by a lesion invading the cavernous sinus or by the acute compression of the cavernous sinus itself in case of pituitary apoplexy. Facial pain or facial numbness caused by trigeminal ganglion or to V1, V2, or V3 irritation is rare for sellar lesion. Such symptoms, diplopia and facial pain, may attest to the presence of an aggressive tumor with a significant size that extends beyond the limit of the sella.[24]

NEUROIMAGING

Neuroradiology provides to the surgeons crucial information regarding the nature of the lesion and its relationships to neurovascular structures, its epicenter, and its extension into the surrounding tissues. MRI stands as the primary diagnostic tool for the diagnosis and assessment of sellar and parasellar lesions.[25] However, CT scan can be a useful complement. It may show some calcifications (craniopharyngiomas [CPs], meningioma, chordoma, aneurysm) and bony erosion or destruction (floor of the sellae, clivus).

In preparation for surgery, it is also useful to study the bony anatomy and its relationship with the tumor and important structures, such as the internal carotid artery. CT angiography helps to rule out life-threatening diagnoses, such as sellar aneurysm, preoperatively and to study more precisely the shape and trajectory of the paracavernous segment of the ICA. Cerebral angiography and extracranial imaging studies must be considered for specific etiologies (aneurysm, hypophysitis, malignant tumor, metastasis).

BIOLOGICAL WORKUP

In all patients with sellar tumors, the pituitary function should be evaluated with a complete biochemical workup (gonadal, adrenal, and thyroid function and PRL and GH secretion). Specific stimulation and suppression tests for pituitary hormones are required in selected cases to evaluate some pituitary hypersecretion or pituitary deficiency.

NEOPLASTIC LESIONS
Pituitary Lesions

Anterior pituitary lesions
Benign lesions

Hyperplasia Hyperplasia is defined as a cell proliferation of one or more specific anterior pituitary cell types induced by a known stimulus. It is a process that stops when the stimulus is removed. Pituitary hyperplasia is classified as primary (idiopathic) or secondary hyperplasia in the case of absent or negative feedback stimulation accompanying end-organ failure (particularly primary hypothyroidism). Hyperplasia can be physiologic, for example, when lactotroph cells proliferate during pregnancy, or pathologic, as when induced by an excess of hypophysiotropic hormones. It may cause clinical endocrine syndrome, such as acromegaly or Cushing disease. Hyperplasia appears as a pituitary enlargement on MRI and can be clinically indistinguishable from adenomas. A complete endocrinologic evaluation should be performed. The suppression of the promoting factors is usually sufficient. Close follow-up is required.[26]

Adenomas PAs are the most common intracranial neoplasm with a population prevalence of 0.1% and autopsy prevalence of around 15%.[11] Most PAs are sporadic. Rare hereditary conditions, such as multiple endocrine neoplasia type 1, are associated with the development of PAs. PAs are composed of adenohypophyseal cells. Any kind of cell types encountered in the adenohypophysis may be found in PAs.

According to their size, PAs are classified into microadenomas (<1 cm in diameter), macroadenomas (>1 cm), and giant adenomas (>4 cm) (**Fig. 3**). Clinically, PAs are classified as functioning adenomas and nonfunctioning adenomas. Approximately 65% of adenomas secrete hormones (PRL, 48%; GH, 10%; ACTH, 6%; thyrotropin-releasing hormone, 1%) causing hypersecretory syndromes. In addition to the hypersecretion syndromes, large tumor with compression of the surrounding normal pituitary tissue can alter the production of other hormones.

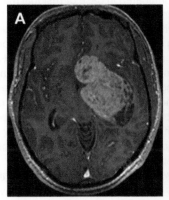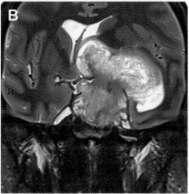

Fig. 3. Giant macroadenoma in a patient presenting with blindness on the left side (optic atrophy), intracranial hypertension, and cognitive deficit. (*A*) Coronal T2-WI. (*B*) Axial T1 gadolinium-enhanced WIs. Note the impressive mass effect on the temporal lobe.

Functioning adenomas **Prolactinomas** are the most frequent functioning PAs.[11] Most of the microprolactinomas are diagnosed in women during the reproductive period and present with oligomenorrhea or amenorrhea, galactorrhea, and infertility. In men and elderly women, prolactinomas are mostly macroadenomas and present with visual symptoms. Impotence and decreased libido are common in men but are usually not the revealing complaint.[27] Most patients presenting with prolactinomas are usually given medical treatment.[28] Therefore, surgery for prolactinomas is considerably reduced, and the candidates for surgery are those patients who did not respond to medical treatment, experienced major adverse effects induced by all of the available dopaminergic agonists, or have persistent masse effects requiring surgery. Prolactinomas resistant to dopaminergic agonists are good candidates for surgery and if complete resection is not achievable, hormonal control helps with surgical debulking.[29] It has also been reported that patients undergoing surgery for a prolactinomas that have been exposed to bromocriptine are more likely to be fibrous during surgery than those in an untreated patient. This was not observed for patients previously exposed to cabergoline.[30] Curative surgical resection as a primary mode of treatment for small lesions when complete resection can be easily achieved has recently gained attention as an alternative to lifelong dopamine agonist treatment.

GH-secreting adenomas account for about 20% of PAs. Acromegaly affects both sexes similarly, and the mean age at diagnosis is 40 to 45 years. Because the symptoms are slowly progressive, the dysmorphic syndrome is usually recognized quite late by the patient and his relatives (swelling of the hands and feet is often an early feature, protrusion of the brow and lower jaw, enlarged nose and inferior lip, wide spacing of the teeth). Therefore, most patients have a macroadenoma at the time of diagnosis, and visual symptoms may also be present. The biochemical workup shows high serum GH and insulinlike growth factor levels. In about 30% to 50% of patients, there is a cosecretion of PRL resulting in associated symptoms of hyperprolactinemia. Surgery is considered the first-line treatment when the tumor is resectable, especially in cases of well-circumscribed adenomas. Severe associated comorbidities associated with severe acromegaly (hypertension, diabetes mellitus, cardiovascular disease, severe sleep apnea) should be ruled out carefully preoperatively, as they may increase the surgical risk.[31] Preoperative treatment with somatostatin receptor ligands may be considered to reduce this risk. When total resection is unlikely, the best treatment strategy is significant debulking if possible followed by medical treatment. Medical treatment options include somatostatin receptor ligands, dopamine agonist, and GH receptor antagonist.[32,33] Radiation therapy is indicated in case of residual mass after surgery and if the medical treatment is unsuccessful or not tolerated.

ACTH-secreting adenomas associated with Cushing disease represent approximately 10% to 15% of all adenomas. Cushing disease has a peak incidence between the ages of 30 and 40 years and tends to be more frequent in women. Most ACTH-secreting adenomas are microadenomas, and approximately 15% are invasive at the time of surgery.[34] Ectopic PA tissue causing Cushing's disease is rare but a potential cause for surgical failure.[35,36] Microadenomas and ectopic adenomas may be extremely difficult to locate on MRI. On the other hand, any lesion that harbors the radiologic features of a microadenoma is not necessarily endocrinologically active. Indeed, as previously mentioned, the prevalence of incidentalomas is high. In complex cases, bilateral inferior petrosal sinus sampling is sometimes required.[37] High-resolution functional imaging along with with high-resolution morphologic MRI improve the detection of intrasellar or ectopic microadenomas.[38]

TSH-secreting adenomas are the least frequent PAs. Clinically, they may present with hyperthyroidism, but they can also arise in the setting of hypothyroidism or in clinically euthyroid patients.[39] Most TSH-secreting adenomas are invasive macroadenomas.

Nonfunctioning adenomas Approximately one-third of PAs are not associated with clinical evidence of hormone hypersecretion. However, most nonfunctioning PAs are actually gonadotropin-secreting adenomas. They present rarely with clinical evidence of hormone excess and are considered silent adenomas. In 10% of nonfunctioning PAs, immunostaining is negative. Exceptionally, nonfunctioning PAs may be positive for GH, PRL, TSH, or ACTH despite no secretion being identified clinically; such cases are known as *silent somatotroph, lactotroph, thyrotroph,* or *corticotroph* adenomas.

Nonfunctioning PAs, because they have usually reached a significant size at the time of diagnosis, most often present with visual symptoms and signs of hypopituitarism (**Fig. 4**). Hypopituitarism is related to the compression caused by the adenoma on the normal pituitary the function of which is secondarily impaired. At time of diagnosis,

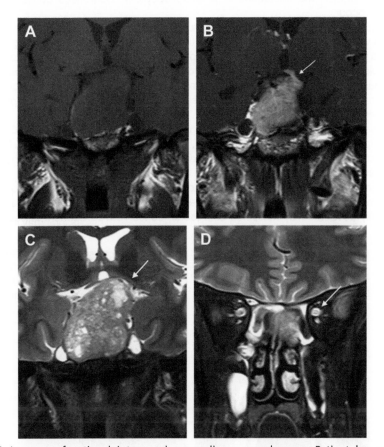

Fig. 4. Large nonfunctional intra- and suprasellar macroadenoma. Patient has a light perception on the left side and an optic atrophy. (*A*) Coronal T1-WI without gadolinium. (*B*) Coronal T1-WI shows homogenous enhancement after gadolinium. The pituitary stalk is deviated (*white arrow*). (*C*) Coronal T2-WI shows more clearly the compression of the chiasma and optic nerve on the left side (*white arrow*). (*D*) Coronal T2-WI at the level of the orbital apex shows atrophy and hypersignal of the Optic Nerve (*white arrow*).

60% to 85% of patients present at least 1 pituitary deficiency.[40] They also sometimes present with mild hyperprolactinemia caused by pituitary stalk compression.

Surgery is required in cases of visual disorders. Hypopituitarism may be an indication for surgery, but recovery is uncertain (30%) and surgery by itself carries a risk of hypopituitarism of 5% to 10 %.[41] Careful follow-up is advocated for incidentalomas.

To evaluate the risk of recurrence or progression, it is advocated to test 3 proliferation markers: proliferation index assessed on Ki-67 antibody, mitotic activity, and p53 expression.[41] Recent studies have found that a Ki-67 greater than 3% predicts recurrence/progression with high specificity (89%).[42,43] However, even in cases of recurrent tumors, the Ki-67 may be low so it is recommended to test the 3 proliferative markers.[41]

Pituitary apoplexy Pituitary apoplexy is a serious acute complication of PAs, most often nonfunctioning. They usually present with acute symptoms characterized by a sudden onset of headache. It is frequently associated with nausea and vomiting. Visual symptoms such as diplopia, ptosis, visual acuity, and visual field impairment are also common manifestations of pituitary apoplexy. Decreased consciousness may also occur.

The incidence of pituitary apoplexy is probably around 2% of all surgically treated patients with pituitary adenoma.[44,45] The etiology is an infarct in a pre-existing lesion, usually a macroadenoma, followed by hemorrhage or necrosis. Promoting factors may be low blood pressure (cardiac surgery, myocardial infarction, trauma with shock) with an increased demand of the lesion or treatments (anticoagulants, dopamine agonists), and it has been described as the consequence of stimulation test of pituitary hormones.[40,44]

MRI is highly sensitive for the detection of acute or old hemorrhage (**Fig. 5**). Subarachnoid hemorrhage may also be seen. Angiographic MRI should be performed to rule out any associated aneurysm (differential diagnosis) or vasospasm of the anterior communicating complex.[46]

Pituitary apoplexy is frequently associated with hypopituitarism, and hydrocortisone replacement should be initiated immediately after diagnosis. Although surgery was historically advocated by most neurosurgeons, conservative treatment is becoming

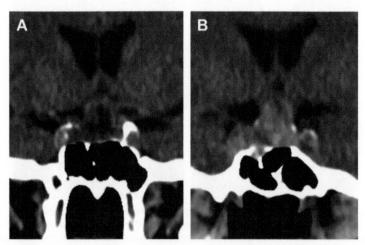

Fig. 5. Pituitary apoplexy in a patient followed up for PAs and presenting in the emergency room with acute headache. (*A*) CT scan before hemorrhage. (*B*) CT scan shows hyperdensity caused by hemorrhage.

more popular and is now advocated in cases of mild stable or long-standing visual symptoms or isolated occulomotor palsy, together with adequate endocrinologic management and close clinical and ophthalmologic follow-up. Early surgical decompression should be considered in cases of visual status worsening.

Atypical adenomas Tumors that show histologic features suggestive of aggressive clinical behavior, a Ki-67 labeling index (LI) greater than 3%, and extensive nuclear p53 positivity on immunohistochemial staining are considered atypical adenomas. In such cases, a close follow-up after surgery is highly recommended.[47] The proliferative marker Ki-67 (MIB-1) has been used to distinguish aggressive tumors but some controversies remain about its real prognosis value.[48,49] Several studies have shown a correlation between the Ki-67 LI and the invasiveness of pituitary carcinomas, and it seems that some of the controversies come from the various criteria used to defined invasiveness.[48,50] In a study of 159 patients from Pizarro and colleagues,[51] the Ki-67 index was not significantly different in adenomas infiltrating the cavernous sinus, which supports the hypothesis that the medial wall of the cavernous sinus is a weak barrier. Although the Ki-67 LI does not seem to provide independent information to predict tumor recurrence, it does seem to provide valuable prognostic information, and in the case of high Ki-67 labeling index, a closer follow-up is advocated. However, new markers are certainly needed to help clinicians.[50]

Malignant lesions: primary pituitary carcinomas Pituitary carcinomas are rare, accounting for less than 1% of all pituitary neoplasms. The diagnosis of pituitary carcinoma requires the demonstration of distant metastasis (**Fig. 6**). Most of them are

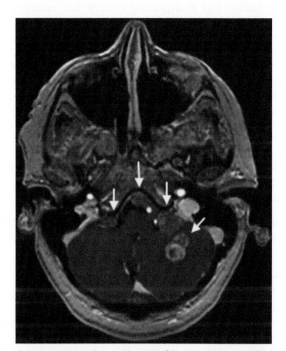

Fig. 6. Pituitary carcinoma metastasis in a 70-year-old woman operated on 10 years before for a prolactinoma with subsequent irradiation (50 Gy). Axial T1-enhanced gadolinium-weighted image shows multiple lesions at the level of the cranio-cervical junction (*white arrows*). Histology confirmed the diagnosis of pituitary carcinoma metastasis with a Ki-67 LI of 10%.

functionally active and most produce ACTH and PRL. Usually the initial course cannot be distinguishable from the one of a benign pituitary adenoma. Multiple local recurrences and finally metastatic dissemination usually occur later in the course of the condition. Only rarely do patients present with metastases concurrent with the initial sellar tumor. On the contrary to metastatic pituitary carcinoma, primary pituitary carcinomas generally do not impair pituitary endocrine function.[52] The latency between the diagnosis of a PA and the diagnosis of metastasis ranges from a few months to almost 20 years. It seems to be shorter for PRL-producing tumors than for ACTH-producing lesions. Once the diagnosis is made, the survival is poor, and 66% of patients die within 1 year.[52] Standard morphologic features associated with malignancy (hypercellularity, nuclear and cellular pleomorphism, increased mitotic activity, necrosis, and dural/osseous invasion) are commonly present but are not necessarily diagnostic of carcinoma. Ki-67 labeling indices are quite variable and show considerable overlap with common PAs; however, they are often higher, and it may help to alert the clinicians about the possibility of a pituitary carcinomas.[53] Treatment strategies include dopamine agonists for PRL-secreting tumors, radiation therapy, and chemotherapy (Temozolomide) but are only palliative.[54]

Posterior pituitary lesions

Pituicytomas Pituicytes are cells that may exceptionally transform into pituicytomas. Pituicytes are rare low-grade astrocytic tumors,[55,56] and their histogenesis is debated. The most accepted theory is that they arise from pituicytes, which are specialized glial cells located in the stalk or posterior pituitary. Recent studies suggest that they may originate from folliculostellate cell located in the adenohypophysis.[57]

Pituicytomas are benign and slow-growing tumors that usually occur in young to middle-age women. They are ubiquitarious in the hypothalamic-pituitary axis and can be entirely intrasellar or suprasellar or involve both compartments. Clinical presentation is similar to that of other regional masses; headache and hypopituitarism are the most common manifestations for intrasellar lesions. Visual symptoms can occur in cases of suprasellar location. Despite their neurohypophyseal origin, diabetes insipidious (DI) is rare. MRI shows a solid, demarcated, enhancing sellar or suprasellar mass usually isointense to gray matter on T1 and hyperintense on T2-weighted image (WI). They usually mimic an adenoma but occasionally the enhanced adenohypophysis might be displaced anteriorly. The diagnosis is confirmed by histologic examination. Microscopy shows bipolar or spindle cell morphology. Immunohistochemistry displays diffuse S-100 protein staining with variable glial fibrillary acidic protein immunopositivity (**Fig. 7**). Epithelial membrane antigen is negative.[58] Surgery is advocated when the lesion is symptomatic.

Granular cell tumor Granular cell tumor arises from granular cell pituicytes. They are extremely rare and similar to pituicytomas.

NONPITUITARY TUMORS
Benign Nonpituitary Tumors

Craniopharyngiomas

CPs are rare microcystic benign epithelial lesions arising from the pituitary itself or the pituitary stalk. Most of them occur in the sellar and parasellar region. The incidence of CPs is 0.5 to 2 per million habitants per year. It has a bimodal age distribution at presentation with peaks of incidence, respectively, between 5 to 14 years and 55 to 70 years of age. Around 40% present during childhood or adolescence. Sex ratio is equal to 1. CPs are thought to originate from ectodermal remnant of Rathke's pouch

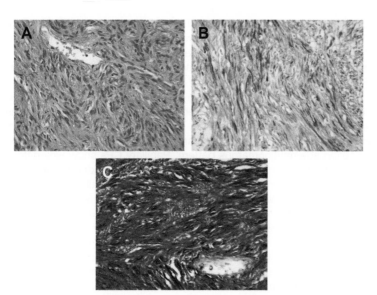

Fig. 7. Pituicytoma in a young man complaining of headache and decreased libido. Surgery was performed. (*A*) Microscopy shows elongated spindle cells. (*B*) Immunohistochemistry exhibits mild glial fibrillary acidic protein staining. (*C*) Strong diffuse positivity for PS-100.

along the craniopharyngeal duct (embryogenetic theory) or from metaplasia of the adenohypophyseal cells in the pars tuberalis of the adenohypophysis, resulting in the formation of squamous cell nests (metaplastic theory). CPs commonly infiltrate surrounding structures such as the hypophysis, pituitary stalk, and hypothalamus, which explains the initial symptoms but which may lead to postoperative complications. Thus, despite high survival rates (87%–95% in recent series), the long-term quality of life is frequently impaired because of complications related to the close relationship with those important structures. Malignant transformation is extremely rare.[59] CPs can be divided into 2 histologic subtypes: the adamantinomatous type is predominantly found in children and young adults, whereas the papillary type is more frequent in adults. CPs are most often located in the suprasellar and sellar regions (53%–75%), purely in the suprasellar region (20%–41%), and rarely only in the sellar region (5%–6%). Most importantly, CPs are opportunistic tumors that grow along the path of least resistance and spread along cerebrospinal fluid (CSF) road maps. The 3-dimensional variations of the arachnoid that forms the basal cisterns certainly have to some extent an influence on the extension of CPs. They can extend in the supra and infrachiasmatic region, behind the infundibulum in the interpedoncular cistern, in the prepontine cistern, and into the third ventricle. They can also be located purely into the third ventricle, growing into the floor of the third ventricle or exceptionally, above the floor. Several classifications are available based on their extension and their relationship with the chiasm, the pituitary stalk, and the third ventricle.[60]

There are slow-growing tumors and symptoms usually occur insidiously. Presenting signs are highly variable depending on the age of the patient, the size of the lesion, and its extension. Intracranial hypertension is not infrequent, especially in children, and is either caused by the tumor itself or caused by hydrocephalus secondary to the obstruction of the foramen of Monroe, the third ventricle or the aqueduct of Sylvius itself. Other manifestations are visual impairment and endocrine dysfunction, which result much more frequently in hyposecretion(s) (short stature in childhood, diabetes insipidus, amenorrhea, hypothyroidism) than in hypersecretion (precocious puberty).[61] Weight gain is also a common symptom, and its etiology is not yet fully understood. It concerns 75% of survivors after therapy.[62]

Macroscopically CPs typically show calcifications, solid tissue, and cysts. Pure cystic CPs may be encountered in 15% of the cases. Its outside membrane may be thin with eggshell calcification. In 15%, the tumor can be only solid. In 70% CPs are a mix of solid and cystic parts. Cystic content is often described as motor oil and contains a large amount of cholesterol crystals. Microscopically, adamantinomatous CPs are composed of pseudostratified columnar cells palisade around stellate cells forming the so-called adamantinomatous pattern. Papillary CPs show well-differentiated squamous epithelium, which may be separated to form pseudopapillae.

Most adamantinomatous CPs express nuclear β-catenin antibody in relation with its tumorogenesis. Survivin, which is an inhibitor of apoptosis, is positive in most and could be a potential indicator for assessing CPs aggressiveness.[63]

CT and MRI usually show a polylobular lesion with solid or cystic parts. Calcifications are usual and better seen on CT scan. Three-dimensional constructive interference in steady state (with a high T2/T1 ratio) is interesting to analyze the relationship of the tumor with the different cisterns, vessels, nerves, floor of the third ventricles, and hypothalamus, which is essential to define the best surgical strategy (**Fig. 8**).

Prognosis is variable according to the type, size, and extension of the lesion. For lesions easily accessible and well circumscribed, complete resection is the treatment of choice. In case of incomplete resection, the recurrence rate is high. Thus, for more complex lesion with tight relationship with the hypothalamus, there are still ongoing debates between supporters of a primary gross total resection and supporters of a partial resection followed by irradiation.[64] The significant morbidity (severe hypothalamic dysfunction, altered neuropsychological status) owing to aggressive surgical resection to achieve gross total resection has led to a more conservative strategy combining partial resection and fractionated radiation therapy for the lesions with suspected infiltration of the hypothalamus, especially in children.[65–67]

Concerning the surgical approach, it is clear from the recent literature that endoscopic endonasal approach has become one of the approaches of choice for most CPs.[68,69] Surgery offers the advantage for a more logical line of sight that provides an access to the multiple areas of the basal cistern where CPs usually extend. For sellar lesions, the advantages are not in doubt. For complex lesions with suprasellar extension, it seems that the endoscopic approach offers better ophthalmologic results, but its advantage is not as obvious in terms of endocrinologic outcome, and the higher risk of CSF leak has not been overcome yet. Thus, there is certainly still some room for the transcranial approach, and the respective indication of transcranial and endoscopic approach has to be clarified. CPs are complex lesions to treat and require multidisciplinary management by experienced teams that include an endocrinologist, pediatrician, neurosurgeon, and radiation oncologist.

Chordomas, chondrosarcomas, and chondromas
The preoperative distinction between chordomas, chondrosarcomas, and chondromas may be challenging. Chordomas, chondrosarcomas, and chondromas belong to a rare variety of skull base tumors that arise from the bony and cartilaginous structures. These tumors are usually grouped together because of some similarities in terms of location, radiologic appearance, and histology. Their treatment strategies also share common features. However, chondrosarcomas are generally treated more conservatively, and the long-term prognosis is better.

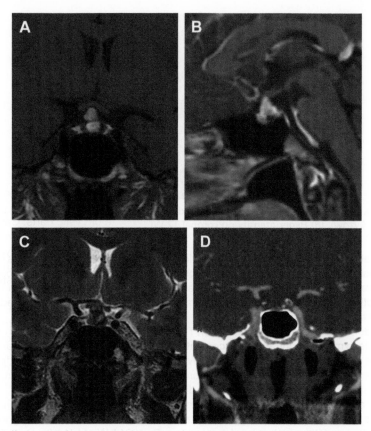

Fig. 8. Sellar craniopharyngioma. (*A*) Coronal T1-WI shows a hyperintense lesion developed inside the stalk with a downward extension in the pituitary gland. (*B*) Sagittal T1-WI with contrast. (*C*) The lesion has a heterogeneous signal on coronal T2-WI. (*D*) CT angiography performed for preoperative planning shows no calcifications of the lesion.

Chordomas Chordoma is a rare neoplasm considered to be of low to intermediate malignancy. It originates from the notochord cells. The incidence of chordomas is estimated around 0.51 to 0.80 cases per million accounting for 1% to 5.2% of all malignant bone tumors.[70,71] Chordomas represent less than 0.1% of all skull base tumors.[72] Because of the topographic distribution of the notochord cells, chordomas are mostly midline tumors, which usually occur along the spinal column or in the skull base. A total of 25% to 36% of the tumors are found in the skull base, but strictly intrasellar chordomas are rare (**Fig. 9**). Sellar invasions are most often associated with clival chordomas.

Clinical presentation depends on the size and extension of the lesion. The most common presenting symptoms are visual complaints, mainly diplopia. Intermittent or partial abducens nerve palsy is a common initial symptom of clival chordomas, related to posterior cavernous sinus extension. However, depending on the epicenter of the lesion and its size at the time of diagnosis (the lesion can reach a considerable size before being symptomatic), other cranial nerve deficits can be seen: third and fourth cranial nerve palsy in the case of cavernous infiltration, trigeminal nerve for petrous apex extension (facial numbness), lower cranial nerves, and hypoglossal

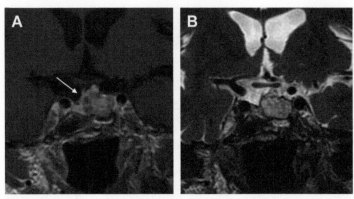

Fig. 9. Sellar chordomas. (*A*) The pituitary gland is displaced laterally on coronal T1-WI with contrast (*arrow*). (*B*) Hyperintensity on coronal T2-WI.

nerve palsy for lower clivus and craniocervical junction chordomas. Symptoms related to brainstem compression are less common but not exceptional (ataxia, hemiparesis). Compression of the OC leads to visual defect like any other sellar lesion. Endocrine dysfunction is unusual, but hypopituitarism or mild hyperprolactinemia, related to pituitary stalk compression, can be seen.

Chordomas are usually hypointense on T1-WI and hyperintense on T2-WI. There is a moderate to marked contrast enhancement. CT shows bony remnant rather than calcifications and is needed preoperatively to evaluate the bony erosion. Apparent diffusion coefficient has shown to be useful to differentiate chordomas and chondrosarcomas; the latest harboring the highest apparent diffusion coefficient values.[73]

From a pathologic standpoint, chordomas is usually classified as a benign tumor because of the absence of malignant features, although this lesion has an aggressive local behavior with a high rate of recurrence. The 2014 World Health Organization (WHO) classification splits chordomas into well-differentiated chordomas (classical myxoid chordoma, chondroid or mixed types) and dedifferentiated chordomas. Vacuolated physaliferous cells, surrounded by a myxoid matrix, are usually seen on microscopy. Recently, brachyury expression proved to be a unique specific diagnostic marker for chordomas, both sensitive and specific, particularly helpful to differentiate chordomas from chondrosarcomas.[74]

Chordomas tend to recur, and metastasis may also occur; its long-term prognosis is poor. Several studies emphasized the importance of radical resection and aggressive adjuvant radiation therapy.[72,75–77] An endonasal endoscopic approach is becoming the gold standard to resect skull base chordomas.[78,79] However, because of their location and extension, radical resection is not always achievable. Proton beam therapy is the type of radiation therapy that is most often recommended for chordomas.[80] Chemotherapy can be proposed in cases of recurrences but have shown until now only limited results.

Chondrosarcomas Chondrosarcomas develop from the chondrocytes usually located laterally from the sella at the level of the different synchondrosis. Even if the histologic grading takes into account the malignant potential of the chondrosarcoma (grade I, well differentiated to grade III, poorly differentiated), most chondrosarcomas are classified as low grade and are slow growing tumors. They appear histologically as large cells with single or multiple nuclei in a variable amount of chondroid matrix. Calcifications are frequent (**Fig. 10**). Brachyury is crucial for the differential diagnosis of

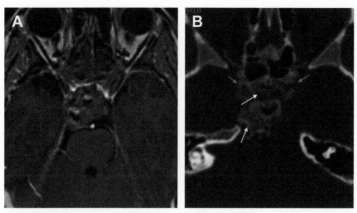

Fig. 10. Sellar chondrosarcoma in a young woman complaining of intermittent diplopia caused by abducens nerve palsy. (*A*) The signal is also heterogeneous on axial T1-WI with gadolinium. The hyposignal is explained by the presence of calcifications. (*B*) Calcifications are well demonstrated on CT angiography. Red arrows point to the intracavernous internal carotid arteries. White arrow shows intrasellar calcification. Yellow arrow indicates the epicenter of lesion on the spheno-petrous synchondrosis.

mimickers such as chordomas; immunostaining for brachyury is negative for chondrosarcomas.[81]

Surgery is the main treatment modality. However, complex locations associated with important calcifications usually make the complete removal technically challenging. Complementary radiation therapy has proven to be effective treatment for chondrosarcomas, reducing the recurrence rate. Because of its less aggressive nature compared with chordomas, radiation therapy may reduce the need for complete resection in challenging location.

Chondromas Few cases of skull base chondromas are described in the literature. However, histologic distinction between low-grade chondrosarcomas and chondromas is still an ongoing debate.[82]

Meningiomas

Meningiomas are benign tumors derived from arachnoid cells and attached to the dura mater. Meningiomas of the sellar region usually originate from the surrounding regions and secondarily extend toward the sellar compartment. Among them, one classically distinguishes suprasellar meningiomas (tuberculum meningiomas, diaphragm sellae meningioma, and anterior clinoid meningiomas) and cavernous sinus meningiomas. Purely intrasellar meningiomas are rare and may be difficult to distinguish from adenoma (**Fig. 11**).

Meningiomas have morphologic features consistent with their arachnoid origin and are classified into 3 grades according the WHO classification, which is based on their histologic appearance but also on the Ki-67/MIB-1 proliferative index.

Most meningiomas are almost always WHO grade 1 meningiomas, which are benign tumors with a low recurrence rate. On the other hand, grade II and III are associated with a more aggressive natural history and a high risk of recurrence.

Tuberculum sellae meningioma Tuberculum sellae meningioma accounts for 5% to 10% of all intracranial meningiomas.[83] They arise from the tuberculum, the chiasmatic

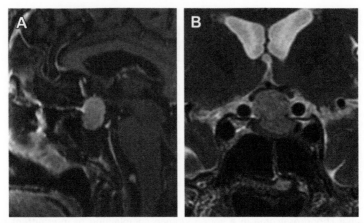

Fig. 11. Intrasellar meningioma. Patient complaining of a visual deficit on the left eye. (*A*) Sagittal T1-WI with gadolinium shows a homogenous enhancement of an intra- and suprasellar lesion mimicking a pituitary adenoma. (*B*) The lesion lies on the hypophysis on coronal T2-WI.

sulcus, and the limbus sphenoidale. As they enlarge they usually displace the optic nerve laterally and the chiasma superiorly. Visual impairment is usually the first symptom that leads to the diagnosis. Pituitary function has to be assessed but is usually normal. Posterior and downward extension into the sella is frequent. Posterior extension may reach the basilar artery and the floor of the third ventricle and may be responsible for a mass effect on the pituitary stalk. Contrast enhancement on MRI is usually intense and shows a dural tail that is suggestive of a meningioma but nonspecific (**Fig. 12**). The sella turcica has usually a normal volume compared with macroadenomas. Hyperostosis seen on CT scan, corresponding histologically to infiltrated bone, is also helpful for the diagnosis.

Surrounding neurovascular structures are progressively stretched as the tumor enlarges. There is usually no invasion of the neural structures and the arachnoid plane is most often intact. However, some nerves or arteries may be encased in between lobes

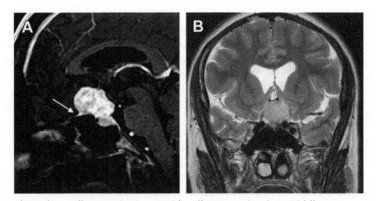

Fig. 12. Tuberculum sellae meningioma with sellar extension in a middle-age woman complaining of visual deficit. (*A*) Dural tail (*white arrow*) sagittal T1-WI with gadolinium. (*B*) Coronal T2-WI is crucial to assess the relation with the optic chiasma and arteries in the surroundings.

of the tumor. Because of the frequent optic nerve and chiasma compression, surgery remains the treatment of choice. To optimize visual outcome, the identification of an optic canal extension of the tumor, usually along the medial aspect of the optic nerve; the localization of the optic nerves and chiasma related to the tumor on the preoperative MRI; and the results of the ophthalmologic examination are essential to define the optimum line of sight and surgical approach (endoscopy vs classic open craniotomy, side of the approach in case of open surgery, unroofing of the optic canal).

Cavernous sinus meningiomas Cavernous sinus meningiomas arise from the lateral wall of the cavernous sinus or may originate within the cavernous sinus itself. They can extend laterally in the middle fossa, superiorly toward the supraclinoid carotid artery, optic nerve, and optic chiasm, posteriorly in the petroclival angle via the porous trigeminal, medially into the sphenoid sinus or toward the sella turcica. A narrowing of the intracavernous internal carotid artery can be seen.[84] In case of intracavernous meningiomas, histologic studies have found an infiltration of the wall of the internal carotid artery and infiltration of the cranial nerves.[85] Patients commonly present with headaches (retro or periorbital), occulomotor nerve deficit (third nerve deficit is more frequent than abducens nerve deficit), facial paresthesia or numbness, or impaired visual acuity or visual field. In case of sellar involvement, a complete endocrinologic evaluation should be done but pituitary dysfunction is not common and usually occurs late. Cavernous sinus meningiomas are complex lesions to treat, and multidisciplinary management is required. Surgery is targeted to the extracavernous part of the lesion to decompress the brainstem, the optic pathway, or the temporal lobe. The remaining part of the tumor inside the cavernous sinus is usually followed or treated with radiation therapy.

Hemangioblastomas
Exceptional capillary hemangioblastomas located in the sella turcica have been described.[86,87] In 84% of the cases they occur in association with a von Hippel-Lindau (vHL) disease. MRI shows hypervascularization of the tumor seen as a dense enhancement on T1-weighted sequence after gadolinium injection. An enhancement of the dura mater may lead to the misdiagnosis of a meningioma.

Differential histopathologic diagnosis includes angioblastic meningioma and metastasis of renal cell carcinoma in the context on vHL disease. Immunohistochemical studies confirm the diagnosis with positive immunoreactivity for neuron-specific enolase, vimentin, and S100 protein and negative immunoreactivity to epithelial membrane antigen and glial fibrillary acidic protein. The preoperative diagnosis is extremely difficult, especially for patients who do not have any features of vHL disease. However, any suspicion of a hemangioblastomas should warn the surgeons not to choose an extended endoscopic resection because of the risk of massive intraoperative hemorrhage, which interferes with a safe endoscopic dissection in this region.

Malignant Nonpituitary Tumors

Metastatic lesions
Metastatic lesions of the pituitary gland are rare and occur in 1% to 3.6% of malignant tumors. However, if both the pituitary and surrounding regions are considered, the rates are significantly higher. Breast and lung are the most frequent primary sites. Most of the lesions are asymptomatic. However, symptoms from the pituitary metastasis are quite frequently the first manifestation of the metastatic disease. Most commonly reported symptoms are DI, ophthalmoplegia from infiltration of the cavernous sinus, decreased visual acuity and visual field defects from compression and infiltration of the optic nerves and chiasma, anterior pituitary insufficiency, and headache/pain. DI is a frequent symptom related to the infiltration of the posterior pituitary.

In case of resection, the tumor is usually highly vascular, and infiltration of the optic nerves, chiasma, and hypothalamus are not unusual if there is a significant suprasellar extension (**Fig. 13**). The prognosis is poor and related to the systemic disease. The role for surgery is limited and does not improve survival. In most series, radiation therapy is the most frequently used treatment either with limited radiation to the sellar and parasellar region or with whole-brain irradiation. Surgery may be considered to improve quality of life and to save vision in cases of rapid decrease visual acuity. In such cases, careful debulking for decompression should be the goal, as there is a frequent infiltration of the visual apparatus and engulfment of the small vessels that vascularize the optic nerves, chiasma, and pituitary stalk. Because of heavy bleeding and infiltration of surrounding structures, a transcranial approach may be a better option than the endoscopic endonasal approach.[88]

Lymphomas

Primary sellar lymphomas are sparsely reported in the literature. Pituitary involvement leads to hypopituitarism or DI. MRI shows isointense signal on T1-WI with dense

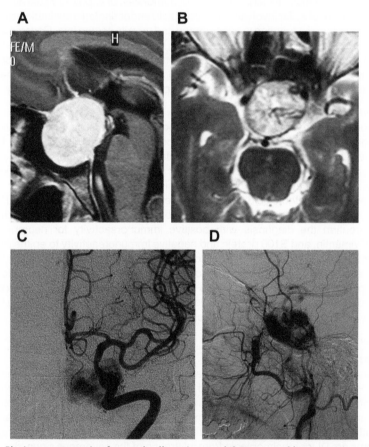

Fig. 13. Pituitary metastasis of a renal cell carcinoma. (*A*) Dense and homogeneous contrast enhancement on sagittal T1-WI with contrast. (*B*) Hyperintense on axial T2-WI. (*C*) Intense tumor blush from the internal carotid artery on AP angiogram. (*D*) Intense tumor blush from the external carotid artery.

gadolinium enhancement that overlaps with many other lesions. Histology and immunostaining confirm the diagnosis.

Germ cell tumor

Intracranial germinomas derived from residual germ cells and are willingly located in the suprasellar and pineal region. Exceptional intrasellar locations have been described. Bifocal pineal and sellar locations are even more unusual but suggest the diagnosis. A pineal region tumor associated with a DI also suggests the diagnosis of germinoma.[89] Germinomas usually have massive contrast enhancement, which make these tumors difficult to differentiate from the most frequent lesion in the region, PAs.

If the diagnosis is not done before the surgery, MRI of the spine should be performed after surgery to identify CSF dissemination, which is common. Treatment is based on radiation therapy and chemotherapy.

DEVELOPMENTAL LESIONS
Rathke's Cleft Cyst

Rathke's cleft cysts (RCCs) are derived from the remnants of Rathke's pouch and belong to the spectrum of cystic epithelial lesions. After the formation of the pituitary gland, the residual lumen between the anterior and intermediate lobe constitutes Rathke's cleft. Further enlargement of the Rathke's cleft with proliferation of the cell lining and accumulation of its secretions leads to RCCs.

Reported incidence of RCCs at autopsy is quite high (2%–26 %) and, with the wide use of MRI, many asymptomatic RCCs are diagnosed.[90,91] They are mostly intrasellar or intrasuprasellar. Pure suprasellar lesions are rare at the time of diagnosis. When clinically eloquent, main symptoms are headaches, visual impairment, and endocrine dysfunction, which may concern one-third of patient each.[92] Hyperprolactinemia is the most frequent ante hypophysis dysfunction, followed by gonadotropin deficiency, pan-hypopituitarism, hypothyroidism, and hypocortisolism. Pre-existing DI may be encountered in RCC.

On MR imaging, an RCC is a well-circumscribed spherical or ovoid cyst. Most lesions are intra and/or suprasellar with an epicenter located at the level of the pars intermedia.

The MRI signal intensity of the cyst content shows high variability on T1- and T2-weighted sequences depending on the cystic contents.[93] Gadolinium enhancement of the pituitary around the cyst wall may be observed leading to the classical aspect of "the egg in the cup" (**Fig. 14**).

Histology confirms the diagnosis of RCCs showing a simple cuboidal or columnar epithelium with ciliated or mucinous goblet cells. Pseudostratified epithelium may be observed. Squamous metaplasia may also be encountered, which tends to prove that this lesion belongs to the spectrum of cystic epithelial lesions of the sellar region.[94] Complete resection of the peripheral membrane is not recommended to avoid any postoperative hypopituitarism or DI.[95] Biopsy of the cyst wall via an endonasal endoscopic route to confirm the diagnosis and large drainage of the cyst content to release the mass effect is the most reasonable surgical management. Transcranial approaches have been advocated for rare pure suprasellar symptomatic lesion.[96]

Dermoid/Epidermoid Cysts

Dermoid and epidermoid cysts are rare congenital nonneoplastic developmental lesions that can occur at any level of the cranio-spinal axis. Originating from the ectoderm, they are slow-growing tumors that usually become symptomatic in the adulthood.

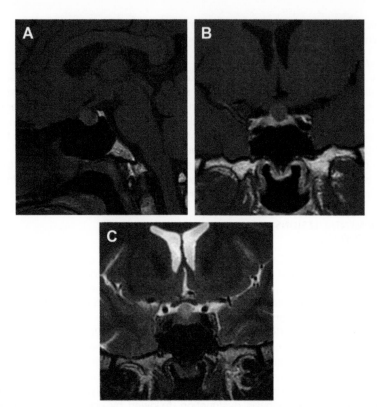

Fig. 14. RCC in a young patient complaining of secondary amenorrhea. (*A*) The lesion appears isointense on sagittal T1-WI. (*B*) Gadolinium injection leads to a homogenously pituitary gland enhancement. The lesion appears as the classical egg in the cup (*C*) The lesion is hyperintense on coronal T2-WI.

Dermoid cysts

Dermoid cysts are congenital inclusion cysts that appear as well-circumscribed heterogeneous extra-axial masses. They are composed of dermal derivatives such as hair follicles and fat. Dermoid cysts are reported to be more frequent in childhood. Even if they occur preferentially along the midline, the sellar or parasellar locations are rare. Dermoid cysts may rupture in the subarachnoid space, causing aseptic meningitis, which is seen on MRI by T1 hyperintense fillings in the cortical sulci.

Epidermoid

Epidermoids are rare cystic tumors arising from ectodermal remnants. Their wall has a multilayered squamous epithelium that contains epidermis and dry keratin. They are slow-growing tumors that tend to mold and dilate the subarachnoid spaces. Malignant transformations have been exceptionally described.[97]

The preponderant location of epidermoid cyst in the paramedian space in contrast to strictly median dermoid cysts explains the rarity of the sellar region location. However, sellar and parasellar location have been described. Mass effect of these slow-growing tumors may lead to headache and vision loss. They may also rupture with their caustic content flowing into the subarachnoid space: meningitis (septic or aseptic), vasospasm, hypophysitis, and pituitary apoplexy have been described.[98] The diagnosis is confirmed by restricted diffusion on diffusion-WI.

Surgery remains the standard treatment. Complete removal is difficult and most often part of the capsule, which is quite adherent to the surrounding neurovascular structures, have to be left in place. Because of the slow-growing nature of this lesion and the risk of long-term recurrence, a long-term follow-up is required.

Arachnoid Cysts

Arachnoid cysts are benign lesions containing CSF and whose wall is formed by arachnoid. They vary widely in size and location, and intrasellar arachnoid cysts are rare. Etiopathogenesis is not completely understood. Because normally arachnoid tissue is not present below the diaphragma sella, one of the major hypotheses is that an arachnoid fold coming from above makes its way through a large diaphragma (or a defect of the diaphragma) to reach the sella. The pouch will secondarily increased in size because of unidirectional flow, which is usually explained by a ball valve effect.[99] Other pathologic conditions such as intracranial hypertension or pituitary atrophy may favor or initiate this mechanism. The clinical presentation may be similar to that of a nonfunctioning adenoma. On MRI, arachnoid cysts appear as a round, well-marginated lesions that are isointense to CSF on all sequences. Cyst wall is very thin. Calcifications are absent, and no rim enhancement can be visualized after gadolinium injection. Content signal may sometimes be slightly different from the CSF (intra-cystic micro-hemorrhage); thus, it may be difficult to differentiate them from RCCs, cystic adenomas, and cystic CPs. However preoperative diagnosis is of importance before surgery. If needed, surgical treatment (either fenestration or derivation of the cyst) is the only therapeutic option. The risk of postoperative CSF leak would favor a classical approach rather than a transsphenoidal route. However, recent teams have shown some good result with an extended endoscopic approach.[100,101] They typically displace the adenohypophysis anteriorly and the infundibulum posteriorly.[102]

Empty Sella Syndrome

Empty sella is a herniation of the subarachnoid space within the sella turcica associated with stretching of the pituitary stalk and flattening of the pituitary gland against the sellar floor.[103]

This syndrome is classified in primary (patients with no history of pituitary tumor surgery or radiotherapy) and secondary empty sella syndrome. Main risk factors are obesity, pseudotumor cerebri (both associated with elevated intra-intracranial hypertension), and pregnancy (because of the stretching of the diaphragma caused by pituitary hyperplasia).[104]

Empty sella syndrome is most often an incidental radiologic finding. Clinical symptoms such as headache and visual disturbances are reported in 1.6% to 16% of the cases.[104] Visual symptoms are explained by the optic tract ptosis. Endocrine dysfunctions do exist but are usually mild. Rhinorrhea has been reported, which is a strong argument for the intracranial hypertension theory.[105] If the diagnosis of pseudotumor cerebri is suspected, careful MRI exploration of the lateral sinuses has to be done to rule out any stenosis that could be treated by stenting.[106] Surgical treatment is generally not necessary except when clear-cut campimetric or visual defects are present.

INFLAMMATORY AND INFECTIOUS LESIONS
Hypophysitis

Inflammation of the pituitary is classified into primary and secondary hypophysitis. Etiologies are listed in **Table 2**. Common features on MRI are swelling of the adenohypophysis, posthypophysis, and stalk. Special attention must be brought on the

Table 2
Classification of hypophysitis

Primary	Lymphocytic autoimmune	
	Granulomatous	
	Xanthomatous	
Secondary	Infectious	Tuberculosis
		Bacterial
		Fungal
		Viral
	Noninfectious	Wegener's
		Sarcoidosis
		Crohn's
		Takayasu's
		Ruptured cyst

sphenoid sinus: its involvement of both pituitary and sphenoidal tissue suggest the diagnosis of hypophysitis (**Fig. 15**). Surgery may be needed to confirm the diagnosis. Histology and immunochemistry vary according to the origin of the hypophysitis.

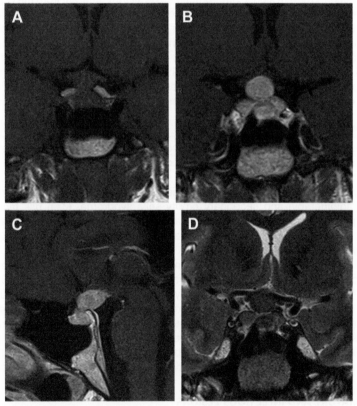

Fig. 15. IgG4-related hypophysistis in a 45-year-old man presenting with headache and decreased libido. (*A*) The lesion is isointense to gray matter. (*B*) T1-WI with contrast shows a homogenous gadolinium enhancement. (*C*) Sagittal T1-WI with contrast: The lesion involves the pituitary gland and the stalk is thickened. (*D*) Close relationships with neurovascular structures is well demonstrated on coronal T2 WI.

Mucocele

Intrasellar mucoceles are very rare and are an extension of mucoid retention caused by chronic obstruction of the sphenoid sinus. They are usually hyperintense on T1- and T2-weighted sequences. A previous sinus surgery could contribute to delayed mucocele.[107]

VASCULAR LESIONS: ANEURYSMS

An intrasellar aneurysm must be appropriately recognized before any surgical procedure to prevent a catastrophic bleeding situation. Hanak and colleagues[108], in an extensive review, reported 40 cases of aneurysms in the literature in 2012. Aneurysms with intrasellar extension usually originate from the cavernous or supraclinoid portion of the ICA in 90% of the cases and from the anterior communicating complex in the remaining 10%.[109,110] The mean diameter of the aneurysms was greater than 14.5 mm. When nonruptured, the most common presenting symptoms are visual deficit, headache, and endocrine dysfunction. Cranial nerve palsies caused by compression of the cranial nerve III and VI are not uncommon.

A patent aneurysm is suggested by the presence of a round flow void on T2-weighted sequences. Diagnosis is then confirmed with a CT angiography or magnetic resonance angiography that clearly locates the neck and defines the relationship between the

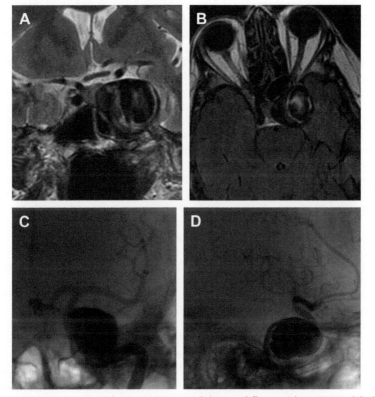

Fig. 16. Intracavernous carotid giant aneurysm. (*A*) Round flow void on T2-WI. (*B*) Flowing blood appears also as high-intensity signal on gradient sequences. (*C*) AP angiogram shows the filling of the aneurysm. (*D*) Lateral view shows the relationship with the parent vessel.

aneurysm and the parent artery. Thrombosed aneurysms need a more careful analysis. Positive diagnosis relies essentially on MRI features. Thrombus inside the sac usually presents as a multilamellated area with mixed signal intensity (T1 hyperintensity and heterogeneous T2 hypointensity) representing the various stage of the clots.

If incompletely thrombosed, flowing blood through the patent portion of the sac appears also as a flow void on T2-WI and high-intensity signal on gradient sequences (**Fig. 16**). CT scan is useful to assess the presence of calcification.

Even if it is extremely rare, it is mandatory to know that a pituitary adenoma may be associated with an intrasellar aneurysm. Preoperative diagnosis of this condition is essential.[111]

Collision Sellar Lesions

Collision sellar lesions are defined by the concomitant presence of a pituitary adenoma with a second sellar lesion.[112] Although rare, the possibility of coexisting lesions has to be kept in mind particularly by pituitary surgeons.

REFERENCES

1. Freda PU, Post KD. Differential diagnosis of sellar masses. Endocrinol Metab Clin North Am 1999;28(1):81–117, vi.
2. Kelberman D, Dattani MT. Hypothalamic and pituitary development: novel insights into the aetiology. Eur J Endocrinol 2007;157(Suppl 1):S3–14.
3. Kerr RG, Tobler WD, Leach JL, et al. Anatomic variation of the optic strut: classification schema, radiologic evaluation, and surgical relevance. J Neurol Surg B Skull Base 2012;73(6):424–9.
4. Guthikonda B, Tobler WD Jr, Froelich SC, et al. Anatomic study of the prechiasmatic sulcus and its surgical implications. Clin Anat 2010;23(6):622–8.
5. Rhoton AL Jr. The sellar region. Neurosurgery 2002;51(4 Suppl):S335–74.
6. Kehrli P, Ali M, Reis M Jr, et al. Anatomy and embryology of the lateral sellar compartment (cavernous sinus) medial wall. Neurol Res 1998;20(7):585–92.
7. Dietemann JL, Kehrli P, Maillot C, et al. Is there a dural wall between the cavernous sinus and the pituitary fossa? Anatomical and MRI findings. Neuroradiology 1998;40(10):627–30.
8. Yasuda A, Campero A, Martins C, et al. The medial wall of the cavernous sinus: microsurgical anatomy. Neurosurgery 2004;55(1):179–89 [discussion: 189–90].
9. Cebula H, Kurbanov A, Zimmer LA, et al. Endoscopic, endonasal variability in the anatomy of the internal carotid artery. World Neurosurg 2014;82(6):e759–64.
10. Orija IB, Weil RJ, Hamrahian AH. Pituitary incidentaloma. Best Pract Res Clin Endocrinol Metab 2012;26(1):47–68.
11. Ezzat S, Asa SL, Couldwell WT, et al. The prevalence of pituitary adenomas: a systematic review. Cancer 2004;101(3):613–9.
12. Vernooij MW, Ikram MA, Tanghe HL, et al. Incidental findings on brain MRI in the general population. N Engl J Med 2007;357(18):1821–8.
13. Arita K, Tominaga A, Sugiyama K, et al. Natural course of incidentally found nonfunctioning pituitary adenoma, with special reference to pituitary apoplexy during follow-up examination. J Neurosurg 2006;104(6):884–91.
14. Yamada S, Ohyama K, Taguchi M, et al. A study of the correlation between morphological findings and biological activities in clinically nonfunctioning pituitary adenomas. Neurosurgery 2007;61(3):580–4 [discussion: 584–5].
15. Chamoun R, Layfield L, Couldwell WT. Gonadotroph adenoma with secondary hypersecretion of testosterone. World Neurosurg 2013;80(6):900.e7–11.

16. Vidal S, Horvath E, Kovacs K, et al. Reversible transdifferentiation: interconversion of somatotrophs and lactotrophs in pituitary hyperplasia. Mod Pathol 2001; 14(1):20–8.
17. Meij BP, Lopes MB, Vance ML, et al. Double pituitary lesions in three patients with Cushing's disease. Pituitary 2000;3(3):159–68.
18. Raverot G, Assié G, Cotton F, et al. Biological and radiological exploration and management of non-functioning pituitary adenoma. Ann Endocrinol (Paris) 2015;76(3):201–9.
19. Abe T, Matsumoto K, Kuwazawa J, et al. Headache associated with pituitary adenomas. Headache 1998;38(10):782–6.
20. Levy MJ, Matharu MS, Meeran K, et al. The clinical characteristics of headache in patients with pituitary tumours. Brain 2005;128(Pt 8):1921–30.
21. Gondim JA, de Almeida JP, de Albuquerque LA, et al. Headache associated with pituitary tumors. J Headache Pain 2009;10(1):15–20.
22. Grochowicki M, Vighetto A, Berquet S, et al. Pituitary adenomas: automatic static perimetry and Goldmann perimetry. A comparative study of 345 visual field charts. Br J Ophthalmol 1991;75(4):219–21.
23. Chiu EK, Nichols JW. Sellar lesions and visual loss: key concepts in neuro-ophthalmology. Expert Rev Anticancer Ther 2006;6(Suppl 9):S23–8.
24. Feiz-Erfan I, Rao G, White WL, et al. Efficacy of trans-septal trans-sphenoidal surgery in correcting visual symptoms caused by hematogenous metastases to the sella and pituitary gland. Skull Base 2008;18(2):77–84.
25. Pinker K, Ba-Ssalamah A, Wolfsberger S, et al. The value of high-field MRI (3T) in the assessment of sellar lesions. Eur J Radiol 2005;54(3):327–34.
26. De Sousa SM, Earls P, McCormack AI. Pituitary hyperplasia: case series and literature review of an under-recognised and heterogeneous condition. Endocrinol Diabetes Metab Case Rep 2015;2015:150017.
27. Wong A, Eloy JA, Couldwell WT, et al. Update on prolactinomas. Part 1: Clinical manifestations and diagnostic challenges. J Clin Neurosci 2015;22(10):1562–7.
28. Wong A, Eloy JA, Couldwell WT, et al. Update on prolactinomas. Part 2: Treatment and management strategies. J Clin Neurosci 2015;22(10):1568–74.
29. Vroonen L, Jaffrain-Rea ML, Petrossians P, et al. Prolactinomas resistant to standard doses of cabergoline: a multicenter study of 92 patients. Eur J Endocrinol 2012;167(5):651–62.
30. Menucci M, Quiñones-Hinojosa A, Burger P, et al. Effect of dopaminergic drug treatment on surgical findings in prolactinomas. Pituitary 2011;14(1):68–74.
31. Chanson P, Timsit J, Harris AG. Heart failure and octreotide in acromegaly. Lancet 1992;339(8787):242–3.
32. Katznelson L, Laws ER Jr, Melmed S, et al. Acromegaly: an endocrine society clinical practice guideline. J Clin Endocrinol Metab 2014;99(11):3933–51.
33. Giustina A, Chanson P, Kleinberg D, et al. Expert consensus document: a consensus on the medical treatment of acromegaly. Nat Rev Endocrinol 2014; 10(4):243–8.
34. Bertagna X, Guignat L, Groussin L, et al. Cushing's disease. Best Pract Res Clin Endocrinol Metab 2009;23(5):607–23.
35. Flitsch J, Schmid SM, Bernreuther C, et al. A pitfall in diagnosing Cushing's disease: ectopic ACTH-producing pituitary adenoma in the sphenoid sinus. Pituitary 2015;18(2):279–82.
36. Seltzer J, Lucas J, Commins D, et al. Ectopic ACTH-secreting pituitary adenoma of the sphenoid sinus: case report of endoscopic endonasal resection and systematic review of the literature. Neurosurg Focus 2015;38(2):E10.

37. Lad SP, Patil CG, Laws ER Jr, et al. The role of inferior petrosal sinus sampling in the diagnostic localization of Cushing's disease. Neurosurg Focus 2007;23(3):E2.

38. Chittiboina P, Montgomery BK, Millo C, et al. High-resolution(18)F-fluorodeoxy-glucose positron emission tomography and magnetic resonance imaging for pituitary adenoma detection in Cushing disease. J Neurosurg 2015;122(4): 791–7.

39. Wang EL, Qian ZR, Yamada S, et al. Clinicopathological characterization of TSH-producing adenomas: special reference to TSH-immunoreactive but clinically non-functioning adenomas. Endocr Pathol 2009;20(4):209–20.

40. Chanson P, Raverot G, Castinetti F, et al. Management of clinically non-functioning pituitary adenoma. Ann Endocrinol (Paris) 2015;76(3):239–47.

41. Castinetti F, Dufour H, Gaillard S, et al. Non-functioning pituitary adenoma: When and how to operate? What pathologic criteria for typing? Ann Endocrinol (Paris) 2015;76(3):220–7.

42. Jaffrain-Rea ML, Di Stefano D, Minniti G, et al. A critical reappraisal of MIB-1 labelling index significance in a large series of pituitary tumours: secreting versus non-secreting adenomas. Endocr Relat Cancer 2002;9(2):103–13.

43. Righi A, Agati P, Sisto A, et al. A classification tree approach for pituitary adenomas. Hum Pathol 2012;43(10):1627–37.

44. Verrees M, Arafah BM, Selman WR. Pituitary tumor apoplexy: characteristics, treatment, and outcomes. Neurosurg Focus 2004;16(4):E6.

45. Nielsen EH, Lindholm J, Bjerre P, et al. Frequent occurrence of pituitary apoplexy in patients with non-functioning pituitary adenoma. Clin Endocrinol (Oxf) 2006;64(3):319–22.

46. Suzuki H, Muramatsu M, Murao K, et al. Pituitary apoplexy caused by ruptured internal carotid artery aneurysm. Stroke 2001;32(2):567–9.

47. DeLellis RA. Pathology and genetics of tumours of endocrine organs. IARC Press; 2004.

48. Prevedello DM, Jagannathan J, Jane JA Jr, et al. Relevance of high Ki-67 in pituitary adenomas. Case report and review of the literature. Neurosurg Focus 2005;19(5):E11.

49. Mete O, Ezzat S, Asa SL. Biomarkers of aggressive pituitary adenomas. J Mol Endocrinol 2012;49(2):R69–78.

50. Salehi F, Agur A, Scheithauer BW, et al. Ki-67 in pituitary neoplasms: a review—part I. Neurosurgery 2009;65(3):429–37 [discussion: 437].

51. Pizarro CB, Oliveira MC, Coutinho LB, et al. Measurement of Ki-67 antigen in 159 pituitary adenomas using the MIB-1 monoclonal antibody. Braz J Med Biol Res 2004;37(2):235–43.

52. Ragel BT, Couldwell WT. Pituitary carcinoma: a review of the literature. Neurosurg Focus 2004;16(4):E7.

53. Heaney AP. Clinical review: Pituitary carcinoma: difficult diagnosis and treatment. J Clin Endocrinol Metab 2011;96(12):3649–60.

54. Raverot G, Sturm N, de Fraipont F, et al. Temozolomide treatment in aggressive pituitary tumors and pituitary carcinomas: a French multicenter experience. J Clin Endocrinol Metab 2010;95(10):4592–9.

55. Huang BY, Castillo M. Nonadenomatous tumors of the pituitary and sella turcica. Top Magn Reson Imaging 2005;16(4):289–99.

56. Brat DJ, Scheithauer BW, Staugaitis SM, et al. Pituicytoma: a distinctive low-grade glioma of the neurohypophysis. Am J Surg Pathol 2000;24(3):362–8.

57. Furtado SV, Ghosal N, Venkatesh PK, et al. Diagnostic and clinical implications of pituicytoma. J Clin Neurosci 2010;17(7):938–43.

58. Phillips JJ, Misra A, Feuerstein BG, et al. Pituicytoma: characterization of a unique neoplasm by histology, immunohistochemistry, ultrastructure, and array-based comparative genomic hybridization. Arch Pathol Lab Med 2010;134(7):1063–9.
59. Sofela AA, Hettige S, Curran O, et al. Malignant transformation in craniopharyngiomas. Neurosurgery 2014;75(3):306–14 [discussion: 314].
60. Pascual JM, Prieto R, Castro-Dufourny I, et al. Classification systems of adult craniopharyngiomas: the need for an accurate definition of the hypothalamus-tumor relationships. Arch Med Res 2012;43(7):588–90 [author reply: 591].
61. Muller HL. Craniopharyngioma. Endocr Rev 2014;35(3):513–43.
62. Iughetti L, Bruzzi P. Obesity and craniopharyngioma. Ital J Pediatr 2011;37:38.
63. Zhu J, You C. Craniopharyngioma: survivin expression and ultrastructure. Oncol Lett 2015;9(1):75–80.
64. Karavitaki N. Management of craniopharyngiomas. J Endocrinol Invest 2014; 37(3):219–28.
65. Sughrue ME, Yang I, Kane AJ, et al. Endocrinologic, neurologic, and visual morbidity after treatment for craniopharyngioma. J Neurooncol 2011;101(3): 463–76.
66. Garnett MR, Puget S, Grill J, et al. Craniopharyngioma. Orphanet J Rare Dis 2007;2:18.
67. Zada G, Kintz N, Pulido M, et al. Prevalence of neurobehavioral, social, and emotional dysfunction in patients treated for childhood craniopharyngioma: a systematic literature review. PLoS One 2013;8(11):e76562.
68. Komotar RJ, Roguski M, Bruce JN. Surgical management of craniopharyngiomas. J Neurooncol 2009;92(3):283–96.
69. Cavallo LM, Solari D, Esposito F, et al. The role of the endoscopic endonasal route in the management of craniopharyngiomas. World Neurosurg 2014;82(6 Suppl):S32–40.
70. Eriksson B, Gunterberg B, Kindblom LG. Chordoma. A clinicopathologic and prognostic study of a Swedish national series. Acta Orthop Scand 1981;52(1): 49–58.
71. McMaster ML, Goldstein AM, Bromley CM, et al. Chordoma: incidence and survival patterns in the United States, 1973-1995. Cancer Causes Control 2001; 12(1):1–11.
72. Tzortzidis F, Elahi F, Wright D, et al. Patient outcome at long-term follow-up after aggressive microsurgical resection of cranial base chordomas. Neurosurgery 2006;59(2):230–7 [discussion: 230–7].
73. Yeom KW, Lober RM, Mobley BC, et al. Diffusion-weighted MRI: distinction of skull base chordoma from chondrosarcoma. AJNR Am J Neuroradiol 2013; 34(5):1056–61. S1.
74. Miettinen M, Wang Z, Lasota J, et al. Nuclear Brachyury Expression Is Consistent in Chordoma, Common in Germ Cell Tumors and Small Cell Carcinomas, and Rare in Other Carcinomas and Sarcomas: An Immunohistochemical Study of 5229 Cases. Am J Surg Pathol 2015;39(10):1305–12.
75. Samii M, Tatagiba M. Surgical management of craniopharyngiomas: a review. Neurol Med Chir (Tokyo) 1997;37(2):141–9.
76. Tamaki N, Nagashima T, Ehara K, et al. Surgical approaches and strategies for skull base chordomas. Neurosurg Focus 2001;10(3):E9.
77. George B, Bresson D, Bouazza S, et al. Chordoma. Neurochirurgie 2014;60(3): 63–140 [in French].
78. Chibbaro S, Cornelius JF, Froelich S, et al. Endoscopic endonasal approach in the management of skull base chordomas–clinical experience on a large series,

technique, outcome, and pitfalls. Neurosurg Rev 2014;37(2):217–24 [discussion: 224–5].

79. Koutourousiou M, Gardner PA, Tormenti MJ, et al. Endoscopic endonasal approach for resection of cranial base chordomas: outcomes and learning curve. Neurosurgery 2012;71(3):614–24 [discussion: 624–5].

80. Noel G, Feuvret L, Calugaru V, et al. Chordomas of the base of the skull and upper cervical spine. One hundred patients irradiated by a 3D conformal technique combining photon and proton beams. Acta Oncol 2005;44(7):700–8.

81. Barresi V, Ieni A, Branca G, et al. Brachyury: a diagnostic marker for the differential diagnosis of chordoma and hemangioblastoma versus neoplastic histological mimickers. Dis Markers 2014;2014:514753.

82. McLoughlin GS, Sciubba DM, Wolinsky JP. Chondroma/Chondrosarcoma of the spine. Neurosurg Clin N Am 2008;19(1):57–63.

83. Chi JH, McDermott MW. Tuberculum sellae meningiomas. Neurosurg Focus 2003;14(6):e6.

84. O'Sullivan MG, van Loveren HR, Tew JM Jr. The surgical resectability of meningiomas of the cavernous sinus. Neurosurgery 1997;40(2):238–44 [discussion: 245–7].

85. Larson JJ, van Loveren HR, Balko MG, et al. Evidence of meningioma infiltration into cranial nerves: clinical implications for cavernous sinus meningiomas. J Neurosurg 1995;83(4):596–9.

86. Mills SA, Oh MC, Rutkowski MJ, et al. Supratentorial hemangioblastoma: clinical features, prognosis, and predictive value of location for von Hippel-Lindau disease. Neuro Oncol 2012;14(8):1097–104.

87. Amelot A, Bouazza S, Polivka M, et al. Sporadically second localization of cerebellar hemangioblastoma in sella turcica mimicking a meningioma with no associated von Hippel-Lindau disease. Br J Neurosurg 2015;29:1–3.

88. Fassett DR, Couldwell WT. Metastases to the pituitary gland. Neurosurg Focus 2004;16(4):E8.

89. Ballesteros MD, Durán A, Arrazola J, et al. Primary intrasellar germinoma with synchronous pineal tumor. Neuroradiology 1997;39(12):860–2.

90. Sanno N, Oyama K, Tahara S, et al. A survey of pituitary incidentaloma in Japan. Eur J Endocrinol 2003;149(2):123–7.

91. Teramoto A, Hirakawa K, Sanno N, et al. Incidental pituitary lesions in 1,000 unselected autopsy specimens. Radiology 1994;193(1):161–4.

92. Oyama N, Tahara S, Oyama K, et al. Assessment of pre- and postoperative endocrine function in 94 patients with Rathke's cleft cyst. Endocr J 2013; 60(2):207–13.

93. Choi SH, Kwon BJ, Na DG, et al. Pituitary adenoma, craniopharyngioma, and Rathke cleft cyst involving both intrasellar and suprasellar regions: differentiation using MRI. Clin Radiol 2007;62(5):453–62.

94. Zada G, Lin N, Ojerholm E, et al. Craniopharyngioma and other cystic epithelial lesions of the sellar region: a review of clinical, imaging, and histopathological relationships. Neurosurg Focus 2010;28(4):E4.

95. Aho CJ, Liu C, Zelman V, et al. Surgical outcomes in 118 patients with Rathke cleft cysts. J Neurosurg 2005;102(2):189–93.

96. Fan J, Peng Y, Qi S, et al. Individualized surgical strategies for Rathke cleft cyst based on cyst location. J Neurosurg 2013;119(6):1437–46.

97. Vellutini EA, de Oliveira MF, Ribeiro AP, et al. Malignant transformation of intracranial epidermoid cyst. Br J Neurosurg 2014;28(4):507–9.

98. Tuna H, Torun F, Torun AN, et al. Intrasellar epidermoid cyst presenting as pituitary apoplexy. J Clin Neurosci 2008;15(10):1154–6.

99. Hornig GW, Zervas NT. Slit defect of the diaphragma sellae with valve effect: observation of a "slit valve". Neurosurgery 1992;30(2):265–7.
100. Oyama K, Fukuhara N, Taguchi M, et al. Transsphenoidal cyst cisternostomy with a keyhole dural opening for sellar arachnoid cysts: technical note. Neurosurg Rev 2014;37(2):261–7 [discussion: 267].
101. McLaughlin N, Vandergrift A, Ditzel Filho LF, et al. Endonasal management of sellar arachnoid cysts: simple cyst obliteration technique. J Neurosurg 2012; 116(4):728–40.
102. Nomura M, Tachibana O, Hasegawa M, et al. Contrast-enhanced MRI of intrasellar arachnoid cysts: relationship between the pituitary gland and cyst. Neuroradiology 1996;38(6):566–8.
103. Giustina A, Aimaretti G, Bondanelli M, et al. Primary empty sella: why and when to investigate hypothalamic-pituitary function. J Endocrinol Invest 2010;33(5): 343–6.
104. Guitelman M, Garcia Basavilbaso N, Vitale M, et al. Primary empty sella (PES): a review of 175 cases. Pituitary 2013;16(2):270–4.
105. De Marinis L, Bonadonna S, Bianchi A, et al. Primary empty sella. J Clin Endocrinol Metab 2005;90(9):5471–7.
106. Ding D, Starke RM, Durst CR, et al. Venous stenting with concurrent intracranial pressure monitoring for the treatment of pseudotumor cerebri. Neurosurg Focus 2014;37(1 Suppl):1.
107. Herman P, Lot G, Guichard JP, et al. Mucocele of the sphenoid sinus: a late complication of transsphenoidal pituitary surgery. Ann Otol Rhinol Laryngol 1998;107(9 Pt 1):765–8.
108. Hanak BW, Zada G, Nayar VV, et al. Cerebral aneurysms with intrasellar extension: a systematic review of clinical, anatomical, and treatment characteristics. J Neurosurg 2012;116(1):164–78.
109. Murai Y, Kobayashi S, Mizunari T, et al. Anterior communicating artery aneurysm in the sella turcica: case report. Surg Neurol 2004;62(1):69–71 [discussion: 71].
110. Hornyak M, Hillard V, Nwagwu C, et al. Ruptured intrasellar superior hypophyseal artery aneurysm presenting with pure subdural haematoma. Case report. Interv Neuroradiol 2004;10(1):55–8.
111. Seda L Jr, Cukiert A, Nogueira KC, et al. Intrasellar internal carotid aneurysm coexisting with GH-secreting pituitary adenoma in an acromegalic patient. Arq Neuropsiquiatr 2008;66(1):99–100.
112. Koutourousiou M, Kontogeorgos G, Wesseling P, et al. Collision sellar lesions: experience with eight cases and review of the literature. Pituitary 2010;13(1): 8–17.

Principles of Pituitary Surgery

Christopher J. Farrell, MD[a],*, Gurston G. Nyquist, MD[b], Alexander A. Farag, MD[b], Marc R. Rosen, MD[b], James J. Evans, MD[a]

KEYWORDS

- Pituitary tumors • Pituitary surgery • Transnasal • Transsphenoidal
- Endoscopy versus microscopy

KEY POINTS

- The principles of pituitary surgery involve extensive surgical planning and decision making.
- Various technical nuances distinguish the endoscopic from the microscopic transsphenoidal approach.
- Strategies can be used during the nasal, sphenoidal, and sellar stages of surgery to maximize tumor resection, minimize complications, and preserve sinonasal anatomy/function.

INTRODUCTION
Evolution of Transsphenoidal Surgery

Since the initial description of a transnasal approach for the treatment of pituitary tumors in 1907, transsphenoidal surgery has undergone continuous evolution marked by close collaboration between neurosurgeons and otolaryngologists. Oskar Hirsch developed a lateral endonasal approach in 1910 that he initially performed as a 5-step procedure over a period of several weeks before simplifying the procedure to a single-step submucosal transseptal approach.[1] Contemporaneously, Harvey Cushing began approaching pituitary tumors using a transsphenoidal approach but transitioned to the transcranial route because of his concern that an endonasal approach provided restricted access and poor illumination, compromising adequate decompression of the optic apparatus.[2] Most neurosurgeons followed Cushing's lead and transsphenoidal surgery was not "rediscovered" until Jules Hardy introduced the surgical microscope in the 1960s.[3]

[a] Department of Neurological Surgery, Thomas Jefferson University, 909 Walnut Street, 2nd Floor, Philadelphia, PA 19107, USA; [b] Department of Otolaryngology, Thomas Jefferson University, Philadelphia, PA, USA
* Corresponding author.
E-mail address: christopher.farrell@jefferson.edu

Otolaryngol Clin N Am 49 (2016) 95–106
http://dx.doi.org/10.1016/j.otc.2015.09.005
0030-6665/16/$ – see front matter © 2016 Elsevier Inc. All rights reserved.

The first completely endoscopic transsphenoidal approach for pituitary tumors was reported in 1992 by Jankowski, and further advanced by the collaborative teams of Jho and Carrau in Pittsburgh and Sethi and Pillay in Singapore.[4,5] Over the last 20 years, the endoscopic technique has been adopted by a multitude of surgeons who have favored the dynamic panoramic view afforded by the endoscope, allowing for improved visualization and better resection of tumors extending into the suprasellar area and cavernous sinuses. In addition, the advent of extended endoscopic endonasal approaches, such as the transplanum and lateral transcavernous approaches, has facilitated resection of large, invasive pituitary tumors that were previously deemed unresectable or requiring transcranial surgery.

Critics of the endoscopic approach have rightfully focused on the loss of stereoscopic vision as a major limitation, with mastery of the procedure demanding a steep learning curve. Prospective studies directly comparing the microscopic and endoscopic approaches for pituitary tumors have not been performed; however, an increasing body of literature has established the safety and noninferiority of endoscopic endonasal techniques, and several studies have demonstrated improvement in the extent of tumor resection. McLaughlin and colleagues[6] reported that, after microsurgical resection of pituitary adenomas, endoscopy revealed residual tumor leading to further resection in 36% of cases. Messerer and colleagues[7] found their gross total resection rate increased from 50% using the microscope to 76% on initial conversion to the endoscopic approach. In this review, we describe the principles of pituitary surgery, including the key elements of surgical decision making, and discuss the technical nuances distinguishing the endoscopic from the microscopic approach.

PRINCIPLES OF SURGERY
Indications for Surgery

Pituitary adenomas are most frequently categorized as functional or nonfunctional depending on their hormonal secretory pattern. Prolactinomas represent the most common functional adenoma, and the mainstay of treatment is dopamine-agonist medical therapy, with surgical treatment reserved for patients who fail to respond despite dose escalation or are intolerant to the medications. Transsphenoidal surgery remains the primary treatment for adenomas secreting adrenocorticotropic hormone (ACTH, Cushing disease) and growth hormone (acromegaly) with biochemical remission rates significantly correlated with tumor size and invasiveness.[7]

Nonfunctional pituitary adenomas (NFPA) are extremely common. Autopsy and radiographic studies reveal the presence of NFPA in 11% to 27% of the population.[8,9] Although most NFPAs are microadenomas (<1 cm) and clinically asymptomatic, macroadenomas may present with compressive symptoms including headache, visual impairment, hormonal insufficiency, and cranial nerve palsies caused by cavernous sinus extension. Surgery is generally indicated for patients with macroadenomas causing visual compromise or exhibiting growth on serial imaging studies. Approximately 5% of patients with pituitary adenomas present with apoplexy caused by intratumoral hemorrhage or infarction.[10]

Preoperative Surgical Planning

The main goal in endoscopic pituitary surgery is to maximize tumor resection while avoiding complications such as visual deterioration, cerebrospinal fluid (CSF) leakage, endocrinopathy, vascular injury, and sinonasal morbidity. Although pituitary adenomas are typically benign lesions, recurrences are common after incomplete surgical removal, and thorough preoperative surgical planning is essential to achieve optimal outcomes.

MRI studies reliably delineate the size and extension of pituitary tumors, with the notable exception of some ACTH-secreting microadenomas that may be radiographically occult. Inspection of the preoperative MRI provides an assessment of the likelihood of gross total resection primarily based on cavernous sinus extension as well as a prediction of the surgical challenges that will be encountered, such as intraoperative CSF leakage and a narrow surgical corridor because of reduced distance between the parasellar carotid arteries. Large tumors that extend vertically within the suprasellar area may significantly compromise the diaphragma sellae, or even invade the ventricular system resulting in high-flow CSF leaks requiring more extensive repairs such as nasoseptal flap (NSF) placement, lumbar drainage, or use of autologous tissues (eg, fascia lata or adipose tissue). As discussed in more detail later, preoperative anticipation of the need for an NSF is critical because the flap must be either harvested during the initial nasal stage of the approach or the vascular pedicle to the flap preserved such that a viable flap can be harvested later should it prove necessary. In addition, detection of the position of the normal compressed pituitary gland on the preoperative MRI assists with the preservation of hormonal function as intraoperative distinction of the gland from the tumor based on color and consistency differences is frequently subtle.

Computed tomography (CT) studies provide complementary information helpful in surgical planning. Coronal and sagittal reconstructions reveal bony changes, such as erosion of the sellar floor and dorsum, and can be used intraoperatively for image guidance, especially in patients with altered sinonasal anatomy related to previous surgery. Similarly, we have found preoperative nasal endoscopy helpful to optimize our surgical plan and avoid complications related to paranasal sinus disease or anatomic variability. Typically, chronic rhinosinusitis does not represent an absolute contraindication to transsphenoidal surgery; however, patients with acute rhinosinusitis, especially those with fungal disease, should be treated appropriately before elective surgery[11] Preoperative otolaryngologic evaluation is critical in patients with acromegaly who frequently present challenges for airway management during surgery because of soft tissue hypertrophy and bony abnormalities[12]

Surgical Approach: Nasal Stage

The endoscopic surgical approach for pituitary tumors can be divided into the nasal, sphenoidal, and sellar stages. Since the inception of our endoscopic skull base program at Thomas Jefferson University in 2005, we have advocated for a team approach between otolaryngology and neurosurgery. The complementary skill of experienced sinus and pituitary surgeons has enabled us to optimize oncologic outcomes and minimize complications, both minor and major. Our approach to pituitary surgery has evolved and we have adopted a tailored approach to these tumors based on their size, invasiveness, and secretory pattern, allowing us to minimize sinonasal disruption without compromising tumor resection.

Patients are positioned supine with the head on a gel headrest. Neuronavigation is used routinely to help guide the surgical approach and assess the adequacy of tumor resection with co-registration of the preoperative CT and MRI using facemask fiducials. Although neuronavigation is valuable, over-reliance on this adjunct and a failure to correlate with anatomic landmarks can lead the surgeon off course. The head is slightly elevated to reduce mucosal congestion and bleeding during the approach. We do not routinely prepare the skin of the face or nasal cavity with antiseptic solution, but graft sites such as the lateral thigh for fascia lata or adipose tissue should be prepared in a sterile standard fashion.

The turbinates are gently lateralized with a blunt instrument. Although routine resection of the middle turbinates is favored by some surgeons to increase the nasal working corridor, we have found that turbinate lateralization combined with a limited posterior septectomy provides more than sufficient access to the sella for pituitary tumor resection and minimizes postoperative patient sinonasal morbidity.[13,14] A binarial approach is typically performed allowing 2 surgeons to work simultaneously with up to 4 instruments in the field, including the endoscope. In our experience, a pedicled NSF is rarely necessary for cranial base repair during standard transsellar pituitary adenoma resection; however, in certain cases the need for an NSF is unanticipated or may become necessary during future surgeries.[15] As such, we advocate at least unilateral preservation of the NSF whenever possible and have described a variety of tailored approaches to the sphenoid sinus that enable NSF preservation applicable to endoscopic pituitary surgery. Our standard approach, termed the "1.5 approach," involves an ipsilateral wide sphenoidotomy ("1") on the working instrument side with a limited contralateral sphenoidotomy ("0.5") on the endoscope side (**Fig. 1**A). The limited sphenoidotomy is performed by extending the natural sphenoid os superiorly with Kerrison rongeurs, thus preserving the more inferiorly located sphenopalatine artery supply to the nasal septal mucoperiosteum and mucoperichondrium. Addition of a limited posterior septectomy (typically 1 cm) allows communication of the binarial sphenoid exposures and provides ample working room and maneuverability (unpublished data). In patients with nasal obstruction caused by septal deviation or large spurs, a "tunnel approach" is performed involving a septoplasty and submucosal "tunnel" with a wide contralateral sphenoidotomy (**Fig. 1**B). The approach begins with a standard hemi-transfixion incision used for septoplasty, and the septal mucoperichondrium is raised and extended posteriorly over the vomer and laterally along the sphenoid rostrum. A septoplasty or spur removal is then performed, with the resultant unilateral "tunnel" analogous to the standard microscopic transseptal approach with preservation of the NSF ipsilaterally. On the contralateral side, a wide sphenoidotomy is performed. If NSF harvest proves necessary, the superior and inferior incisions for the flap can be performed and elevation completed on the "tunnel" side. The NSF harvest and replacement ("raise and return") approach involves a standard harvest of the NSF combined with a wide contralateral sphenoidotomy. We typically reserve this

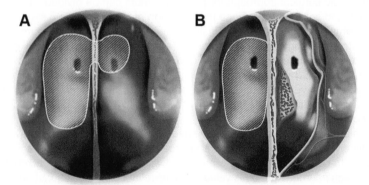

Fig. 1. Nasal stage. (*A*) "1.5" approach to the sphenoid sinus with wide ipsilateral sphenoidotomy and limited contralateral sphenoidotomy with preservation of inferiorly located sphenopalatine arterial supply to the nasoseptal flap. (*B*) "Tunnel" approach for patients with septal spurs with ipsilateral wide sphenoidotomy and submucosal elevation of septal mucoperichondrium.

approach for cases in which there is a high likelihood of NSF use, such as tumors with very significant vertical suprasellar extension or that extend anteriorly over the planum where, depending on tumor consistency, an extended endonasal approach may become necessary for complete tumor resection. This approach is also used for cases with potential for a high-flow CSF leak. If cranial base repair with the NSF proves unnecessary, the flap can be returned to its native position along the septum. These "raised and returned" flaps tend to heal quite well with minimal crusting and postoperative discomfort. We do not advocate routine harvest of the NSF, however, as this technique is associated with increased sinonasal morbidity including the possibility of olfactory dysfunction, septal perforation, and sensory loss because of superior alveolar nerve injury. A variety of investigators have described "rescue flap" modifications where the NSF is partially raised during the nasal stage such that the vascular pedicle is preserved, although these modifications have been associated in some cases with increased risk of olfactory loss.[16,17]

Surgical Approach: Sphenoid Stage

The anatomy of the sphenoid sinus is highly variable in regard to its bony septa and pneumatization. The configuration of sphenoid sinus pneumatization can significantly affect access to the sella. The pneumatization of the sphenoid sinus is usually completed by 10 years of age and most adults possess the well-pneumatized sellar pattern.[18] The sellar floor lies along the posterior wall of the sphenoid sinus within the midline and the importance of maintaining a midline orientation cannot be overstated. In addition to the sellar prominence, anatomic landmarks along the posterior sphenoid wall include the medial and lateral opticocarotid recesses, parasellar carotid prominences, and clival recess. Frequently, the entirety of these landmarks may not be plainly apparent and careful attention to the preoperative imaging combined with judicious use of neuronavigation will prevent inadvertent complications. The intrasphenoidal septa should be taken down with use of the high-speed drill or Thru-cutting instruments, avoiding any fracturing or rotational maneuvers as these septa often have posterior attachments along the carotid prominences. In addition, anticipating the presence of Onodi air cells will prevent injury to the optic nerves. Endoscopic transsphenoidal pituitary approaches can be safely performed in children and adults with the conchal and presellar variant patterns, but prolonged drilling will be required along with an increased reliance on neuronavigation.

The sella is typically expanded in the presence of macroadenomas and the bony floor may be thinned or absent. Conversely, microadenomas do not cause expansion or thinning of the sellar floor, often requiring bone removal with a diamond burr to access the dura. The sphenoid mucosa should be stripped from the sellar floor bluntly or with gentle bipolar cautery before drilling the sella. Monopolar cautery may lead to optic nerve or carotid injury and its use is highly contraindicated along the posterior sphenoid wall. If an NSF is placed for repair, further mucosal stripping should be performed to prevent delayed mucocele development by trapping mucosa under the flap. Bony removal of the sellar floor is usually performed with rotatable Kerrison rongeurs after a pilot bony opening has been created with the drill or Cottle elevator. As opposed to the microscopic approach, where all but the central portion of the intrasellar tumor is removed based on "feel," bony removal for the endoscopic approach needs to be more extensive to maximize the visualization benefits of the endoscope and allow for tumor dissection. In the endoscopic approach, the anterior wall of the sella should be removed to the medial edges of the cavernous sinuses bilaterally and extended superiorly to the intracavernous sinus in the region of the tuberculum sella (**Fig. 2A**). The amount of bony removal of the sellar floor is variable. More extensive removal should

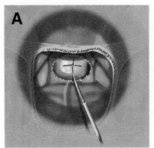
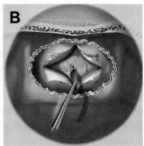
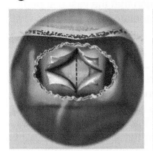
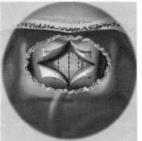
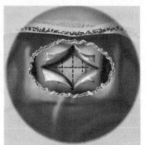

Fig. 2. Microadenoma removal. (*A*) Bony removal of sellar floor to medial extent of cavernous sinuses bilateral and cruciate dural opening performed with retractable blade. (*B*) En bloc resection of pituitary microadenoma with extracapsular dissection. (*C*) Pituitary gland exploration for occult microadenoma with staged vertical and horizontal gland incisions.

be performed for tumors with significant suprasellar extension as this additional bony removal allows for introduction of more vertically angled instruments helpful in removing tumor that fails to descend into the sella after debulking. For tumors that clearly invade the cavernous sinuses, further lateral bony removal across the anterior face of the parasellar carotid arteries can be performed.

Surgical Approach: Sellar Stage

The exposed dura of the sella is then opened in a cruciate fashion with a retractable knife and angled scissors. Horizontal cuts should be made in a lateral-to-medial direction to avoid carotid injury, while the vertical incision should be made in a superior-to-inferior direction to avoid inadvertent entry into the anterior arachnoid cistern with resultant CSF leakage (see **Fig. 2**A). The principles of tumor removal differ for micro- and macro-adenomas. Historically, pituitary adenomas have been resected in a piecemeal fashion using a variety of blunt ring curette-type instruments. Oldfield and colleagues,[19] however, demonstrated the advantages of dissection of the histologic pseudocapsule surrounding pituitary adenomas, allowing microadenomas to be ideally resected in an en bloc extracapsular fashion (**Fig. 2**B). When feasible, en bloc resection reduces the likelihood of tumor remnants and increases biochemical remission for functional adenomas.[20] Rarely, in patients with Cushing disease, a pituitary microadenoma may not be visible on MRI, but the diagnosis confirmed by ACTH-dependent increase of cortisol levels and high-dose dexamethasone suppression. In these cases, ACTH levels are measured from the inferior petrosal sinuses using invasive catheters to determine the likely side of the adenoma within the sella. The pituitary gland is then explored systematically using a series of horizontal and vertical incisions to identify the adenoma beginning on the presumptive side (**Fig. 2**C).

En bloc resection of macroadenomas is rarely possible and we advocate a strategy of systematic internal debulking, followed by extracapsular dissection along the cavernous sinus walls and diaphragm. As shown in **Fig. 3**, the inferior aspect of the tumor is first debulked with ring curettes in the midline before extending posteriorly to the dorsum sella and laterally toward the medial cavernous sinus walls. Pituitary adenomas are frequently soft tumors and overzealous interior debulking can lead to premature diaphragma sellae herniation, with subsequent trapping of the tumor within the folds of the collapsed arachnoid. Manipulation of the diaphragm in order to complete tumor removal from these folds often leads to compromise and intraoperative CSF leakage. To avoid this, the lateral superior recesses should be debulked before continued midline debulking. Once the tumor has been adequately debulked, the interface between the dura and the tumor pseudocapsule is defined with angled curettes and developed in an extracapsular fashion toward the medial cavernous sinus wall. For tumors without true cavernous sinus invasion, this pseudocapsule can be dissected circumferentially and then brought down away from the diaphragm. The transition zone between the normal gland and the tumor must be anticipated and carefully developed to avoid injury to the gland and resultant pituitary insufficiency.

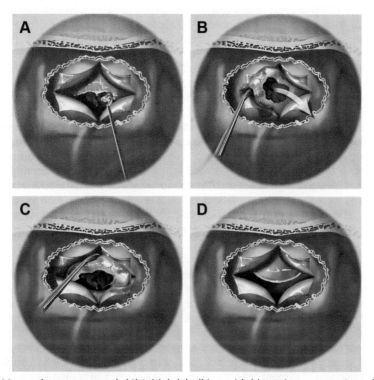

Fig. 3. Macroadenoma removal. (*A*) Initial debulking with blunt ring curettes is performed within the midline inferior extent of the pituitary macroadenoma. (*B*) After interior debulking, extracapsular dissection of the lateral aspect of tumor is performed with separation of the tumor pseudocapsule from the medial wall of the cavernous sinus. (*C*) Superior extracapsular dissection of the tumor away from the diaphragma sellae. (*D*) Symmetric descent of the diaphragm after complete macroadenoma removal.

Infrequently, pituitary macroadenomas may be extremely fibrous and resection of these tumors can be considerably more dangerous because of the need for sharp debulking, placing the carotid arteries and optic apparatus at increased risk for injury. We have found use of ultrasonic aspirators and side-cutting rotatable microdebriders (NICO Myriad System; NICO Corp., Indianapolis, IN) extremely helpful in performing tumor debulking, with location of the carotid arteries repetitively confirmed with neuronavigation and the micro-Doppler. In rare cases where adequate decompression cannot be safely performed through a standard transsphenoidal transsellar opening, we convert to an extended endoscopic approach (EEA) with drilling of the tuberculum sella and planum. The additional bony removal and more anterior dural opening enables tumor to be dissected from the optic nerves and chiasm under direct visualization but requires more extensive skull base repair.

The most frequent areas of residual tumor after transsphenoidal resection of pituitary macroadenomas are the cavernous sinuses and suprasellar area.[21,22] Once tumor resection is believed to be completed, the sellar cavity is directly inspected with 30° to 70° endoscopes, with careful attention to these areas for detection of tumor remnants adherent to the normal pituitary gland. Symmetric descent of the diaphragm into the sella usually indicates optic chiasm decompression and failure of the diaphragm to descend, or asymmetric descent, should prompt further search for residual tumor. After final confirmation of complete tumor resection, meticulous hemostasis is achieved with the use of hemostatic matrix agents and gentle packing with cottonoids. In our experience, the most common reason for postoperative hemorrhage has been incomplete tumor resection, and absolute hemostasis is necessary when residual tumor is expected.

Once tumor removal has been completed, we advocate a graded approach to dural reconstruction. In the absence of any intraoperative CSF leakage as confirmed by Valsalva maneuver, the dura is simply covered with a layer of absorbable hemostatic cellulose to promote epithelialization. Small dural defects resulting in low-flow CSF leakage are repaired with a synthetic dural substitute inlay graft placed under the leaflets of the dural opening and supplemented with a thin layer of dural sealant (**Fig. 4**). For larger diaphragmatic defect, the arachnoid is directly repaired with a dural substitute covering the site of leakage, followed by placement of an inlay dural graft and sealant. For EEA and high-flow leaks related to entry into the ventricular system, an NSF is used to buttress the synthetic dural graft repair or a fascia lata "button" graft repair is performed as previously described.[23] Lumbar drain placement and nasal packing are rarely necessary for CSF leak avoidance.

Cavernous Sinus Invasion

The cavernous sinuses are paired thin-walled venous channels located lateral to the sella. The internal carotid artery (ICA) and its branches course within the center of the channel with the oculomotor, trochlear, abducens, and trigeminal cranial nerves located more laterally. Pituitary adenomas commonly invade the medial wall of the cavernous sinus within the carotid siphon, with the extent of invasion predicting the likelihood of gross total tumor resection. Although the endoscopic approach provides improved visualization of tumor within the cavernous sinus, complete resection remains challenging.[24] In most patients, the presence of residual benign adenoma within the cavernous sinuses can be managed expectantly or with radiation therapy (eg, stereotactic radiosurgery or stereotactic radiotherapy) with control rates for nonfunctional tumors typically around 90%.[25] Tumor control rates after radiosurgery are significantly reduced, however, for larger volume tumors demonstrating the importance of maximal surgical debulking before radiation treatment. Biochemical

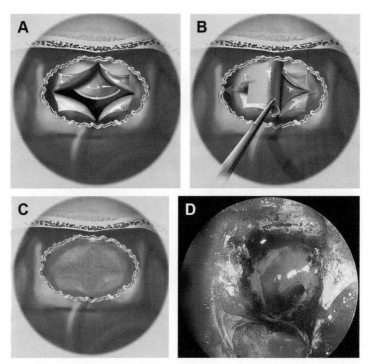

Fig. 4. Dural reconstruction. (*A*) Intrasellar cavity after tumor resection with incompetent diaphragma sellae and low-flow CSF leakage. (*B*) Placement of "inlay" synthetic dural substitute beneath leaves of dura. (*C*) Supplementation of dural graft with tissue sealant. (*D*) Intraoperative view after dural reconstruction with watertight closure.

remission rates for functional adenomas are significantly lower than tumor control rates, with remission achieved in only approximately half of patients with Cushing disease and acromegaly.[23] More aggressive resection of functional tumors invading the cavernous sinus is often appropriate with the goal of either achieving complete resection or reduction of the residual tumor volume for subsequent radiosurgery.

Surgical approaches to the cavernous sinus include the medial and lateral approaches. The medial approach (**Fig. 5**A) is a continuation of the standard transsphenoidal approach but involves following the adenoma through the cavernous sinus medial wall breach. To increase access to the cavernous sinus, the sellar bony opening is extended laterally across the anterior face of the carotid artery. Intrasellar tumor resection is completed before entry into the cavernous sinus. The cavernous sinus should be approached through the contralateral nare using angled ring curettes and suctions to optimize the angle of attack with visualization performed using a 30° to 70° endoscope. Further opening of the medial cavernous wall may be required to allow for instrument entry and is done using sharp dissection after the exact position of the carotid artery has been confirmed with Doppler ultrasonography. Vigorous venous bleeding is expected after removal of tumor from the cavernous sinus and is usually easily controlled with hemostatic matrix agents.

A lateral cavernous sinus approach may be considered in patients harboring functional adenomas or who have failed prior radiation with the bulk of their cavernous sinus tumor volume lateral to the carotid artery, although the risk of cranial nerve and ICA injury are significantly increased with this approach (**Fig. 5**B). Fortunately, most

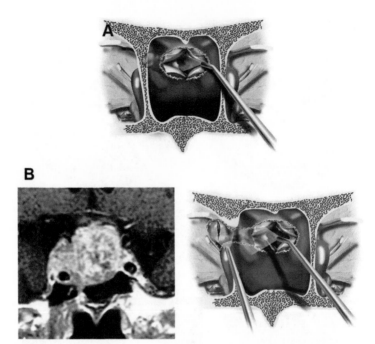

Fig. 5. Cavernous sinus approaches. (*A*) Medial cavernous sinus approach with widened bony opening over carotid prominence and tumor debulking through the medial cavernous sinus wall with angled endoscopes and curettes. (*B*) Lateral cavernous sinus approach with removal of pterygoid process after ipsilateral ethmoidectomies. After maximal debulking of the tumor within the sella and medial aspect of the cavernous sinus, the carotid artery is localized with the micro-Doppler and the lateral cavernous sinus wall opened sharply for further macroadenoma removal.

cranial nerve palsies are transient, resolving within several weeks or months, and use of electrophysiologic monitoring of the oculomotor, trochlear, and abducens nerves may further reduce the likelihood of permanent injury. To access the region lateral to the carotid artery, a wide lateral sphenoid sinus exposure is necessary, often with a transpterygoid extension. During the nasal stage, a complete unilateral anterior and posterior ethmoidectomy is performed after removal of the middle turbinate. The vidian canal is identified in the lateral floor of the sphenoid sinus and the superomedial aspect of the pterygoid process is removed to expose the lateral aspect of the cavernous sinus. Careful evaluation of the preoperative CT images helps determine the access to the lateral cavernous sinus and in some patients with large, well-pneumatized sphenoid sinuses, access may be achieved through the lateral sphenoid sinus recess without extensive pterygoid drilling. After carotid artery localization with the micro-Doppler, the dura is opened sharply and the tumor resected. A multilayered closure with NSF coverage is then performed.

The most feared and potentially devastating morbidity with the cavernous sinus approaches is ICA rupture, with the likelihood of injury increased with fibrous tumors and previous irradiation. Management of carotid artery injury is discussed more extensively in other articles in this issue, but typically requires intraoperative control using direct compression followed by vessel sacrifice in the interventional angiography suite.[26–31]

SUMMARY

Endoscopy represents the most recent evolution of transsphenoidal surgery. Although the endoscopic approach has not been proved to be superior to the classic microscopic approach for resection of pituitary adenomas, the benefits of endoscopy become most apparent during removal of large, invasive tumors where the panoramic visualization afforded by the endoscope allows for more complete resections to be performed. As neurosurgeons continue to take on the challenge of endoscopy and surmount their learning curve, endoscopic transsphenoidal surgery for pituitary adenomas will certainly become the standard.

REFERENCES

1. Lanzino G, Laws ER. Pioneers in the development of transsphenoidal surgery: Theodor Kocher, Oskar Hirsch, and Norman Dott. J Neurosurg 2001;95(6): 1097–103.
2. Liu JK, Cohen-Gadol AA, Laws ER, et al. Harvey Cushing and Oskar Hirsch: early forefathers of modern transsphenoidal surgery. J Neurosurg 2005;103(6): 1096–104.
3. Patel SK, Husain Q, Eloy JA, et al. Norman Dott, Gerard Guiot, and Jules Hardy: key players in the resurrection and preservation of transsphenoidal surgery. Neurosurg Focus 2012;33(2):E6.
4. Jankowski R, Auque J, Simon C, et al. Endoscopic pituitary tumor surgery. Laryngoscope 1992;102(2):198–202.
5. Jho HD, Carrau RL. Endoscopic endonasal transsphenoidal surgery: experience with 50 patients. J Neurosurg 1997;87(1):44–51.
6. McLaughlin N, Eisenberg AA, Cohan P, et al. Value of endoscopy for maximizing tumor removal in endonasal transsphenoidal pituitary adenoma surgery. J Neurosurg 2013;118(3):613–20.
7. Messerer M, De Battista JC, Raverot G, et al. Evidence of improved surgical outcome following endoscopy for nonfunctioning pituitary adenoma removal. Neurosurg Focus 2011;30(4):E11.
8. Naidich MJ, Russell EJ. Current approaches to imaging of the sellar region and pituitary. Endocrinol Metab Clin North Am 1999;28(1):45–79, vi.
9. Molitch ME, Russell EJ. The pituitary "incidentaloma". Ann Intern Med 1990; 112(12):925–31.
10. Nawar RN, AbdelMannan D, Selman WR, et al. Pituitary tumor apoplexy: a review. J Intensive Care Med 2008;23(2):75–90.
11. Nyquist GG, Friedel ME, Singhal S, et al. Surgical management of rhinosinusitis in endoscopic-endonasal skull-base surgery. Int Forum Allergy Rhinol 2015;5(4): 339–43.
12. Friedel ME, Johnston DR, Singhal S, et al. Airway management and perioperative concerns in acromegaly patients undergoing endoscopic transsphenoidal surgery for pituitary tumors. Otolaryngol Head Neck Surg 2013;149(6):840–4.
13. Schmitt H, Buchfelder M, Radespiel-Tröger M, et al. Difficult intubation in acromegalic patients: incidence and predictability. Anesthesiology 2000;93(1):110–4.
14. Cavallo LM, Messina A, Cappabianca P, et al. Endoscopic endonasal surgery of the midline skull base: anatomical study and clinical considerations. Neurosurg Focus 2005;19(1):E2.
15. Nyquist GG, Anand VK, Brown S, et al. Middle turbinate preservation in endoscopic transsphenoidal surgery of the anterior skull base. Skull Base 2010; 20(5):343–7.

16. Hadad G, Bassagasteguy L, Carrau RL, et al. A novel reconstructive technique after endoscopic expanded endonasal approaches: vascular pedicle nasoseptal flap. Laryngoscope 2006;116(10):1882–6.

17. Griffiths CF, Cutler AR, Duong HT, et al. Avoidance of postoperative epistaxis and anosmia in endonasal endoscopic skull base surgery: a technical note. Acta Neurochir (Wien) 2014;156(7):1393–401.

18. Otto BA, Bowe SN, Carrau RL, et al. Transsphenoidal approach with nasoseptal flap pedicle transposition: modified rescue flap technique. Laryngoscope 2013; 123(12):2976–9.

19. Hong SD, Nam D-H, Park J, et al. Olfactory outcomes after endoscopic pituitary surgery with nasoseptal "rescue" flaps: electrocautery versus cold knife. Am J Rhinol Allergy 2014;28(6):517–9.

20. Hamid O, El Fiky L, Hassan O, et al. Anatomic variations of the sphenoid sinus and their impact on trans-sphenoid pituitary surgery. Skull Base 2008;18(1):9–15.

21. Reittner P, Doerfler O, Goritschnig T, et al. Magnetic resonance imaging patterns of the development of the sphenoid sinus: a review of 800 patients. Rhinology 2001;39(3):121–4.

22. Luginbuhl AJ, Campbell PG, Evans J, et al. Endoscopic repair of high-flow cranial base defects using a bilayer button. Laryngoscope 2010;120(5):876–80.

23. Hofstetter CP, Nanaszko MJ, Mubita LL, et al. Volumetric classification of pituitary macroadenomas predicts outcome and morbidity following endoscopic endonasal transsphenoidal surgery. Pituitary 2012;15(3):450–63.

24. Oldfield EH, Vortmeyer AO. Development of a histological pseudocapsule and its use as a surgical capsule in the excision of pituitary tumors. J Neurosurg 2006; 104(1):7–19.

25. Monteith SJ, Starke RM, Jane JA, et al. Use of the histological pseudocapsule in surgery for Cushing disease: rapid postoperative cortisol decline predicting complete tumor resection. J Neurosurg 2012;116(4):721–7.

26. Woodworth GF, Patel KS, Shin B, et al. Surgical outcomes using a medial-to-lateral endonasal endoscopic approach to pituitary adenomas invading the cavernous sinus. J Neurosurg 2014;120(5):1086–94.

27. Ceylan S, Koc K, Anik I. Endoscopic endonasal transsphenoidal approach for pituitary adenomas invading the cavernous sinus. J Neurosurg 2010;112(1): 99–107.

28. Ding D, Starke RM, Sheehan JP. Treatment paradigms for pituitary adenomas: defining the roles of radiosurgery and radiation therapy. J Neurooncol 2014; 117(3):445–57.

29. Dallapiazza RF, Jane JA. Outcomes of endoscopic transsphenoidal pituitary surgery. Endocrinol Metab Clin North Am 2015;44(1):105–15.

30. Shakir HJ, Garson AD, Sorkin GC, et al. Combined use of covered stent and flow diversion to seal iatrogenic carotid injury with vessel preservation during transsphenoidal endoscopic resection of clival tumor. Surg Neurol Int 2014;5:81.

31. Koitschev A, Simon C, Löwenheim H, et al. Management and outcome after internal carotid artery laceration during surgery of the paranasal sinuses. Acta Otolaryngol 2006;126(7):730–8.

Reconstruction of Skull Base Defects

Cristine N. Klatt-Cromwell, MD[a], Brian D. Thorp, MD[a,*],
Anthony G. Del Signore, MD[a], Charles S. Ebert, MD, MPH[a], Matthew G. Ewend, MD[b],
Adam M. Zanation, MD[a,b,*]

KEYWORDS

- Skull base reconstruction • Nasoseptal flap • Pericranial flap • Temporoparietal flap
- CSF leak • Endoscopic skull base surgery

KEY POINTS

- This article describes an array of options for skull base reconstruction.
- Techniques used for acellular grafting, cellular grafting, and vascularized flap reconstruction are described, as well as benefits and limitations of each.
- A standard approach to patient management, from preoperative evaluation to postoperative care is also described.

INTRODUCTION

Endoscopic skull base surgery has become increasingly complex over recent years. As approaches to the skull base have expanded, reconstructive options have broadened and diversified. A multitude of reconstruction techniques are discussed in the literature. Most recently, vascularized grafts have been used for reconstruction. As endoscopic techniques have expanded to include large intradural and even intra-arachnoidal surgery, combinations of these reconstructive options have been used in tandem.

TREATMENT GOALS AND PLANNED OUTCOMES

The primary goal of the reconstructive surgeon is to provide a watertight separation between the sinonasal tract and intradural space to prevent postoperative

Financial Conflict of Interest Disclosure: None.
[a] Department of Otolaryngology—Head and Neck Surgery, University of North Carolina at Chapel Hill, 170 Manning Drive, CB# 7070, Chapel Hill, NC 27599-7070, USA; [b] Department of Neurosurgery, University of North Carolina at Chapel Hill, 170 Manning Drive, CB# 7060, Chapel Hill, NC 27599, USA
* Corresponding authors. 170 Manning Drive, CB# 7070, Chapel Hill, NC 27599-7070.
E-mail addresses: brian_thorp@med.unc.edu; adam_zanation@med.unc.edu

cerebrospinal fluid (CSF) leak, thereby decreasing the risk of devastating sequelae like pneumocephalus and/or meningitis while promoting timely and uncomplicated wound healing.

PREOPERATIVE PLANNING AND PREPARATION

Before surgery, careful consideration of the tumor characteristics, including its type, proximity to other structures, and expected surgical defect, must be undertaken. In addition, patient factors that could affect postoperative healing must be considered, including other underlying health problems, smoking history, prior radiotherapy, and obesity.

PATIENT POSITIONING

Patients undergoing endoscopic endonasal skull base surgery, either extradural or intradural, are largely managed in a standardized fashion with few very specific modifications that are outside the scope of this discussion. Once general anesthesia has been established, meticulous positioning and preparation are undertaken before the commencement of the procedure. In a select group of patients, including those with known elevated intracranial pressures, morbid obesity, and/or those in whom large dural defects with resultant high-flow CSF leaks are expected, consideration for placement of a lumbar drain before starting the procedure should be undertaken. With the evolution of skull base surgery over the past decade, it became common to have lumbar drains placed before surgery for CSF diversion.[1] It was thought, from experience with open cranial cases, that diversion would relieve pressure in the setting of postoperative edema. However, like all interventions, lumbar drains came with a unique and separate set of risks and complications, including headache, meningitis, tension pneumocephalus, and herniation. The literature reports a 3% risk of major complications, and 5% risk of minor complications associated with lumbar drains.[2] Because of this, several recent studies have been performed to assess the need for lumbar drains in the preoperative period for endoscopic skull base resections. Garcia-Navarro and colleagues[3] reviewed 46 cases in which 67% of patients had lumbar drains placed. Only 2 patients had postoperative CSF leaks, and they found no significant relationship between lumbar drain usage and postoperative CSF leak rate. Ransom and colleagues[4] retrospectively reviewed 65 patients who had lumbar drains placed at the time of surgery. They found a postoperative CSF leak rate of 6.2%, whereas their lumbar drain complication rate was 12.3%, and recommended very judicious us of lumbar drains to avoid further complications. Because of this, the use of lumbar drains should be restricted to only very specific patients at the discretion of the surgeon.

Once the decision for lumbar placement has been made and performed, the bed is then turned 90° away from the anesthesia team. Next, at the discretion of the surgeon, the patient may remain flat or be placed in a modified beach chair position, with the head of bed elevated and feet lowered. A degree of reverse Trendelenberg also may be used to optimize positioning. It is our standard practice to not place the patient in pin immobilization, but scenarios exist when this immobilization is used, particularly when a combined endonasal and transcranial approach is required. Finally, depending on the proposed reconstruction, additional required surgical sites (eg, abdomen, lateral thigh, and scalp) are prepped and draped in the standard fashion to facilitate surgical access. Once this is completed, the image guidance system is brought into the field and positioned in the standard fashion following patient registration.

RECONSTRUCTION
Grafts

Skull base defects may be repaired using acellular or cellular free grafts. Acellular grafts, such as those composed of a noncellular dermal matrix, and cellular grafts, such as mucoperichondrium/mucoperiosteum, fat, dermal fat, or fascia, have been described. These techniques were initially adopted from work that repaired CSF leaks resulting from endoscopic sinus surgery or trauma.[5] As endoscopic endonasal surgery developed, free grafts were expanded to be used for larger dural defects.

Acellular grafts may be used in an inlay and/or onlay fashion. In cases with dural resection, a collagen matrix (Duragen; Integra Life Sciences, Plainsboro, NJ) is often used as an inlay graft. This graft, laid either between dura and the osseous skull base (epidural plane) or brain and dura (subdural plane), should extend approximately 5 to 10 mm beyond the dural margins in all directions and is used to obliterate dead space and in many cases abate any CSF flow. This can be followed by an onlay graft or flap. For ease of discussion in this section, we focus on onlay grafts, recognizing that the surgeon's preference dictates onlay technique. Acellular dermal matrix (Allo-Derm Life Cell, Branchburg, NJ) also may be placed in the epidural plane or subdural plane. The graft is prepared by hydration in normal saline and is sized to extend beyond the edges of the defect. If the size of the defect prevents an inlay graft or prior inlay technique has already been used, the acellular dermal matrix may be used as an onlay graft after complete removal of underlying mucosa. It is vital that all mucosa be removed to prevent any mucocele formation.

Cellular grafts may be derived from a multitude of locations. Free mucosal grafts may be taken from any site in the nose, but in our practice is typically taken from the middle turbinate that is often removed during the initial approach to the skull base to facilitate a bimanual technique. Used as an onlay graft, this is placed onto the skull base defect after mucosa has been cleared from the bony ledges. The graft provides an excellent scaffold for wound healing; however, the small size limits its use in larger skull base resections. Other cellular grafting techniques include the abdominal free fat graft. To harvest, a small incision is made in the periumbilical region, right or left lower abdominal quadrant, or the lateral hip. The required volume of fat is then circumferentially dissected, removed, and placed in saline solution until the completion of the extirpative portion of the procedure. Fat is typically used to help obliterate space, thereby creating a laminar skull base defect. It may be used in conjunction with other reconstructive techniques further described in other portions of this article. Recently, dermal fat grafts have come into more frequent use. To harvest, an elliptical incision is performed and carried through the dermis. Before proceeding with fat removal, the epidermis is removed, thereby leaving the dermis attached to the underlying fat. The required volume of fat is then circumferentially removed while keeping the dermis in continuity. The use of dermis with fat allows for improved manipulation of the graft in situ and the ability to create a more laminar surface for the use of subsequent multilayered reconstruction. The harvest of fat or dermal fat grafts adds a second surgical site and adds potential donor site complications, including hematoma formation, seroma formation, and/or wound infection; therefore, meticulous sterile technique and multilayer closure should be used.

Flaps

More robust repair of large intradural and intra-arachnoidal defects often requires vascularized flap reconstruction. Vascularized reconstructive techniques began with the development of the Hadad-Bassagasteguy flap in 2006. This flap, more commonly known as the nasoseptal flap (NSF), has become the workhorse of large skull base defect repair. Pedicled on the posterior septal artery, the NSF is composed of muco-periosteum and mucoperichondrium and is characterized by a long robust pedicle, making it extensively mobile along the skull base.[6] The size of the NSF also can be enlarged with extension onto the nasal floor, allowing it to span from orbit to orbit and from sella to frontal sinus. In some cases, the need for a nasoseptal flap for recon-struction is not known at the beginning of the case. In these cases, to preserve the vascular supply to the NSF before sphenoidotomy, a nasoseptal "rescue" flap may be elevated. This technique has also been shown to reduce healing time and overall postoperative recovery.

NASOSEPTAL FLAP

After standard positioning, the nasal cavity is prepared with the placement of 0.05% oxymetazoline-soaked pledgets and thorough decongestion is allowed to take place. To assist in the approach, the inferior turbinates are outfractured bilaterally and the middle turbinate ipsilateral to the side of NSF harvest is removed. Attention is then turned to the flap elevation. The flap is harvested based on the anticipated size of the defect and is typically overestimated to ensure proper coverage. Using needle tip electrocautery, 2 parallel incisions are made. The superior incision is made 1 to 2 cm from the most superior portion of the septum to preserve the olfactory epithe-lium. The inferior incision is made across the posterior choana below the floor of the sphenoid sinus, and extends along the nasal floor (**Fig. 1**) This incision can be modified to make a larger flap. A vertical incision is then placed to connect the 2 previous inci-sions at the level of the head of the inferior turbinate. This can be extended as far as the mucocutaneous junction. All incisions should be completed before undertaking eleva-tion of the NSF to prevent tearing. Elevation of the NSF is performed using a Cottle elevator or suction dissector, and is started anteriorly. This is done with care to main-tain the integrity of the flap without creating perforations. The flap is elevated posteri-orly back to the sphenoid face with preservation of the vascular pedicle (**Fig. 2**) The flap is then placed in the nasopharynx or ipsilateral maxillary sinus for preservation until the reconstruction portion of the procedure. Should the need for the NSF be un-known at the beginning of the case, a nasoseptal "rescue" flap may be performed. For the rescue flap, partial harvest is done at the beginning of the case.[7] In these cases, the superior incision is performed extending from the sphenoid os to the superior

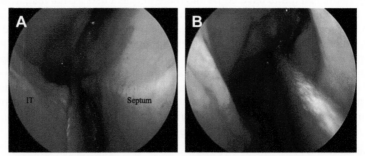

Fig. 1. NSF incision. (*A*) Inferior longitudinal incision about the right nasal septum at the junction of the septum and nasal floor. (*B*) Superior longitudinal incision about the right nasal septum. Care is taken to ensure an adequate distance from the olfactory groove. The right middle turbinate has been removed before performing the noted incisions. IT, inferior turbinate.

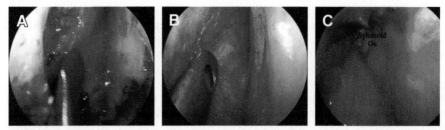

Fig. 2. Progressive NSF elevation. (*A*) Elevation and exposure of the caudal septal mucosa. During this dissection, care is taken to ensure that a broad plane is developed before proceeding posteriorly. (*B*) Progressive posterior septal elevation. (*C*) Visualization of the right sphenoid os as the flap is reflected inferiorly and laterally.

aspect of the septum, approximately 1 cm below the cranial-most aspect to prevent damage to olfactory filaments. This incision is extended 2 cm anteriorly, in contrast to the NSF previously described. A Cottle elevator is then used to reflect the flap inferiorly to expose the sphenoid rostrum, while protecting the vascular pedicle should a flap be required for reconstruction later in the case.[8] Once protected, a posterior septectomy may be performed and the skull base surgery may be completed. On completion of the extirpative portion of the procedure, attention is then turned to multilayer reconstruction of the skull base defect (**Fig. 3**) If a rescue flap was used and the flap is required for reconstruction, completion of the flap is undertaken as detailed previously.[7,8]

ENDOSCOPIC-ASSISTED PERICRANIAL FLAP

The pericranial flap (PCF) has long been used as a reconstructive option for skull base defects. This very robust flap is based on the supraorbital and supratrochlear arteries, and offers a reconstructive option for the entire skull base.[9] As with all developments in endoscopic skull base surgery, an endoscopic technique was developed to further use this flap in larger reconstructions or as a secondary option when the NSF is not available.[10] This technique allows endoscopic-assisted harvest and introduction through a bony window at the nasion. Because of its pedicle location, this flap serves as an ideal option to use for the most anterior of defects, including those in the cribriform or ethmoid. Because of its large size, the PCF may be used with extensive

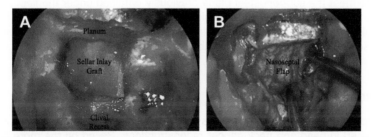

Fig. 3. Sellar reconstruction. (*A*) Following the extirpative portion of the procedure, the resultant sellar defect is reconstructed first with an inlay graft, which obliterates the potential space in this location while also creating a laminar surface for further reconstructive efforts. (*B*) The previously harvested nasoseptal flap is mobilized from the nasopharynx (not pictured) then placed over the sellar defect with full defect coverage noted. Packing material is then placed (not pictured).

versatility. Patel and colleagues[11] studied a group of 10 patients who underwent endonasal reconstruction with the PCF and used preoperative computed tomography scans for operative planning. Using these radiological studies, defect distance locations and size estimates of the PCF needed to fill these defects were performed. The average length from the nasion to the anterior wall of the sphenoid sinus, nasion to the posterior wall of the sella turcica, and nasion to the inferior point of the clivus were measured, revealing an average distance of 4.51 cm, 7.57 cm, and 12.10 cm, respectively. These distances were termed anterior fossa defects, sellar defects, and clival defects. Using these radiographic measurements and an average external pedicle length measurement of 4.36 cm, derived from the sum of the distances from lateral to the supraorbital notch/foramen in a horizontal plane to the mid-forehead plus the mid-forehead to the nasion, average PCF lengths required from reconstruction were obtained. Then using a 3-cm correction factor to account for flap transposition through the nasionectomy and retraction, the following length estimates were obtained: 11.31 to 12.44 cm for anterior fossa defects, 14.31 to 15.57 cm for sellar defects, and 18.3 to 20.42 for clival defects. All patients in this study had no evidence of postoperative CSF leak, including those with preoperative radiation therapy.

The patient is positioned in the same fashion as previously described. In addition, the face is prepped for the skin incisions both at the nasion and in the scalp. The scalp incision in planned as an ipsilateral hemicoronal incision, and in our institution is placed at the hairline near the midline then transition to the temporal hair tuft as a standard hemicoronal incision. The Doppler ultrasound also can be used to find the supraorbital and supratrochlear vessels, and a 3-cm flap pedicle is marked with the pedicle in the midline. The skin incision is then performed and often limited to only the most superior aspect of the hemicoronal incision, recognizing that this incision can be lengthened as needed for flap exposure. The dissection is then carried out in a subgaleal plane. This is first performed posteriorly and can be aided by the endoscope. Once completed, anterior dissection is carried out and this also can be aided by the endoscope. Once this degree of dissection has been adequately performed, a horizontal incision is made in the pericranium at the posterior aspect of the dissection, and bilateral incisions are made after ensuring adequate flap width. These bilateral incisions are tapered toward the pedicle ensuring maintenance of the noted 3-cm pedicle width. The pericranial flap is then meticulously elevated (**Fig. 4**) Once this is complete, attention is then turned to the glabella. Here, a skin incision is made and dissection is carried to the periosteum at the level of the nasion. Subperiosteal dissection is then carried to meet the subperiosteal plane previously obtained under the flap. A drill is then used to open the bone at the nasion to enter the nasal cavity (**Fig. 5**) The flap is carefully introduced through the nasionectomy into the nasal cavity and used for skull base reconstruction. Should a glabellar incision need to be avoided, a coronal incision may be used.

TEMPOROPARIETAL FASCIA FLAP

The temporoparietal fascia flap (TPFF) is a well-known reconstructive technique traditionally used in head and neck cancer reconstructions. Based on the more anterior branch of the superficial temporal artery (STA) from the external carotid artery, this strong fascial flap provides a multitude of advantages.[10] It is used in endoscopic endonasal reconstruction when other options, such those described previously, are not available.[12] Advantages to this flap include predictable and robust vascular anatomy, large size, and pliability with sufficient bulk. Additionally, in patients with a history

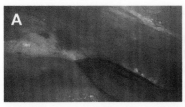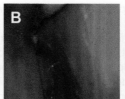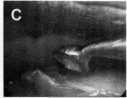

Fig. 4. Progressive endoscopic-assisted pericranial flap development. (*A*) Following superficial skin incisions, a subgaleal plane is accessed and then developed. Sharp dissection is favored to allow development of the thickest pericranial flap possible. (*B*) Monopolar cautery using a needle tip bent at 90 degrees facilitates pericranial incisions that are tapered toward the pedicle while maintaining 3 cm of width, which protects the vascular pedicle. (*C*) Progressive elevation of the dissected flap is performed with a periosteal elevator.

of skull base malignancies, this flap also offers the opportunity for nonirradiated tissue to be used for reconstruction. Because of the orientation of its vascular pedicle, it is not preferred for use in the anterior skull base. Patient selection is important in cases in which the TPFF may be used for reconstruction, as history of temporal artery biopsy or previous scalp radiation may lead to complications at the harvest or donor site, respectively. Complications for this flap include donor site necrosis or alopecia. Facial nerve anatomy also must be considered, as the dissection places the frontal branch of the facial nerve at risk for damage. In addition, because of the need for infratemporal

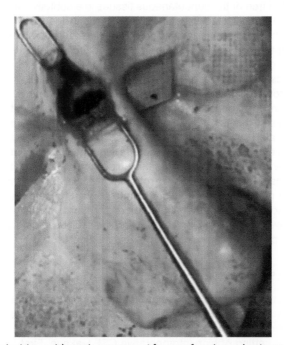

Fig. 5. Glabellar incision with nasionectomy. After performing a horizontal glabellar incision and carrying it to the level of the nasal bones and nasal processes of the frontal bones, the overlying periosteum is dissected and this plane is developed to the previously developed subperiosteal plane. A nasionectomy is then performed allowing access to the nasal cavity.

fossa dissection for transposition of the flap, the internal maxillary artery is also at risk for injury.

To properly size the TPFF, it is vital that the extirpative portion of the procedure be completed before harvest. The patient is prepped for endoscopic endonasal surgery and on the ipsilateral scalp, a hemicoronal incision is marked in the sterile fashion. Of note, the laterality of the donor site is typically ipsilateral to the expected defect; however, donor site risk factors must be considered before selection and either side may be used. Before making scalp incisions, a completed anterior and posterior ethmoidectomy and maxillary antrostomy are performed on the side of the flap. The sphenopalatine (SPA) artery and posterior nasal artery are then identified and clipped. The pterygopalatine fossa (PPF) is then exposed with dissection of the SPA into this area. The posterior and lateral walls of the maxillary sinus are then removed to expose the infratemporal fossa. The internal maxillary artery is then visualized, and its branch, the descending palatine artery, is then identified and dissected free. Once this has been completed, the entire contents of the PPF then may be moved laterally to visualize the pterygoid plates. Here, the pterygopalatine ganglion is identified and preserved, often requiring sacrifice of the vidian nerve to provide adequate displacement. Meticulous understanding of the anatomy in this area is vital for flap transposition and preservation of vital structures.

After endoscopic preparation for flap transposition is complete, the external flap harvest is then performed. A hemicoronal incision is made down to the level of the hair follicles, with meticulous care to not injure the vascular pedicle during this incision, as the STA lies in the subcutaneous tissues in this area. The fibrous septa of the TPFF are then dissected free of the subcutaneous tissues in a subfollicular plane. Once the required flap size is dissected free, an incision through the fascia is placed at the lateral aspect, and the flap is elevated from the deep temporal fascia down to its pedicle requiring the periosteum from the zygomatic arch be elevated. A wide tunnel for transposition of the flap into the nasal cavity is then formed from this site to the infratemporal fossa into the nose. This is done with commercially available percutaneous tracheostomy dilators. In some cases, a lateral canthotomy incision may be made at this point to expose the pterygomaxillary fissure to assist in transposition of the flap; however, this is not always required. Once this tunnel is developed, the tract is serially dilated using commercially available percutaneous tracheostomy dilators. Once complete, a guide wire is passed through the largest dilator, which is then removed, and the flap is then attached to this guide wire and pulled into the nasal cavity with external assistance to avoid over-rotation of the flap. The external incisions are then closed after placement of a suction drain to prevent hematoma or serum formation. Within the nose, standard reconstruction of the skull base includes inlay grafting techniques followed by the TPFF onlay overlying the skull base defect. The remainder of the multilayer closure is described in the next section.

MULTILAYER BOLSTER/CLOSURE

Following reconstructive efforts, the surgeon must appropriately bolster the repair to facilitate support during the initial healing phases. The described technique is most applicable to vascularized flaps, but may be used for grafting techniques especially when used in the setting of high intraoperative CSF leakage. First, Surgicel (Ethicon US, LLC, Somerville, NJ) is placed circumferentially about the margins of the reconstruction. Following placement of Surgicel, key regions of the repair may be bolstered with firm Nasopore (Polyganics, Groningen, The Netherlands) For example, the clival recess may be bolstered to ensure adequate approximation of the repair to the defect.

Once this is complete, Duraseal (Confluent Surgical Inc, Waltham, MA) is then placed over the entire repair to achieve a 3-dimensional bolster. Nasopore is then packed in layers to completely cover the reconstruction, thereby providing further bolstering to the repair. This is vital for both adequate healing to occur as well as to prevent any movement during removal of any nondissolvable bolstering packs that may be placed. Once adequately bolstered, nondissolvable packs, such as a Foley balloon or expandable tamponlike sponges, may be used if additional bolstering is required. If a 12-French Foley catheter is used it may be placed under direct visualization. The balloon is inflated with saline and helps provide gentle pressure to the skull base reconstruction. Instead of the Foley catheter, 10-cm expandable sponges, cut to size, may be used to stabilize the underlying repair. These are typically placed bilaterally under direct visualization and provide similar support of the underlying repair. Expandable sponges are often favored in the setting of defects of the planum or ethmoid roof where direct cranial pressure against the gravity field with the patient in the upright position is required. Either nondissolvable packing technique is typically removed 3 to 5 days after surgery.

POTENTIAL COMPLICATIONS AND MANAGEMENT

Following endoscopic endonasal surgery with skull base reconstruction, complications, including postoperative CSF leak, pneumocephalus, intracranial infection, and/or graft/flap failure or displacement, may occur.[13] In a recent meta-analysis of 38 studies on endonasal techniques used to reconstruct large skull base defects, the overall postoperative CSF leak rate was 11.5% (70/609) Subset analysis of this study revealed that patients reconstructed with free grafts had a CSF leak rate of 15.6% (51/326), whereas those reconstructed with vascularized flaps had a rate of 6.7%.[14] In a study of 152 flaps performed by Thorp and colleagues,[15] 5 (3.3%) cases of CSF leak were noted. Of these, 3 were NSF, 1 PCF, and 1 inferior turbinate flap. All cases were in the setting of high-flow intraoperative CSF leak. The average duration from the original procedure until the leak was 43.6 days, although with the removal of one outlier in the set, the average was 32 days. Symptoms include patient-reported salty or metallic taste and clear rhinorrhea that can be confirmed with a beta-2 transferrin test. CSF leaks also can be visualized on sinonasal endoscopy, but inspection can be obscured by packing material placed in the initial operative procedure.

CSF leaks infrequently present more than 6 weeks from surgery with similar symptoms. These complications can be associated with further therapies, such as radionecrosis during, or more commonly, after completion of postoperative radiation therapy. Rarely, complications may occur because of patient noncompliance, highlighting the importance of extensive patient counseling and routine follow-up to include sinonasal endoscopy. Although much of immediate postoperative concern focuses on reconstruction, pneumocephalus may also occur and presents typically with headache, nausea/vomiting, and/or changes in mental status. Careful questioning, appropriate radiographic studies, and endoscopic examination, coupled with a low index of suspicion will identify these patients.

OUTCOMES

Ongoing research in the area of endoscopic endonasal skull base surgery has served as the driving force to improve patient care and has provided a multitude of viable reconstructive options for the reconstructive surgeon. The literature reflects multiple studies that show excellent results using an array of techniques, even in the setting of high-flow CSF leaks.[16,17] After the description of the NSF in 2006, vascularized repairs shifted into the standard of care for complex skull base reconstructions. With its use, the rate of postoperative CSF leak dropped to less than 5% for skull base defects. In a prospective study assessing 70 skull base reconstructions for high-flow CSF leaks, the rate was found to be 5.7%. In this study, all patients underwent NSF reconstruction of high-flow leaks with dural defects.[17] Research also has demonstrated that the NSF may be revised, taken down, and reused, with similar postoperative CSF leak rates and no evidence of flap death.[18] Moreover, a recent review evaluating 152 vascularized flaps found that the overall leak rate was 3.3%, emphasizing the high rate of success using vascularized reconstructive techniques.[15] Several systematic reviews in the literature have compared endoscopic skull base reconstructions and the use of free grafts versus vascularized flaps. In a study by Harvey and colleagues, 609 patients with large dural defects were included. Patients in this study underwent either free graft reconstruction or vascularized repairs. They assessed these groups separately and calculated CSF leaks for both groups. The leak rate in the free graft group was found to be 15.6% (51/326), whereas the leak rate in the vascularized repair group was 6.7% (51/326), a difference that was found to be statistically significant. With the advancement of endoscopic surgery and the undertaking of larger more complex reconstructions, this difference in CSF leak rate is important to consider in preoperative planning and patient discussions.[3,14] Although the NSF remains the primary option for vascularized skull base repair, a review of secondary flaps used for skull base reconstruction beyond the NSF (including the PCF and TPFF), revealed the success rate was 97% and comparable to that of the NSF (95%)[10] In a separate, study by Patel and colleagues,[11] 34 endoscopic endonasal skull base reconstructions were assessed in which the NSF was unavailable for reconstruction. The study found only 1 patient (3.6%) who had a postoperative CSF leak. It is clear that vascularized skull base reconstruction confers a success rate of greater than 95% with a multitude of techniques available for the ever-increasing complexity of pathology assessed with endoscopic endonasal techniques.

REFERENCES

1. Stoken J, Recinos PF, Woodard T, et al. The utility of lumbar drains in modern endoscopic skull base surgery. Curr Opin Otolaryngol Head Neck Surg 2015; 23(1):78–82.
2. Governale LS, Fein N, Logsdon J, et al. Techniques and complications of external lumbar drainage for normal pressure hydrocephalus. Neurosurgery 2008;63: 379–84 [discussion: 384].
3. Garcia-Navarro V, Anand VK, Schwartz TH. Gasket seal closure for extended endonasal endoscopic skull base surgery: efficacy in a large case series. World Neurosurg 2013;80:563–8.
4. Ransom ER, Palmer JN, Kennedy DW, et al. Assessing risk/benefit of lumbar drain use for endoscopic skull-base surgery. Int Forum Allergy Rhinol 2011;1: 173–7.
5. Hegazy HM, Carrau RL, Snyderman CH, et al. Transnasal endoscopic repair of cerebrospinal fluid rhinorrhea: a meta-analysis. Laryngoscope 2000;110: 1166–72.
6. Hadad G, Bassagasteguy L, Carrau RL, et al. A novel reconstructive technique after endoscopic expanded endonasal approaches: vascular pedicle nasoseptal flap. Laryngoscope 2006;116:1882–6.

7. Rivera-Serrano CM, Snyderman CH, Gardner P, et al. Nasoseptal "rescue" flap: a novel modification of the nasoseptal flap technique for pituitary surgery. Laryngoscope 2011;121(5):990–3.

8. Rawal RB, Kimple AJ, Dugar DR, et al. Minimizing morbidity in endoscopic pituitary surgery: outcomes of the novel nasoseptal rescue flap technique. Otolaryngol Head Neck Surg 2012;147:434–7.

9. Zanation AM, Snyderman CH, Carrau RL, et al. Minimally invasive endoscopic pericranial flap: a new method for endonasal skull base reconstruction. Laryngoscope 2009;119:13–8.

10. Patel MR, Taylor RJ, Zanation AM, et al. Beyond the nasoseptal flap: outcomes and pearls with secondary flaps in endoscopic endonasal skull base reconstruction. Laryngoscope 2014;124:846–52.

11. Patel MR, Shah RN, Zanation AM, et al. Pericranial flap for endoscopic anterior skull-base reconstruction: clinical outcomes and radioanatomic analysis of preoperative planning. Neurosurgery 2010;66(3):506–12.

12. Fortes FS, Carrau RL, Snyderman CH, et al. Transpterygoid transposition of a temporoparietal fascia flap: a new method for skull base reconstruction after endoscopic expanded endonasal approaches. Laryngoscope 2007;117:970–6.

13. Kassam AB, Thomas A, Carrau RL, et al. Endoscopic reconstruction of the cranial base using a pedicled nasoseptal flap. Neurosurgery 2008;63:ONS44–52.

14. Harvey RJ, Parmar P, Sacks R, et al. Endoscopic skull base defects: a systematic review of published evidence. Laryngoscope 2012;122:452–9.

15. Thorp BD, Sreenath SB, Ebert CS, et al. Endoscopic skull base reconstruction: a review and clinical case series of 152 vascularized flaps used for surgical skull base defects in the setting of intraoperative cerebrospinal fluid leak. Neurosurg Focus 2014;37(4):1–7.

16. Zanation AM, Thorp BD, Parmar P, et al. Reconstructive options for endoscopic skull base surgery. Otolaryngol Clin North Am 2011;44:1201–22.

17. Zanation AM, Snyderman CH, Carrau RL, et al. Nasoseptal flap reconstruction of high flow intraoperative CSF leaks during endoscopic skull base surgery. Am J Rhinol Allergy 2009;23:518–21.

18. Zanation AM, Carrau RL, Snyderman CH, et al. Nasoseptal flap takedown and reuse in revision endoscopic skull base reconstruction. Laryngoscope 2011;121(1):42–6.

Cerebrospinal Fluid Diversion in Endoscopic Skull Base Reconstruction

An Evidence-Based Approach to the Use of Lumbar Drains

Duc A. Tien, MD[a], Janalee K. Stokken, MD[b], Pablo F. Recinos, MD[a,c],
Troy D. Woodard, MD[a,c], Raj Sindwani, MD[a,c],*

KEYWORDS

- Endoscopic skull base reconstruction • Minimally invasive skull base surgery
- Cerebrospinal fluid leak • Cerebrospinal fluid diversion • Lumbar drains
- Subarachnoid drains

KEY POINTS

- Lumbar drains are not necessary in most low-flow or high-flow CSF leaks encountered during endoscopic skull base surgery.
- Placement of a lumbar drain is an invasive procedure and has a 5% minor and 3% major complication rate.
- Use of a lumbar drain can be advantageous in selected high-risk settings in which a high-flow leak is anticipated and the patient has significant risk factors that make closure of the leak more challenging.
- Risk factors for postoperative cerebrospinal fluid leak include intracranial hypertension, previous radiation therapy to the skull base or sinonasal cavity, unusually large or complex defects, certain aggressive or extensive tumors, and in settings in which preferred reconstructive options (ie, pedicled flaps) are not available.

Disclosures: Funding Sources: None.
[a] Section of Rhinology, Sinus and Skull Base Surgery, Head and Neck Institute, Cleveland Clinic, 9500 Euclid Avenue, A71, Cleveland, OH 44195, USA; [b] Department of Otolaryngology, Head and Neck Surgery, Mayo Clinic, 200 First St. SW, Rochester, MN 55905, USA; [c] Minimally Invasive Cranial Base and Pituitary Surgery Program, Rose Ella Burkhardt Brain Tumor & Neuro-Oncology Center, Cleveland Clinic, 9500 Euclid Avenue, S73, Cleveland, OH 44195, USA
* Corresponding author. Head & Neck Institute, Cleveland Clinic Foundation, 9500 Euclid Avenue #A-71, Cleveland, OH 44195.
E-mail address: sindwar@ccf.org

INTRODUCTION

Endoscopic skull base surgery has evolved dramatically over the past decade, and so have techniques for skull base reconstruction. Lumbar drain (LD) placement was initially routinely performed for cerebrospinal fluid (CSF) diversion in the setting of CSF leak and skull base reconstruction because there was uncertainty about how the dural repair would heal. In open cranial procedures, LDs are used to provide brain relaxation to minimize retraction-related cerebral edema. With the endoscopic endonasal approach, retraction is not an issue and the drain is used primarily to reduce stress on the skull base repair. The LD is often kept in place postoperatively to reduce intracranial pressure by continuous CSF drainage, which is believed to facilitate wound healing and improve the success rate of the reconstruction in obtaining a watertight closure.

The size and anatomic site of the defect are factors that are predictive of postoperative CSF leaks.[1,2] For example, larger defects that span the tuberculum sellae and the planum sphenoidale are inherently more complex to reconstruct than smaller defects involving only a small portion of the sella. Most pituitary tumors are resected either without a CSF leak or with a resulting low-flow CSF leak and should be considered as a separate category. Low-flow CSF leaks, as a rule, are easier to control than high-flow leaks. Low-flow CSF leaks can be defined as leaks that occur after dural opening but do not involve an opening into the ventricle or arachnoid cistern (such as the basilar or suprasellar cistern). In contrast to most pituitary tumors, other tumor types, such as meningiomas and craniopharyngiomas, may also be at increased risk for intraoperative and postoperative CSF leak; however, this may be more related to tumor size rather than to disease type.[1,3]

CSF diversion has been considered of particular importance when a high-flow CSF fistula is encountered during a procedure, because these are inherently more challenging to manage. In the setting of endoscopic endonasal surgery, high-flow CSF leaks, as defined by Patel and colleagues,[2] are an instance in which there is violation of a cistern or ventricle. Although debated by some, we strongly agree with this definition of CSF leaks because it is the most clinically relevant and meaningful. With the increased dependability of vascularized pedicled flaps for skull base reconstruction, the need for routine LDs in skull base reconstruction is being challenged, even when there is a high-flow fistula. There is an increasing body of evidence to suggest that LDs are not necessary in the setting of endoscopic skull base reconstruction. Proponents argue that there is no significant difference in the postoperative CSF leak rate when a vascularized pedicled flap is used. In this article, the complications associated with LDs and the evidence on the usefulness of LDs in preventing postoperative CSF leaks after endoscopic skull base reconstruction are reviewed. A rational framework for the use of LDs in endoscopic skull base surgery is also proposed.

CEREBROSPINAL FLUID PHYSIOLOGY AND PRINCIPLES OF DIVERSION

Total CSF volume is estimated to average about 125 to 150 mL in adults.[4] The choroid plexuses of the ventricles produce most CSF. About 20% of CSF is in the ventricles at 1 time and the remainder is within the subarachnoid space. It circulates from the lateral ventricles to the third ventricle and then into the fourth ventricle via the cerebral aqueduct. It then exits the fourth ventricle through the foramen of Magendie (medially) and the 2 foramen of Luschka (laterally) into the subarachnoid space surrounding the brain and spinal cord. It is then absorbed by the arachnoid granulations into the venous system. CSF is renewed about 4 times within 24 hours in an adult; the secretion rate varies between 15 and 25 mL per hour.

The goal of CSF drainage from the lumbar subarachnoid space is to provide a controlled, low-resistance egress of CSF in the immediate postoperative period. CSF is typically drained at 5 to 10 mL/h for 48 to 72 hours. This strategy allows initial healing to occur under decreased tension and, in theory, decreases the chance of persistent CSF fistula. Although LDs are commonly used for this purpose, there is no set standard for their use in skull base reconstruction.

USE OF LUMBAR DRAINS IN ENDOSCOPIC SKULL BASE SURGERY

There are multiple schools of thought on the role of LD in reconstruction of the skull base after endoscopic transnasal tumor resection. The primary considerations revolve around whether or not LDs have a high complication rate and if the morbidity of placing an LD is necessary if the risk of a postoperative CSF leak is minimal. Hadad and colleagues[5] reported that the use of a pedicled nasal septal flap (PNSF) reduced the rate of postoperative CSF leaks rate by about 50%. Their overall CSF leak rate using the PNSF was approximately 5%, and it has become the mainstay of endoscopic skull base reconstruction at most major institutions.[1,5] Although there is increasing evidence that LDs are not routinely required for repair of iatrogenic and low-flow CSF leaks, the effectiveness of LDs has not been well established in skull base reconstruction and there is a paucity of literature on the topic.

Our review of the literature identified only 9 publications that described the use of LDs in skull base reconstruction after tumor resection using the endoscopic endonasal approach within the past 10 years (**Table 1**). Eight of the studies were either non-randomized prospective or retrospective series, and there was 1 literature review. The size of the studies ranged from 59 to 800 patients, and there were an aggregate total of 2124 cases.

Esposito and colleagues[3] published a retrospective study consisting of 668 cases and described a graded approach for CSF leak repair in the setting of skull base reconstruction from July, 1998 to June, 2006. These investigators analyzed their rates of intraoperative and postoperative leak (failed repair) rates and compared various groups (eg, grade of CSF leak, disease type, etc.). Although they used their own classification system for CSF leaks, they reported postoperative CSF leak of 1.6% for grade 0 to 2 intraoperative leaks (low-flow group) compared with grade 3 intraoperative leaks (high-flow group) with a failure rate of 12.0%. They used LDs only in grade 3 leaks and left them in place for at least 48 hours. This practice was initiated after 2 cases with postoperative leaks resolved after LD placement. The investigators did not use a pedicled flap as part of their reconstruction protocol. Overall, the risk of postoperative leak was 2.5%. This study provides evidence that low-flow CSF leaks do not require routine LD drain placement or a PNSF reconstruction.

In one of the largest published studies, Kassam and colleagues[6] retrospectively reviewed their initial 800 endoscopic skull base cases from July, 1998 to June, 2007 at 1 tertiary-care institution. Specifically, the investigators analyzed the frequency of CSF leak with the degree of difficulty of the resection. No LDs were placed preoperatively or intraoperatively. The investigators found an overall CSF leak failure rate of 15.9%. Extrasellar approaches were significantly more likely to be complicated by a postoperative CSF leak (12.1% vs 19.4%, $P = .005$, odds ratio 1.74 (1.18–2.57 95% confidence interval)). Of these patients, 23.6% were treated with an LD only early in the series; 41.7% were treated with both an endoscopic repair and LD. Thus, 65.4% of patients had an LD placed postoperatively (with or without secondary endoscopic repair), with a success rate of 98.8%. This study did not provide specific data on

Table 1
Publications comparing the effectiveness of LDs in endoscopic skull base reconstruction

Reference	Type of Study	Level of Evidence	Number of Cases	Number of Intraoperative Leaks	Number of Low-Flow CSF Leaks	Number of High-Flow CSF Leaks	Cases with Subarachnoid Drain	Number of Leaks with Subarachnoid Drain	Number of Leaks without Subarachnoid Drain	Overall Postoperative Leak (Failure) Rate
Esposito et al,[3] 2007	Retrospective	4	668	378 (56.6%)	320 (84.7%)	58 (15.3%)	30/668 (4.5%)	2/30 (6.7%)	None	17/668 (2.5% overall). 12.1% leak rate in Grade 3 (high-flow)
Zanation et al,[1] 2009	Prospective, nonrandomized	4	70	100% (all high flow)	None	100%	100.0%	4/65 (6.2%)	0/5 (0%)	4/70 (5.7% overall)
Patel et al,[2] 2010	Literature review and retrospective case series	3	150	All 150 cases in series had intraoperative leak	91 (61%)	59 (39%)	57 cases had LD (38%) Low-flow group = 2/91 (2%) (LD placed after postoperative CSF leak) High-flow group = 55/59 (93%)	4/55 (7.3%)	2/91 (2%)	6/150 (4% overall). 6.8% in the high-flow group
Kassam et al,[6] 2011	Retrospective	4	800	NR	NR	NR	No drains placed preoperatively or intraoperatively 65.4% placed postoperatively	NR	NR	127/800 (15.9% overall). Leak rate decreased to 5.4% after implementing PNSF
Ransom et al,[14] 2011	Retrospective	4	65	NR	NR	NR	100%	4/65 (6.2%)	None	4/65 (6.2% overall)

Eloy et al,[10] 2012	Retrospective	4	59 (41 endoscopic)	100%	None	100%	None	None	0/41 (0% endoscopic)	0/59 (0% overall)
Ackerman et al,[7] 2013	Retrospective	4	93 (23 endoscopic)	NR	NR	NR	100%	2/21 (9.5% endoscopic rate)	0/2 (0%)	2/23 (8.7% endoscopic rate)
Garcia-Navarro et al,[8] 2013	Prospective, nonrandomized	4	46	100%	None	100%	32/46 (70%)	1/32 (3.1%)	1/14 (7.1%)	2/46 (4.4% overall)
Ivan et al,[9] 2015	Retrospective	4	98	60 (61%)	NR	NR	49/98 (50%)	8/65 (12%)	4/33 (12%)	11/98 (11% overall)
Total	—	—	2049 (1961 endoscopic cases)	—	—	—	261/2049 (12.7%)	25/333 (7.5%)	7/204 (3.4%)	173/1961 (8.8% overall)

Abbreviations: NR, not reported; PNSF, pedicled nasal septal flap.
Data from Refs.[1–3,6–10,14]

intraoperative CSF leak at the time of initial resection. This important study highlights how CSF diversion is a key tool in managing CSF leak complications.

Patel and colleagues[1] reviewed their prospective series of 150 patients who underwent endoscopic skull base surgery and were reconstructed with a PNSF because of intraoperative CSF leak. The investigators classified CSF leaks into low-flow versus high-flow. Of these cases, 61% were considered low-flow CSF leaks and 2 cases (2%) were complicated by postoperative CSF leak. The remaining 39% of the cases were considered high-flow CSF leaks, and all but 4 patients had an LD placement, with a 7.3% failure rate. The investigators do not specifically discuss if these 4 cases without intraoperative LD developed postoperative CSF leak. In their proposed skull base reconstruction algorithm, the investigators emphasize the importance of including a vascularized flap to reduce postoperative CSF leak complications, but there is little discussion of the role for CSF diversion in their algorithm.

Zanation and colleagues[2] prospectively evaluated their case series of high-flow intraoperative CSF leak, in which they used a PNSF as part of their skull base reconstruction. Sixty-five of 70 patients had an LD placed intraoperatively. Four patients, who did have an LD placed at the time of surgery developed a CSF leak postoperatively (6.2% failure rate). No leaks occurred in the 5 patients who did not have an LD placed. The investigators performed multivariate analysis of postoperative CSF leak risk factors and found that the pediatric patients were at significantly greater risk ($P = .002$), although a dural opening larger than 2 cm ($P = .14$) and previous radiation therapy ($P = .07$) trended toward higher failure rates. This study reported a comparable failure rate for high-flow CSF leak (6.2%) compared with the study by Esposito and colleagues (6.7%), although their definition for high-flow CSF leak was different. Although all 5 patients without LD placement did not develop postoperative CSF leak, this study was not designed or powered to directly compare the 2 groups.

Ackerman and colleagues[7] retrospectively reviewed the efficacy of preoperative LD placement before elective open cranial and endoscopic anterior skull base surgery in reducing postoperative CSF leak. In their series, 21 patients with preoperative LD placement underwent a transnasal, transsphenoidal endoscopic approach for treatment of anterior skull base disease. Two patients developed postoperative CSF leak (9.5%). Although this study combined open and endoscopic approaches and was not designed to evaluate the efficacy of LD in preventing postoperative CSF leak, the endoscopic leak rate was comparable with other studies with or without CSF diversion, thus challenging the efficacy of LD placement.

Several studies have suggested that LDs may not be necessary in all cases of high-flow leaks. Garcia-Navarro and colleagues[8] reviewed their endoscopic case series requiring reconstruction of large diaphragmatic or dural defects over a 5-year period. They had a total of 46 cases in which the gasket seal closure was used. A PNSF was used in addition to the gasket closure in 21 cases (45.7%). An LD was placed intraoperatively in 67% of patients, and the remaining patients had a lumbar puncture for placement of intrathecal fluorescein (Akorn, Buffalo Grove, IL) only. The LDs were left in place for 24 to 48 hours and drained at 5 mL/h. There were 2 postoperative CSF leaks in the series, 1 in the groups with LD placement (3.1%) and 1 in the group without CSF diversion (7.1%), which was not significantly different.

Ivan and colleagues[9] retrospectively reviewed their series using the expanded endoscopic endonasal approach to identify risk factors for postoperative CSF leak in 98 patients. Half of their patients had an intraoperative CSF leak (flow not graded). Eleven patients (11%) had a postoperative CSF leak, and 8 of these patients failed despite postoperative CSF diversion. Of the patients who developed a CSF leak, 6 developed a leak within 7 days of surgery. In their series, abnormal body mass index (BMI, calculated as weight in kilograms divided by the square of height in meters), whether less than 18.5 or more than 25.0 kg/m^2, was the most important preoperative predictor for CSF leak (Likelihood ratio (LR) = 10.36, P = .01). Other risk factors for postoperative CSF leak included age more than 40 years (LR = 7.0, P = .03), presence of intraoperative CSF leak (LR = 5.51, P = .02), and combined open approaches (LR = 14.6, $P \leq$.01). Although this was not a blinded, randomized, controlled study, these investigators provide additional evidence that CSF diversion may not significantly affect postoperative CSF leak rates after endoscopic skull base surgery.

Eloy and colleagues[10] performed a retrospective analysis of patients who underwent endoscopic repair of high-flow CSF leaks using a PNSF without CSF diversion over a 3-year period. The PNSF was a second layer to either fat, Gelfoam (Pfizer, New York, NY), fascia lata, acellular dermal allograft, or DuraGen (Integra, Plainsboro, NJ). A total of 59 defects with leaks considered high flow were repaired, and no postoperative CSF leaks were reported, although this group had a more lenient definition of high-flow leak (high flow was defined as a leak brisk enough to visualize egress through the skull base defect without Valsalva maneuver at the time of closure). Nonetheless, these investigators' results support that CSF diversion may not be necessary even in the setting of high-flow CSF leaks.

There were an aggregate total of 2049 skull base cases (1961 endoscopic cases) within the 9 studies that we analyzed. The overall postoperative CSF leak rate with CSF diversion was 7.5% and without CSF diversion was 3.4%. There are multiple discrepancies in the literature that should also be considered when evaluating the evidence. The definition of high-flow leak is not standardized and is subjective in nature. After our review of the literature, we agree with Patel and colleagues[2] that the best definition of a high-flow CSF leak is any defect that violates a ventricle or cistern. This definition is more objective and meaningful, in our experience. The criteria for perioperative CSF diversion vary between institutions. High-flow CSF leaks are at increased risk for repair failure and thus most investigators have advocated placement of an LD in these cases. This finding could explain the discrepancy in failure rates for postoperative CSF leaks. Another discrepancy was identified in that some series included pituitary lesions in the same category as large skull base lesions, such as meningiomas or craniopharyngiomas. Clearly, some pituitary lesions are large and their removal can result in high-flow leak, but most pituitary tumors are resected either without a CSF leak or with a resulting low-flow CSF leak and should be analyzed as a separate category. The technique for closure (PNSF, gasket closure, acellular dermal allograft) was not consistent between studies. The aggregation of these inconsistencies makes it difficult to compare outcomes. Nonetheless, the studies by Patel and colleagues, Eloy and colleagues and Garcia-Navarro and colleagues provide compelling evidence that CSF diversion may not be necessary even in the setting of high-flow CSF leak.

COMPLICATIONS OF LUMBAR DRAINS

LD placement is an invasive procedure and has risks of complications. Most of these risks are minor and can be managed with minimal consequence to the patient. The complication rate associated with lumbar drainage has been reported as 5% for minor and 3% for major complications.[11] Headache is common during active CSF diversion via an LD. However, headaches can persist after removal of the LD and are believed to occur from persistent CSF leak from the lumbar subarachnoid space into the soft tissues of the lower back. The ensuing intrathecal hypotension causes traction on the meninges and cranial nerves. An epidural blood patch is indicated in patients with severe or persistent symptoms and is required in 0.004% to 29.6% of patients undergoing lumbar puncture, depending on the size and type of needle used.[12,13]

Infectious risks of LD can include cellulitis at the puncture site, meningitis, or ventriculitis. When these conditions occur, they are treated with oral or intravenous antibiotics and at times may require another procedure. Severe infections extend the patient's hospital stay and recovery time. Retained portions of the drain during insertion or removal have also been reported in the literature.[11] Removal of the retained foreign body can add an additional anesthetic and operation for a patient with all of the corresponding risks. More significant complications have also been reported, including tension pneumocephalus, subdural hemorrhage, and uncal herniation.[11] These complications can result from inadvertent overdrainage and present with an acute decline in neurologic functioning. Tension pneumocephalus is a rare but potentially fatal sequela. There are also practical complications that can occur with daily use and potential miscommunication regarding the management of LDs. For example, overdrainage of CSF can occur if meticulous attention is not given to closing the drainage system between scheduled intervals of CSF removal. When this situation occurs, computed tomography of the brain is often obtained to rule out formation of a subdural hematoma. Another concern includes development of deep vein thrombosis, because patients are typically minimally mobile during the period of CSF diversion. Although the use of prophylactic heparin while an LD is in place is controversial, risk of deep vein thrombosis is further increased if the decision is made to not use prophylactic anticoagulation.

Ransom and colleagues[14] retrospectively reviewed the risks and benefits of LD use with their endoscopic anterior skull base case series over a 5-year span. They compared the rate of complications associated with LD use with the need for revision surgery as a result of postoperative CSF leak. A total of 65 patients had LDs placed preoperatively. The investigators reported an overall revision surgery rate of 6.2% for CSF leak, whereas their LD complication rate was 12.3%. No relationship was found between occurrence of LD-associated complications and patient age, gender, presence of any particular comorbidity (data not provided), or number of comorbidities (<3 vs ≥3). No significant effect on complication risk was found for BMI either. The investigators concluded that the complication rate of lumbar drainage may be greater than practitioners recognize, and they recommend that LDs be used judiciously to avoid potential unnecessary morbidity and cost to patients undergoing endoscopic skull base surgeries.

RECOMMENDATIONS

The literature suggests that LDs are not required for low-flow leaks and infrequently required in skull base reconstruction for a high-flow leak, and we do not use them routinely. In our experience, which is largely supported by the literature, the role for CSF diversion in contemporary skull base reconstruction may include:

a. The management of patients with known or suspected intracranial hypertension
b. The treatment of early postoperative (day 1–7) CSF leaks
c. To permit the use of intraoperative intrathecal fluorescein when obtaining a watertight closure is difficult because of complexly shaped or angled anatomy
d. To augment a repair when typical reconstructive options are poor or limited
e. In settings of high-flow CSF leaks that are also deemed to be high risk for reconstruction failure because of medical or anatomic distinctions

When to use an LD can be nuanced, especially when the decision to place an LD is made a priori, at the start of surgery, because placing an LD at the end of a procedure during which a CSF leak has been encountered is of course more challenging and not advised. It is the anticipation of a high-flow leak or a leak that is difficult to control that is truly at the crux of this issue. Because the decision to place an LD is then made at the outset, careful preoperative planning is critical to effective management of an encountered leak and successful outcomes from endoscopic skull base reconstruction.

In general, we use an LD primarily in 2 settings. First, we use it as a therapeutic modality for CSF diversion in patients with small, early postoperative CSF fistulas in whom a drain was not placed previously. In this setting, we recommend placing the drain as soon as there is a clinical suspicion for a CSF leak. Waiting for laboratory tests results for β_2 transferrin can delay treatment for several days. Other investigators have had success with a trial of CSF diversion in patients with postoperative CSF leaks after skull base surgery in whom a drain was not placed at the initial procedure.[2,6,15,16] Second, we consider placement of an LD when a high-flow CSF leak is expected and the patient has other risk factors that may make the closure of the high-flow leak more challenging. The use of an LD in the setting of a high-risk, high-flow CSF leak is the most common indication for the use of LDs in our practice. High-risk cases in which high-flow leaks are anticipated may include patients undergoing revision surgery with a history of previous high-flow leak or radiation, patients with certain types of aggressive or extensive tumors, cases in which large or complex defects are expected, and patients with significant medical risk factors.

An LD with or without the use of intrathecal fluorescein can be considered in larger defects that span the tuberculum sellae, planum sphenoidale, or anterior cranial fossa (**Fig. 1**). These defects are inherently more complex to reconstruct in a watertight

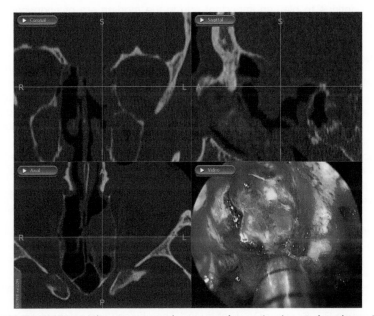

Fig. 1. Intraoperative triplanar computed tomography navigation and endoscopic view showing extravasation of intrathecal fluorescein administered via LD in a high-risk patient with large meningoencephalocele.

manner than smaller defects involving only a small part of the sella. These defects are typically larger, irregular in shape, and angled. The addition of the dye can aid in obtaining a confident closure. Postoperative CSF diversion can then aid in the repair success of these unusually shaped defects. Tumor type, such as meningiomas and craniopharyngiomas, may also be at increased risk for intraoperative and postoperative CSF leak,[1,3] although this may be more related to tumor size rather than disease type. We have also found it judicious to place an LD in pediatric patients undergoing craniopharyngioma resection, because they tend to have multiple risk factors for failure.

Patient risk factors associated with higher risk include intracranial hypertension, previous radiation therapy to the skull base or sinonasal cavity, and previous nasal surgery resulting in inadequate pedicled graft availability. We believe that LDs can augment the effectiveness of endoscopic skull base reconstruction, and their use should be considered in the setting of high-risk, high-flow CSF leaks. Considering each patient individually for their risk of intraoperative high-flow fistula and outlining their contributing risk factors provides a framework that permits the surgical team to use an LD in a rational and systematic manner.

SUMMARY

The role of LD in skull base surgery continues to evolve. LDs are not indicated for routine low-flow CSF leaks, and they are not routinely necessary in skull base reconstructions with high-flow leaks, given the ability of pedicled flaps to minimize the risk of persistent CSF fistulae postoperatively. LD is considered in our institution in settings in which a high-flow leak is anticipated and the patient has other risk factors that may make the closure or healing of the defect more difficult (high-risk, high-flow leak). Although most centers are less reliant on LDs in skull base surgery than in the past, LDs will continue to play an important role in the modern era of endoscopic skull base surgery.

REFERENCES

1. Patel MR, Stadler ME, Snyderman CH, et al. How to choose? Endoscopic skull base reconstructive options and limitations. Skull Base 2010;20(6):397–404.
2. Zanation AM, Carrau RL, Snyderman CH, et al. Nasoseptal flap reconstruction of high flow intraoperative cerebral spinal fluid leaks during endoscopic skull base surgery. Am J Rhinol Allergy 2009;23(5):518–21.
3. Esposito F, Dusick JR, Fatemi N, et al. Graded repair of cranial base defects and cerebrospinal fluid leaks in transsphenoidal surgery. Neurosurgery 2007;60(4 Suppl 1):295–304.
4. Sakka L, Coll G, Chazal J. Anatomy and physiology of cerebrospinal fluid. Eur Ann Otorhinolaryngol Head Neck Dis 2011;128(6):309–16.
5. Hadad G, Bassagasteguy L, Carrau RL, et al. A novel reconstructive technique after endoscopic expanded endonasal approaches: vascular pedicle nasoseptal flap. Laryngoscope 2006;116(10):1882–6.
6. Kassam AB, Prevedello DM, Carrau RL, et al. Endoscopic endonasal skull base surgery: analysis of complications in the authors' initial 800 patients. J Neurosurg 2011;114(6):1544–68.
7. Ackerman PD, Spencer DA, Prabhu VC. The efficacy and safety of preoperative lumbar drain placement in anterior skull base surgery. J Neurol Surg Rep 2013; 74(1):1–9.

8. Garcia-Navarro V, Anand VK, Schwartz TH. Gasket seal closure for extended endonasal endoscopic skull base surgery: efficacy in a large case series. World Neurosurg 2013;80(5):563–8.

9. Ivan ME, Bryan Iorgulescu J, El-Sayed I, et al. Risk factors for postoperative cerebrospinal fluid leak and meningitis after expanded endoscopic endonasal surgery. J Clin Neurosci 2015;22(1):48–54.

10. Eloy JA, Kuperan AB, Choudhry OJ, et al. Efficacy of the pedicled nasoseptal flap without cerebrospinal fluid (CSF) diversion for repair of skull base defects: incidence of postoperative CSF leaks. Int Forum Allergy Rhinol 2012;2(5):397–401.

11. Governale LS, Fein N, Logsdon J, et al. Techniques and complications of external lumbar drainage for normal pressure hydrocephalus. Neurosurgery 2008;63(4 Suppl 2):379–84.

12. De Almeida SM, Shumaker SD, LeBlanc SK, et al. Incidence of post-dural puncture headache in research volunteers. Headache 2011;51(10):1503–10.

13. Hatfield MK, Handrich SJ, Willis JA, et al. Blood patch rates after lumbar puncture with Whitacre versus Quincke 22- and 20-gauge spinal needles. AJR Am J Roentgenol 2008;190(6):1686–9.

14. Ransom ER, Palmer JN, Kennedy DW, et al. Assessing risk/benefit of lumbar drain use for endoscopic skull-base surgery. Int Forum Allergy Rhinol 2011; 1(3):173–7.

15. Tabaee A, Anand VK, Brown SM, et al. Algorithm for reconstruction after endoscopic pituitary and skull base surgery. Laryngoscope 2007;117(7):1133–7.

16. Greenfield JP, Anand VK, Kacker A, et al. Endoscopic endonasal transethmoidal transcribriform transfovea ethmoidalis approach to the anterior cranial fossa and skull base. Neurosurgery 2010;66(5):883–92 [discussion: 892].

Strategies for Improving Visualization During Endoscopic Skull Base Surgery

Janalee K. Stokken, MD[a], Ashleigh Halderman, MD[b],
Pablo F. Recinos, MD[b,c], Troy D. Woodard, MD[b,c],
Raj Sindwani, MD[b,c],*

KEYWORDS

- Hemostasis • Endoscopic • Skull base • Surgery • Paranasal sinus
- Cavernous sinus

KEY POINTS

- A comprehensive preoperative history and review of medications and supplements are important to identify and optimize patients with an increased risk of bleeding.
- Intraoperatively, total intravenous anesthesia, controlled hypotension, controlled heart rate, and a reverse Trendelenburg position can reduce blood loss and improve visibility.
- Hot saline irrigation improves the surgical view, particularly in cases longer than 2 hours.
- Embolization or intraoperative arterial control should be considered preoperatively in vascular tumors.
- Cavernous sinus bleeding can be reliably controlled using FloSeal and pressure applied with a cottonoid.

INTRODUCTION

Minimally invasive skull base surgery is a technique that provides a panoramic view to the surgeon through a 4-mm telescope. This technique has many advantages over open approaches, including the avoidance of an external scar, shortened hospital stays and recovery time, and improved visualization. However, visualization and

Financial Support: None.
Disclosures: None.
[a] Department of Otolaryngology, Head and Neck Surgery, Mayo Clinic, 200 First Street Southwest, Rochester, MN 55905, USA; [b] Section of Rhinology, Sinus and Skull Base Surgery, Head and Neck Institute, Cleveland Clinic Foundation, 9500 Euclid Avenue/A71, Cleveland, OH 44195, USA; [c] Minimally Invasive Cranial Base and Pituitary Surgery Program, Burkhardt Brain Tumor and Neuro-Oncology Center, Neurological Institute, Cleveland Clinic Foundation, 9500 Euclid Avenue, Cleveland, OH 44195, USA
* Corresponding author. Head & Neck Institute, Cleveland Clinic Foundation, 9500 Euclid Avenue/A-71, Cleveland, OH 44195.
E-mail address: sindwar@ccf.org

operative times can be hindered if hemostasis is not optimized. The nasal cavity has a robust vascular supply, and a primary obstacle to the minimally invasive technique is the prevention of blood from obscuring the endoscope and narrowing the surgical field. The risk of serious complications increases when important landmarks cannot be clearly delineated.

Many of the techniques for improving hemostasis are derived from the endoscopic sinus surgery literature and include preoperative evaluation, anesthetic techniques, and intraoperative considerations. Although hemostasis is the primary method for improving visualization, there are other techniques and advances in technology that have allowed for improved visualization and efficiency.

HEMOSTASIS
Preoperative Evaluation

A thorough preoperative patient history is paramount in assessing an increased bleeding risk. Questions about epistaxis, gingival bleeding with brushing, excessive bruising, and severe bleeding with trauma or previous surgery help rule out hereditary disorders. Patients should be asked about medications, supplements, and alternative therapies that may affect coagulation. Medical conditions that inhibit platelet function or cause thrombocytopenia should also be elucidated in the history.

The routine use of coagulation studies is not recommended but should be considered in patients with histories of abnormal bleeding.[1-3] A panel of laboratory tests should be ordered when the history is concerning for a bleeding abnormality and include an activated partial thromboplastin time, prothrombin time, platelet count, fibrinogen, and a von Willebrand panel or thromboelastogram[1,4] If an abnormality is found, further testing and a hematology evaluation are warranted.

The American Society of Anesthesiologists recommends that patients stop all herbal medications 2 to 3 weeks before surgery.[5] Antiplatelet and anticoagulant medications should be stopped before surgery according to the most recent *Chest* guidelines.[6] Bridging with heparin or low-molecular-weight heparin is recommended for patients with a strong indication for anticoagulation (patients who have a mechanical heart valve, atrial fibrillation, or venothromboembolism and high risk for thromboembolism).[7] It is recommended to stop warfarin 5 days, low-molecular-weight heparin 24 hours, and heparin 4 to 6 hours before surgery. Aspirin and nonsteroidal antiinflammatory medications should be stopped 7 to 10 days before but may need to be continued perioperatively in high-risk patients. Thienopyridines (clopidogrel) are stopped 10 days and glycoprotein IIb (GpIIb)/GpIIIa antagonists 24 to 72 hours before surgery. Surgery should be deferred for 6 weeks after bare-metal stent placement and 6 months after drug-eluting stent placement instead of undertaking elective surgery within these periods. Cardiologists should be consulted regarding management of anticoagulation in the perioperative period in high-risk patients; require perioperative antiplatelet therapy may be required in urgent situations.

INTRAOPERATIVE CONSIDERATIONS
Anesthetic Techniques

Total intravenous anesthesia (TIVA) with a combination of propofol and remifentanil has been shown to provide a more optimal surgical field compared with inhalation anesthesia.[8,9] This finding is believed in large part to be related to hemodynamic advantages seen with TIVA compared with inhalation anesthesia. More specifically, TIVA has been associated with lower mean arterial pressures (MAPs), and lower MAP has been shown to affect both blood loss and visibility.[8] MAP and controlled hypotension are discussed in greater detail later. In addition, TIVA has been associated with lower heart rates compared with inhalation anesthesia, and this has been shown to significantly affect surgical field clarity as well.[8,9]

However, in a study by Wormald and colleagues[8] comparing TIVA with inhalation anesthesia, when MAP and heart rate were both held constant, visibility still remained significantly better in the TIVA group, suggesting an additional variable at play. The investigators of this study hypothesized that this additional variable could potentially be vasodilation caused by the inhalational agents, which is not seen with TIVA. Any special requests regarding anesthesia should of course be discussed with the anesthesia team before the start of the case to ensure that the most appropriate and safest anesthesia is given to the patient based on their overall health status. Any other benefit of 1 form of anesthesia over another is a secondary consideration.

PATIENT POSITIONING

The positioning of the patient can have an impact on visualization during surgery. Both Ko and colleagues[10] and Hathorn and colleagues[11] randomized patients into groups to compare the reverse Trendelenburg position (RTP) with a reclined or horizontal position. Ko and colleagues found that a 10° RTP and Hathorn and colleagues found that a 15° RTP significantly decreased total blood loss, blood loss per minute, and improved the surgical field but did not decrease the operative time. Gan and colleagues[12] then compared 5°, 10°, and 20° RTP in a double-blind randomized controlled trial of 75 patients undergoing endoscopic sinus surgery. These investigators found a significant improvement in the Boezaart endoscopic field-of-view score and a decrease in blood loss (1.8, 135 mL) when the head position was at 20° compared with 5° (2.0, 231) and 10° (1.8, 230 mL). There was no significant difference in mean arterial blood pressure, blood loss per minute, or operative time among the 3 groups. Controlled hypotension is a technique often used to help reduce blood loss. A goal MAP between 60 and 70 mm Hg is typically recommended. Some studies have shown that an increased MAP significantly affects the surgical field by increasing blood loss.[8,13,14] Other studies[9,15] have failed to support this finding and suggest that MAP less than 70 mm Hg can increase intraoperative bleeding secondary to vasodilation. Neurologic injury secondary to inadequate cerebral blood flow is also a concern.[16–19] In our experience, visualization is improved when the MAP is safely minimized. The goal MAP is dependent on the patient's preoperative blood pressure control and medical comorbidities.

TOPICAL AND LOCAL VASOCONSTRICTION

Use of topical and injectable vasoconstrictive agents provides 2 major benefits: decongestion of the nasal mucosa and less bleeding. Decongestion of the mucosa alone improves the visual field. It further provides more space through which to pass instruments and can lead to less traumatization to the tissue and thus less bleeding. Anecdotally, it is believed that injection of vasoconstrictive agents leads to less bleeding and better visualization, but this remains to be proved objectively.[20,21]

It is our practice to inject 1% lidocaine with 1:100,000 of epinephrine into the anterior and posterior septum, the lateral nasal wall, middle turbinates, and the sphenopalatine foramen (SPF). We specifically avoid injection at the anatomic location of the posterior septal artery in the interest of preserving the vascular pedicle to the nasoseptal flap.

IRRIGATION

Irrigating with copious amounts of saline washes any fresh or clotted blood from the surgical site and effectively clears the surgical field. Hot saline irrigation (49°C) has been shown to improve visualization in endoscopic sinus surgery for patients with chronic rhinosinusitis when the surgical time was longer than 2 hours.[22] Gan and colleagues[22] also showed a reduced blood loss per minute when irrigating with warm irrigation in longer cases. The mechanism of action is not well understood but is believed to include mucosal and intraluminal edema that narrows and compresses the vessels and thus decreases flow.[23] Hot water irrigation (40–42°C) reduces mucosal bleeding and bleeding from minor intracranial vessels.[24,25]

CONTROL OF ARTERIAL BLEEDING

With many minimally invasive skull base approaches, the internal carotid arteries (ICA) and basilar artery are either in the field or millimeters away (**Figs. 1** and **2**). Injury to the ICA can be devastating and the importance of preparedness for this situation cannot be overstated. The ICA surgical anatomy, mechanisms of injury, management of injury, and outcomes are discussed in greater detail in another section.

EMBOLIZATION

It is our practice for vascular tumors such as juvenile nasopharyngeal angiofibromas (JNAs), and occasionally meningiomas, to perform preoperative embolization. Studies have shown that embolization performed 24 to 48 hours before surgery can be safely carried out with low risk of neurologic complications.[26–28] Two techniques for preoperative embolization of vascular tumors are a transarterial approach (TA) versus direct tumor puncture (DTP). The TA method is effective but has several noted disadvantages. Elhammady and colleagues[28] described these disadvantages as being more time consuming because multiple feeding vessels must be catheterized, less complete embolization given, there may be a need and sometimes

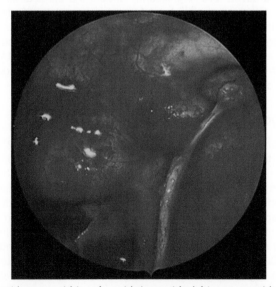

Fig. 1. Opticocarotid recess within sphenoid sinus with dehiscent carotid artery.

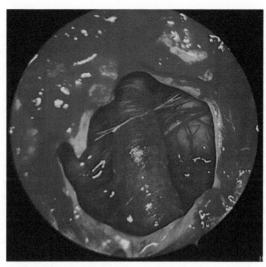

Fig. 2. Exposed basilar artery during endoscopic transclival biopsy of ventral pontine mass.

failure to catheterize these feeding arteries for various reasons (vessel origin angle, diameter of the vessel, tortuosity), and there may be an increased risk of inadvertent embolization into the cerebral circulation. The benefits of DTP were found to be that it is less time consuming and provides better penetration of embolic material into the tumor parenchyma; overall, DTP led to a greater degree of angiographic tumor devascularization.[28]

Various embolic materials exist and are classified into either particulates or liquid embolic material. Particulates tend to have several pitfalls, including coalescence and occlusion of the microcatheter, which then must be exchanged, leading to repeat catheterization of the pedicle and a prolonged operative time. Particulates must also be mixed with contrast dye to be seen on angiography.[29] Particulates also carry a higher risk of inadvertent reflux into the intracranial circulation.[30] Cyanoacrylate and ethylene vinyl alcohol (Onyx, Irvine, CA) are the 2 liquid embolic agents. Overall, the ease of use of Onyx and its properties that allow for more controlled injection with better penetration into the tumor and the ability to pause and restart an injection make it a more popular material than cyanoacrylate.[29] In a study comparing transarterial particulate embolization (TAPE) with direct percutaneous embolization (DPE) with Onyx,[29] the DPE group had significantly less intraoperative blood loss and need for transfusion over the TAPE group, suggesting better clinical outcomes of Onxy over particles.

Endoscopic resection of JNAs has been shown to be appropriate for certain lesions (Andrews stages 1, 2, and some 3a) and has been associated with reduced intraoperative blood loss, shorter hospital stays, and excellent control of disease, with no recurrences after endoscopic resection.[26] Certainly, resection of these tumors can be a challenge given the high volume of blood loss and difficult anatomy of the pterygopalatine or infratemporal fossa. Instituting the techniques discussed within this article along with the 4-handed/2-surgeon technique that has allowed so much success in endoscopic skull base surgery along with careful preoperative planning can provide a more controlled setting and possibly better outcomes.

SURGICAL LIGATION

If significant bleeding from the sphenopalatine artery (SPA) is encountered during any skull base case, then control of that bleeding can be achieved by ligation of the SPA. This procedure was first described by Budrovich and Saetti[31]; an incision is made in the lateral nasal wall roughly 1 cm anterior to the lateral insertion of the middle turbinate. The mucosal flap is elevated posteriorly toward the SPF. Once the SPA is identified posterior to the crista ethmoidalis, it is cauterized or clipped based on surgeon preference (**Fig. 3**).

The anterior ethmoid artery (AEA) is uncommonly involved in skull base lesions but can be encountered during the approach to the skull base. The AEA typically lies along the anterior skull base just posterior to the frontal recess.[32] It is most frequently attached to the skull base but can run in a bony canal 2 to 3 mm below the skull base. This canal is dehiscent in 11.4% to 40% of people.[33,34] Brisk bleeding in the roof of the anterior ethmoids should be considered to be coming from the AEA and this can be addressed with clipping or bipolar cautery (**Fig. 4**). If this procedure fails to achieve hemostasis, an external approach to the AEA where it lies within the orbit can be performed through a Lynch incision. Within the orbit, the AEA lies around 24 mm posterior to the anterior lacrimal crest.[35] Proximal control can be achieved at this location with bipolar cautery or clipping. Any suspected injury to the AEA should prompt immediate evaluation of the ipsilateral eye and orbit and the AEA can retract back into the orbit and create a retrobulbar hematoma. Of course, any concern for the eye or signs of retrobulbar hematoma should be immediately addressed with lateral canthotomy and cantholysis and consultation with an ophthalmologist.

When performing transplanar surgery, the posterior ethmoid artery (PEA) is encountered as you take down the bone of the planum near the face of the sphenoid. Control of this vessel with bipolar cautery is typically enough to obtain adequate hemostasis and reduce the vascular supply to the overlying tumor, which is most commonly a meningioma. However, if the need arises, this vessel can also be proximally controlled via the orbit. In a similar fashion to the AEA, a Lynch incision is made to access the medial wall of the orbit. The PEA is roughly 12 mm posterior to the AEA and 36 mm posterior to the anterior lacrimal crest.

CONTROL OF VENOUS BLEEDING

The most common significant source of venous bleeding during endoscopic skull base surgery is from the cavernous sinus. Bedi and colleagues[36] described the technique of

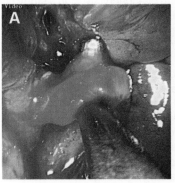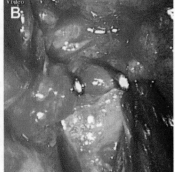

Fig. 3. (*A*) Exposed SPA before clipping. (*B*) SPA after it has been clipped.

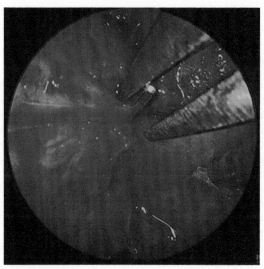

Fig. 4. Endoscopic clipping of AEA.

directly applying FloSeal (Baxter Biosciences, Vienna, Austria) to the site of bleeding followed by tamponade with a cottonoid (**Fig. 5**). This technique controls venous bleeding in seconds. FloSeal is a combination of human-derived thrombin and bovine-derived gelatin matrix that uses the patient's own fibrinogen.[35]

Other options for controlling noncavernous venous bleeding include placement of thrombin-soaked Gelfoam (Pfizer, New York, NY), placement of Surgicel (Ethicon, Somerville, NJ), or bipolar (intradural) and monopolar (extradural) cautery. When persistent focal bleeding from a bony surface does not resolve with warm water irrigation, it can be controlled by drilling with a diamond bur or by applying a small amount of bone

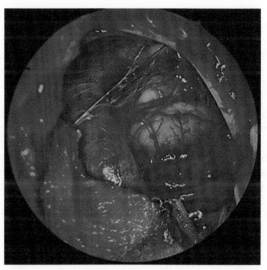

Fig. 5. Venous bleeding during endoscopic transclival biopsy of ventral pontine mass controlled by FloSeal and gentle pressure with cottonoid.

wax with a pledget. However, the most important factors in control of venous bleeding are patience and continued pressure using a cottonoid or nonabsorbable pack.

SURGICAL TECHNIQUES

Middle turbinate resection was initially performed routinely as part of the approach to the sella. At our center, we no longer resect the middle turbinate unless there is not adequate space for instrument maneuvering or endoscope positioning. This strategy may decrease the risk of intraoperative or postoperative hemorrhage from the stump of the resected middle turbinate and leaves an important surgical landmark in place. The middle turbinate should be resected when the nasal cavity is narrow or the septum is deviated, decreasing the visual field or limiting the ability to maneuver instruments. It is our practice to thoroughly cauterize the stump with the suction Bovie to prevent postoperative bleeding from the branches of the SPA.

Maxillary antrostomies can easily be performed at any point during a case to act as an additional reservoir when there is increased mucosal bleeding. Care should be taken not to enlarge the antrostomy too far posteriorly, placing the SPA at risk for injury. Frequent suctioning of the nasopharynx and maxillary antrostomy when they have filled with blood or clot reconstitutes those reservoirs and should be performed frequently throughout the case.

The use of the endoscopic irrigation systems such as the Clearvision (Karl Storz, Tuttlingen, Germany) has become standard practice in minimally invasive skull base surgery. These systems significantly improve the surgical view by rinsing the end of the endoscope and clearing any obstructive debris or blood without having to remove the scope from the nose. In addition, the use of an angled scope provides a wider view of the surgical field than the traditional microscope. In our practice, the combination of an angled scope with continuous use of irrigation provides a hydroscopic view of the surgical bed. This technique has allowed for better visualization for identifying residual tumor around the bony edges of the skull base defect before reconstruction.

SUMMARY

Decreased bleeding during endoscopic skull base surgery leads to improved intraoperative visualization and better outcomes. Control of bleeding during minimally invasive skull base cases begins preoperatively with a thorough history, physical examination, and review of medications. Various intraoperative considerations, including choice of anesthesia, use of topical and local agents, patient positioning, controlled hypotension, and temperature of irrigants, have all been shown to affect blood loss and surgical field visibility. The relevant vascular anatomy and the approaches to perform arterial ligations should be well understood to stop bleeding with inadvertent injury or when necessary during the resection of vascular tumors. It is recommended to consider preoperative embolization for larger vascular tumors, including JNAs and meningiomas. Venous bleeding is most commonly from the cavernous sinus and is easily controlled with pressure and topical hemostatic agents. Using an endoscope irrigation system and opening up additional reservoirs coupled with frequent suctioning of the nasopharynx and maxillary sinuses optimize the surgical field.

REFERENCES

1. Cobas M. Preoperative assessment of coagulation disorders. Int Anesthesiol Clin 2001;39(1):1–15.

2. Howells RC 2nd, Wax MK, Ramadan HH. Value of preoperative prothrombin time/ partial thromboplastin time as a predictor of postoperative hemorrhage in pediatric patients undergoing tonsillectomy. Otolaryngol Head Neck Surg 1997;117(6): 628–32.
3. Zwack GC, Derkay CS. The utility of preoperative hemostatic assessment in adenotonsillectomy. Int J Pediatr Otorhinolaryngol 1997;39(1):67–76.
4. Spiess BD. Coagulation monitoring in the perioperative period. Int Anesthesiol Clin 2004;42(2):55–71.
5. Hodges PJ, Kam PC. The peri-operative implications of herbal medicines [review]. Anaesthesia 2002;57(9):889–99.
6. Douketis JD, Spyropoulos AC, Spencer FA, et al. Perioperative management of antithrombotic therapy: antithrombotic therapy and prevention of thrombosis, 9th ed: American College of Chest Physicians Evidence-Based Clinical Practice Guidelines. Chest 2012;141(2 Suppl):e326S–50S.
7. Samama CM, Bastien O, Forestier F, et al. Antiplatelet agents in the perioperative period: expert recommendations of the French Society of Anesthesiology and Intensive Care (SFAR) 2001–summary statement [Guideline Practice Guideline]. Can J Anaesth 2002;49(6):S26–35.
8. Wormald PJ, van Renen G, Perks J, et al. The effect of the total intravenous anesthesia compared with inhalational anesthesia on the surgical field during endoscopic sinus surgery. Am J Rhinol 2005;19(5):514–20.
9. Eberhart LHJ, Folz BJ, Wulf H, et al. Intravenous anesthesia provides optimal surgical conditions during microscopic and endoscopic sinus surgery. Laryngoscope 2003;113:1369–73.
10. Ko MT, Chuang KC, Su CY. Multiple analyses of factors related to intraoperative blood loss and the role of reverse Trendelenburg position in endoscopic sinus surgery. Laryngoscope 2008;118:1687–91.
11. Hathorn IF, Habib AR, Manji J, et al. Comparing the reverse Trendelenburg and horizontal position for endoscopic sinus surgery: a randomized controlled trial. Otolaryngol Head Neck Surg 2013;148(2):308–13.
12. Gan EC, Habib AR, Rajwani A, et al. Five-degree, 10-degree, and 20-degree reverse Trendelenburg position during functional endoscopic sinus surgery: a double-blind randomized controlled trial. Int Forum Allergy Rhinol 2014;4(1):61–8.
13. Ha TN, van Renen RG, Ludbrook GL, et al. The relationship between hypotension, cerebral flow, and the surgical field during endoscopic sinus surgery. Laryngoscope 2014;124:2224–30.
14. Mengistu AM, Wolf MW, Boldt J, et al. Influence of controlled hypotension using esmolol and sodium nitroprusside on natriuretic peptides in patients undergoing endonasal sinus surgery. Eur J Anaesthesiol 2007;24(6):529–34.
15. Jacobi KE, Bohm BE, Rickauer AJ, et al. Moderate controlled hypotension with sodium nitroprusside does not improve surgical conditions or decrease blood loss in endoscopic sinus surgery. J Clin Anesth 2000;12:202–7.
16. Boezaart AP, van der MJ, Coetzee AR. Comparison of sodium nitroprusside-and esmolol-induced controlled hypotension for functional endoscopic surgery. Can J Anaesth 1995;42:373–6.
17. Lassen NA, Christensen MS. Physiology of cerebral blood flow. Br J Anaesth 1976;48:719–34.
18. Lindop MJ. Complications and morbidity of controlled hypotension. Br J Anaesth 1975;47:799–803.
19. Kim JS, Ko SB, Shin HE, et al. Perioperative stroke in the brain and spinal cord following an induced hypotension. Yonsei Med J 2003;44:143–5.

20. Cohen-Kerem R, Brown S, Villaseñor LV, et al. Epinephrine/lidocaine injection vs. saline during endoscopic sinus surgery. Laryngoscope 2008;118(7):1275–81.
21. Javer AR, Gheriani H, Mechor B, et al. Effect of intraoperative injection of 0.25% bupivacaine with 1:200,000 epinephrine on intraoperative blood loss in FESS. Am J Rhinol Allergy 2009;23(4):437–41.
22. Gan EC, Alsaleh S, Manji J, et al. Hemostatic effect of hot saline irrigation during functional endoscopic sinus surgery: a randomized controlled trial. Int Forum Allergy Rhinol 2014;4(11):877–84.
23. Stangerup SE, Dommerby HO, Lau T. Hot water irrigation in the treatment of posterior epistaxis. Ugeskr Laeger 1996;158(27):3932–4.
24. Snyderman CH, Pant H, Carrau RL, et al. What are the limits of endoscopic sinus surgery? The expanded endonasal approach to the skull base. Keio J Med 2009; 58(3):152–60.
25. Kassam A, Snyderman CH, Carrau RL, et al. Endoneurosurgical hemostasis techniques: lessons learned from 400 cases. Neurosurg Focus 2005;19(1):E7.
26. Bleier BS, Kennedy DW, Palmer JN, et al. Current management of juvenile nasopharyngeal angiofibroma: a tertiary center experience 1999–2007. Am J Rhinol Allergy 2009;23:328–30.
27. Ballah D, Rabinowitz D, Vossough A, et al. Preoperative angiography and external carotid artery embolization of juvenile nasopharyngeal angiofibromas in a tertiary referral paediatric centre. Clin Radiol 2013;68:1097–106.
28. Elhammady MS, Johnson JN, Peterson EC, et al. Preoperative embolization of juvenile nasopharyngeal angiofibromas: transarterial versus direct tumoral puncture. World Neurosurg 2011;76:328–34.
29. Gao M, Gemmete JJ, Chaudhary N, et al. A comparison of particulate and onyx embolization in preoperative devascularization of juvenile nasopharyngeal angiofibromas. Neuroradiology 2013;55:1089–96.
30. Valavanis A, Christoforidis G. Applications of interventional neuroradiology in the head and neck. Semin Roentgenol 2000;35:72–83.
31. Budrovich R, Saetti R. Microscopic and endoscopic ligature of the sphenopalatine artery. Laryngoscope 1992;102:1390–4.
32. Lee WC, Ku PK, Hasselt CA. New guidelines for endoscopic localization of the anterior ethmoidal artery: a cadaveric study. Laryngoscope 2000;110:1173–8.
33. Moon HJ, Kim HU, Lee JG, et al. Surgical anatomy of the anterior ethmoidal canal in ethmoid roof. Laryngoscope 2001;111:900–4.
34. Kainz J, Stammberger H. Das dach des vorderen Siebbeines: ein locus minoris resistnetiae an der Schadelbasis. Laryngol Rhinol Otol 1988;36:162–7.
35. Murr AH, Goldberg AN. External approaches to the paranasal sinuses. In: Kennedy DW, Hwang PH, editors. Rhinology diseases of the nose, sinuses, and skull base. 1st edition. New York: Thieme Medical; 2012. p. 512–25.
36. Bedi AD, Toms SA, Dehdashti AR. Use of hemostatic matrix for hemostasis of the cavernous sinus during endoscopic endonasal pituitary and suprasellar tumor surgery. Skull Base 2011;21(3):189–92.

An Overview of Anterior Skull Base Meningiomas and the Endoscopic Endonasal Approach

Mahmoud Abbassy, MD[a,b], Troy D. Woodard, MD[a,c],
Raj Sindwani, MD[a,c], Pablo F. Recinos, MD[a,c],*

KEYWORDS

- Transsphenoidal • Transcribriform • Transplanum • Tuberculum sellae
- Planum sphenoidale • Olfactory groove

KEY POINTS

- Meningiomas are mostly benign tumors (~95%); however, more aggressive and malignant variants exist.
- The rate of recurrence is directly related to the extent of resection of the tumor, its dural attachment, and pathologic bone.
- The endoscopic endonasal approach provides an optimal corridor for the resection of select anterior midline skull base tumors.
- Reconstruction using vascularized regional flaps, such as the nasal-septal flap, has significantly decrease morbidity, including rates of cerebrospinal fluid leak.
- We recommend a 2-surgeon, 4-hand approach with collaborative expertise in rhinology and neurosurgery.

According to the Central Brain Tumor Registry of the United States, meningiomas are the most common primary brain tumor. Anterior skull base meningiomas represent 6% of all meningiomas.[1] This article provides an overview of meningiomas and

Disclosures: None.
[a] Minimally Invasive Cranial Base and Pituitary Surgery Program, Rose Ella Burkhardt Brain Tumor & Neuro-Oncology Center, Cleveland Clinic, 9500 Euclid Ave, S73, Cleveland, OH 44143, USA; [b] Department of Neurosurgery, Faculty of Medicine, Alexandria University, Champlion Street, El-Azareeta, Alexandria, Egypt; [c] Section of Rhinology, Sinus and Skull Base Surgery, Head and Neck Institute, Cleveland Clinic, 9500 Euclid Ave, A71, Cleveland, OH 44143, USA
* Corresponding author. Skull Base Surgery, Minimally Invasive Cranial Base and Pituitary Surgery Program, CCLCM, CWRU, 9500 Euclid Avenue, S-73, Cleveland, OH 44195.
E-mail address: recinop@ccf.org

Otolaryngol Clin N Am 49 (2016) 141–152
http://dx.doi.org/10.1016/j.otc.2015.08.002
0030-6665/16/$ – see front matter © 2016 Elsevier Inc. All rights reserved.

focuses on the management of anterior skull base meningiomas in which endoscopic endonasal surgery is a treatment option.

EPIDEMIOLOGY

Meningiomas comprise 24% to 30% of all primary intracranial tumors and have an annual incidence of 13 per 100,000.[2–5] The incidence increases in the fourth and fifth decades with a peak in the sixth decade. Female to male ratio is 1.7:1 with an even greater female predisposition in the reproductive age group (3.5:1).[3,4,6–9]

Meningiomas are found incidentally in 1.4% of autopsy cases.[10] Multiple meningiomas represent less than 10% of all sporadic meningiomas; however, they represent a greater cluster in patients with neurofibromatosis type 2 (NF2).[11]

CAUSE AND PATHOPHYSIOLOGY

Meningiomas are thought to grow from the arachnoid cap cells; however, intraosseous and intraventricular meningiomas have been reported.[12] There are several theories regarding the cause and development of meningiomas.[5,12]

Meningiomas and the Female Sex

Meningiomas are most common in women; the female to male ratio tends to be greater in the younger age group. The ratio in postmenopausal women is 1.7:1 compared with 3.5:1 in the reproductive age group. This difference has been explained by the presence of progesterone and estrogen receptors in 88% and 39% of the lesions respectively.[6–9,13,14] In addition, women on estrogen-only hormonal therapy have a slightly increased risk of developing a meningioma, although the same link has not been found for women on estrogen-progestin hormonal therapy.[15]

Meningiomas and History of Radiation

Meningioma development is strongly related to a history of ionizing radiation exposure. This relationship has been witnessed in the survivors of the Hiroshima atomic bombing and later after the delivery of radiation therapy to pediatric patients diagnosed with cancer. The dose of radiation is inversely related to the time to meningioma development. The average interval for meningioma development is 19 to 24 years after exposure to high-dose radiation, compared with 35 years after lower doses of radiation.[5,16–18] Radiation-induced meningiomas tend more to be atypical, multifocal meningiomas, with higher proliferative indices, and they occur at younger ages.[17,19–23]

Genetic Predisposition of Meningiomas

Neurofibromatosis type 2

The pathways that are responsible for the transformation of arachnoid cap cells to meningiomas have been evaluated. One of the common pathways that is affected involves the NF2 gene. Loss of heterozygosity of chromosome 22q results in its inactivation. This gene is thought to encode Merlin, a tumor suppressor gene.[12,24,25]

Non–neurofibromatosis type 2

In families with positive family history and without features of NF2, pathways other than the NF2 gene have been implicated, including vascular endothelial growth factor, Hedgehog gene, and mTORC1 (mammalian target of rapamycin complex 1), which is responsible for tumor suppression.[11,25]

Head Injuries and Meningiomas

Several theories have been proposed regarding the development of meningiomas after head injuries. One hypothesis is that local alteration of the blood-brain barrier as a result of head injury is associated with extravasation of inflammatory mediators. These mediators include cytokines, histamines, and bradykinins, and may predispose patients to meningioma development. In addition, genes that control transcription regulation and signal transduction have been shown to be altered following head injuries.[26] Although reports[27–29] comprising smaller case numbers continue to arise that suggest a link between head injury and meningioma development, a large prospective observational study of 2953 patients with head injuries failed to show a clear link. In addition, women have both a higher incidence of meningiomas and a lower incidence of head trauma compared with men, which goes against this theory.[30]

CLASSIFICATION
According to Grade

Meningiomas are divided into 3 grades according to their histologic features as defined by the World Health Organization (WHO). Grade I meningiomas represent 94.6% of all meningiomas. They are considered benign, tend to grow more slowly, and have a lower risk of recurrence. WHO grade II meningiomas (atypical) are more aggressive and represent 4.2% of all meningiomas, whereas WHO grade III meningiomas (anaplastic) are malignant and represent 1.3%.[31]

According to Site

In addition to the WHO grading system, meningiomas are classified according to the primary dural attachment site of the tumor. Initially proposed by Harvey Cushing and Louise Eisenhardt,[32] this classification helps describe the natural history, including the development of clinical signs and symptoms, and helps in planning the appropriate surgical approach.

Meningiomas have been classified broadly based on supratentorial and infratentorial location, but are commonly subdivided by specific location.[32] Most commonly, meningiomas arise in the convexity (34.7%) and parasagittal locations (22.3%).[33] Infratentorial meningiomas represent 10% of all meningiomas, of which almost 50% are in the cerebellar convexity. The anterior skull base represents the site of origin for 8.8% of all meningiomas. The most common midline anterior skull base dural attachment is the tuberculum sellae (3.6%), followed by the olfactory groove (3.1%).[1,12,34,35]

PATHOLOGY
Gross Pathology

Most meningiomas are firm in consistency, are well demarcated in relation to surrounding tissues, and have a broad dural attachment. It is common for these types of tumor to invade the underlying dura and dural sinuses, and they occasionally involve the bone of the calvarium, causing hyperostosis.[5,36] In addition, meningiomas may invade beyond the bone and even infiltrate the skin and extend to the extracranial compartments such as the orbit.[5] In the midline of the anterior skull base, meningiomas are primarily perfused by the ethmoidal arteries[37]; however, other meningeal and ophthalmic branches can also perfuse them. Although less common, large tumors can obtain perfusion from branches of the frontopolar arteries or other smaller branches from the anterior cerebral arteries. They also may attach or encase the cerebral vessels. Malignant meningiomas can also invade the walls of these vessels.[1]

CLINICAL PRESENTATION OF MIDLINE ANTERIOR SKULL BASE MENINGIOMAS

Olfactory groove meningiomas originate from the meninges that overlie the cribriform plate of the ethmoidal bone and the region bounded by the frontosphenoid, sphenoethmoid, and frontoethmoidal sutures (**Fig. 1**). When these tumors grow large, they can extend posteriorly to the planum sphenoidale. They tend to present at larger sizes than meningiomas arising in different skull base locations. Symptoms tend to develop later in their course because the surrounding structures (ie, the frontal lobes and the olfactory nerves) tolerate compression longer than other neural structures. Symptoms appear gradually and are rarely recognized in the initial stages. In 30% to 40% of patients, early symptoms can include behavioral changes, personality changes, and headaches.[38] Anosmia, despite occurring in 13.3% to 64.5% of patients and being retrospectively noted early in the course, is rarely the symptom leading to tumor discovery. Visual symptoms usually appear as late manifestations because they require a very large tumor to be present.[35,38] Seizures are the presenting sign in 13.3% to 17.8%, whereas in 3.8% to 13.3% of cases the tumors are found incidentally.[38] Foster-Kennedy syndrome refers to unilateral optic atrophy, unilateral anosmia, unilateral central scotoma, and contralateral papilledema. Despite the classic association of Foster-Kennedy syndrome with olfactory groove meningiomas, it is rare given that modern high-quality imaging typically leads to the diagnosis before the meningioma reaches a size large enough to cause this group of symptoms.[1,35]

The planum sphenoidale, which is the portion of the anterior skull base corresponding with the bony roof of the sphenoid sinus, is another common site of origin for anterior skull base meningiomas. Planum sphenoidale meningiomas tend to push the optic

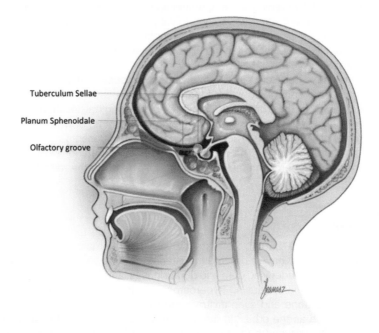

Tuberculum Sellae

Planum Sphenoidale

Olfactory groove

Fig. 1. The 3 origins of anterior skull base midline meningiomas; the green shadow represents the olfactory groove, the blue shadow is the planum sphenoidale, and the yellow shadow is the tuberculum sellae. (*Courtesy of* Cleveland Clinic, Cleveland, OH. CCF ©2014; with permission.)

nerves and chiasm as they grow posteriorly and inferiorly, as well as displacing the frontal lobes laterally.[1] The tumors are initially silent because they rarely involve the pituitary stalk or the visual pathway.[38–40] Usually patients present with headaches (63%) followed by visual impairment (14%); less commonly they present with endocrinopathies caused by impairment of the pituitary stalk.[41]

The tuberculum sellae, which is the junction of the sella turcica with the anterior skull base, gives rise to meningiomas with a distinct presentation compared with the other anterior skull base meningiomas. Their origin lies in the dural attachment at the chiasmatic sulcus, which is just medial to the bilateral optic foramina anterior to the sella.[42] Tuberculum sellae meningiomas can displace the optic nerves and chiasm. The direction of displacement depends on whether the optic chiasm lies anterior to the chiasmatic sulcus (prefixed chiasm, superior displacement) or posterior to the chiasmatic sulcus (postfixed chiasm, posterior and lateral displacement). In addition, tuberculum sellae meningiomas have a propensity to invade the optic canals, resulting in early visual symptoms.[1] Visual deficits are the most common presenting symptoms (84%–89%),[43] followed by endocrinopathies (8.4%–25.9%), headaches (17.1%–23.2%), and seizures (<2.5%). Tuberculum sellae meningiomas are found incidentally in 4.1% to 14.3% of cases.[38]

RADIOLOGY

Meningiomas usually appear isodense on computed tomography unless they have regions of calcifications, in which case those regions are hyperdense.[44] They are isointense on T1-weighted MRI and they uniformly enhance with gadolinium contrast. A dural tail, enhancement of the dural perimeter surrounding the dural attachment, is present in 58% to 72% of cases.[22,45–47]

Given that most meningiomas are benign and grow slowly, the amount peritumoral edema is typically minimal to none on T2 and fluid attenuation inversion recovery MRI sequences. However, edema is frequently observed in atypical and malignant meningiomas. Cyst formation, if present, occurs at the peripheral part of the tumor.[45]

Although meningiomas are the most commonly seen extra-axial tumors, other possibilities must not be discounted in the differential diagnosis, including dural-based metastases, idiopathic hypertrophic pachymeningitis, and granulomas.[45]

MANAGEMENT

Typical benign meningiomas have a slow growth rate and a mean doubling time of 5.2 years. The growth rate tends to be higher in younger patients and lower in the presence of calcification.[48] Therefore initial observation with close imaging follow-up can be considered, especially in elderly patients, those with multiple comorbidities, asymptomatic patients without proven growth, and in those with a calcified meningioma.[48,49] In patients who are symptomatic and/or having demonstrated growth, treatment with surgery or radiation can be considered.

SURGICAL TREATMENT

The surgical approach selected to treat meningiomas differs based on site of dural attachment. A key selection criterion when selecting the surgical approach is the ability to obtain maximum extent of resection, which includes resection of the tumor in addition to the pathologic dural attachment and hyperostotic bone, because this is predictive of rate of recurrence. In 1957, Simpson[50] was the first surgeon to describe the different grades of meningioma resection, with observation of the rate of recurrence of each grade (**Table 1**).

Surgical approaches to skull base meningiomas include traditional open skull base approaches and endoscopic endonasal approaches. Differences in the outcomes of endoscopic endonasal approaches have been debated with regard to extent of resection and safety in comparison with traditional skull base approaches.[38,51–54] Some investigators have limited the use of endonasal approaches to small tumors at the midline of the anterior skull base, whereas others have expanded their endonasal approaches to meningioma involving the cavernous sinus, the clivus, and the petrous ridge.[55–57]

The endonasal approach has several advantages and special anatomic considerations. Apart from the cosmetic aspect of not having external scars, the endonasal corridor is a direct path to the tumor and negates the need for brain retraction.[58,59] As part of the approach, the major vascular supply to the tumor (eg, bony base, ethmoidal arteries, dural base) is addressed before the tumor excision, which results in less blood loss.[59] For tuberculum sellae meningiomas, the endonasal approach allows early medial decompression of the optic nerves, visualization of the optic perforators supplying the optic chiasm, and removal of the tumor in the medial orbital canal.[60–62]

Limitations of the endoscopic endonasal approach include the inability to access tumors with significant lateral extension, specifically those extending laterally to the optic nerves and carotid arteries. A recent meta-analysis by Komotar and colleagues[38] found that open approaches result in more complete resection of anterior skull base meningiomas compared with endoscopic endonasal approaches. However, they concluded that endoscopic endonasal approaches may be safe for certain meningiomas, highlighting the importance of patient selection. Thus, tumors that are medial to the optic nerves and carotid arteries can be good candidates for the endoscopic endonasal approach, whereas tumors that are lateral to the optic nerves or to the carotid arteries should likely be treated via craniotomy. Of particular consideration in olfactory groove meningiomas is the patient's baseline sense of smell. For patients requiring surgery with intact sense of smell, transcranial options such as the supraorbital/eyebrow approach should be considered, to avoid anosmia.[53]

Another major initial criticism, particularly among the neurosurgical community, is that most endoscopes use two-dimensional cameras, resulting in lack of three-dimensional visualization provided by the operating microscope.[53,61] It is important

Table 1		
Grading of meningioma resection by Simpson[50] and the recurrence rate of each grade		
Simpson Grade	Extent of Resection	Rate of Recurrence (%)
I	Gross total resection plus resection of dural attachments and hyperostotic/pathologic bone	9
II	Gross total resection plus coagulation of dural attachments	19
III	Gross total resection with coagulation/resection of dural attachment	29
IV	Subtotal/partial tumor resection	44
V	Biopsy	NA

Abbreviation: NA, not available.

Data from Simpson D. The recurrence of intracranial meningiomas after surgical treatment. J Neurol Neurosurg Psychiatry 1957;20(1):22–39.

to highlight that this same argument was also considered a major limitation in adopting endoscopic techniques for procedures in which the use of endoscopy is now standard (eg, cholecystectomy).[63] With greater numbers of neurosurgical trainees having exposure to endoscopy in residency, the learning curve of mastering endoscopic techniques is now starting at an earlier time, when it can be more easily learned in a supervised, controlled environment.

OUTCOME AND COMPLICATIONS

In a review article by Komotar and colleagues,[38] gross total resection was achieved in 63.2% of patients presenting with olfactory groove meningiomas and 74.7% of patients with planum sphenoidale and tuberculum sellae meningiomas. The main complication was cerebrospinal fluid (CSF) leak, which occurred in 21.3% to 31.6% of cases. However, there was no significant difference in the risk of meningitis compared with studies on cases operated using the traditional open skull base approaches. Although the endoscopic approaches had a greater percentage of patients with improved visual symptoms compared with open approaches (69.1% vs 58.7%), this trend was not statistically significant. No significant difference was found regarding the perioperative mortality compared with the open series. In more recent series, CSF leak rates have been reported in less than 10% of cases owing to better reconstructive techniques using vascularized tissue, including use of the nasoseptal flap based on the septal branch of the sphenopalatine artery (**Fig. 2**).[64–68]

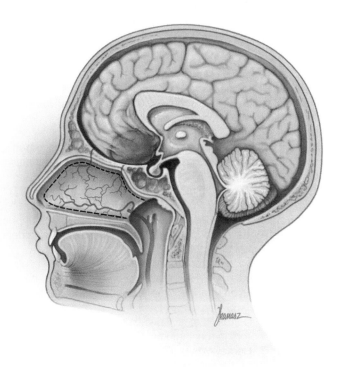

Fig. 2. The vascularized nasoseptal flap (*dotted line*) and its blood supply from the posterior septal branch of the sphenopalatine artery. (*Courtesy of* Cleveland Clinic, Cleveland, OH. CCF ©2014; with permission.)

RADIATION THERAPY AND RADIOSURGERY

Radiotherapy is routinely used for anaplastic meningiomas and the evidence is increasingly favoring the standard use of radiotherapy for atypical meningiomas.[69] It is also done in cases with meningiomas that are either too large or very close to critical structures in patients who are poor surgical candidates.[70]

Radiosurgery is a single fraction of high-dose radiation, delivered with a median marginal dose of 14 Gy. Its advantage compared with radiotherapy is the steep dose decrease beyond the tumor margin. Complications after radiosurgery include headaches, worsening of edema, and temporary or permanent visual field defects secondary to optic nerve injury.[71] Some investigators, such as Pollock and colleagues[72] and Flickinger and colleagues,[71] have shown that local control results are comparable with those of Simpson grade I resection. However, other investigators have questioned the long-term outcome and the potential for malignant transformation of benign meningiomas.[73]

SUMMARY

Meningiomas represent one of the most common primary brain tumors. Anterior skull base midline meningiomas are easily accessible via endoscopic endonasal approaches. Extent of meningioma resection together with the affected dura and pathologic hyperostotic bone is directly related to the rate of the recurrence. Endoscopic anterior skull base approaches allow early devascularization of the tumor, early optic nerve decompression, and the avoidance of excessive brain retraction; all with nonvisible external scars. Careful evaluation of the tumor location and extent is important in selecting the appropriate approach in patients with anterior skull base meningiomas.

REFERENCES

1. Methias Kirsch DK, Schackert G. Anterior midline skull base meningiomas. In: Quinones-Hinojosa A, editor. Schmidek & Sweet operative neurosurgical techniques: Indications, methods and results, vol. 1, 6th edition. Philadelphia: Elsevier; 2012. p. 417–26.
2. Dolecek TA, Propp JM, Stroup NE, et al. CBTRUS statistical report: primary brain and central nervous system tumors diagnosed in the United States in 2005-2009. Neuro Oncol 2012;14(Suppl 5):v1–49.
3. Claus EB, Bondy ML, Schildkraut JM, et al. Epidemiology of intracranial meningioma. Neurosurgery 2005;57(6):1088–95 [discussion: 1088–95].
4. Cordera S, Bottacchi E, D'Alessandro G, et al. Epidemiology of primary intracranial tumours in NW Italy, a population based study: stable incidence in the last two decades. J Neurol 2002;249(3):281–4.
5. Perry A, Louis DN, Scheithauer BW, et al. Meningiomas. In: Louis DN, Hiroko O, Wiestler OD, et al, editors. WHO classification of tumors of the central nervous system. 4th edition. Lyon (France): International Agency for Research on Cancer (IARC); 2007. p. 161–86.
6. Claus EB, Park PJ, Carroll R, et al. Specific genes expressed in association with progesterone receptors in meningioma. Cancer Res 2008;68(1):314–22.
7. Hsu DW, Efird JT, Hedley-Whyte ET. Progesterone and estrogen receptors in meningiomas: prognostic considerations. J Neurosurg 1997;86(1):113–20.
8. Maxwell M, Galanopoulos T, Neville-Golden J, et al. Expression of androgen and progesterone receptors in primary human meningiomas. J Neurosurg 1993;78(3): 456–62.

9. Pravdenkova S, Al-Mefty O, Sawyer J, et al. Progesterone and estrogen receptors: opposing prognostic indicators in meningiomas. J Neurosurg 2006;105(2): 163–73.

10. Rausing A, Ybo W, Stenflo J. Intracranial meningioma–a population study of ten years. Acta Neurol Scand 1970;46(1):102–10.

11. Louis DN, Ramesh V, Gusella JF. Neuropathology and molecular genetics of neurofibromatosis 2 and related tumors. Brain Pathol 1995;5(2):163–72.

12. Raizer J, Sherman Sojka WJ. Meningiomas. In: Rober A, Gross JWM, editors. Neurooncology. 1st edition. Oxford (United Kingdom): Wiley-Blackwell; 2012. p. 115–23.

13. Blaauw G, Blankenstein MA, Lamberts SW. Sex steroid receptors in human meningiomas. Acta Neurochir 1986;79(1):42–7.

14. Korhonen K, Salminen T, Raitanen J, et al. Female predominance in meningiomas can not be explained by differences in progesterone, estrogen, or androgen receptor expression. J Neurooncol 2006;80(1):1–7.

15. Benson VS, Kirichek O, Beral V, et al. Menopausal hormone therapy and central nervous system tumor risk: large UK prospective study and meta-analysis. Int J Cancer 2015;136(10):2369–77.

16. Kleinschmidt-DeMasters BK, Lillehei KO. Radiation-induced meningioma with a 63-year latency period. Case report. J Neurosurg 1995;82(3):487–8.

17. Harrison MJ, Wolfe DE, Lau TS, et al. Radiation-induced meningiomas: experience at the Mount Sinai Hospital and review of the literature. J Neurosurg 1991;75(4): 564–74.

18. Soffer D, Pittaluga S, Feiner M, et al. Intracranial meningiomas following low-dose irradiation to the head. J Neurosurg 1983;59(6):1048–53.

19. Godlewski B, Drummond KJ, Kaye AH. Radiation-induced meningiomas after high-dose cranial irradiation. J Clin Neurosci 2012;19(12):1627–35.

20. Mack EE, Wilson CB. Meningiomas induced by high-dose cranial irradiation. J Neurosurg 1993;79(1):28–31.

21. Yousaf I, Byrnes DP, Choudhari KA. Meningiomas induced by high dose cranial irradiation. Br J Neurosurg 2003;17(3):219–25.

22. Gosztonyi G, Slowik F, Pasztor E. Intracranial meningiomas developing at long intervals following low-dose X-ray irradiation of the head. J Neurooncol 2004;70(1): 59–65.

23. Musa BS, Pople IK, Cummins BH. Intracranial meningiomas following irradiation– a growing problem? Br J Neurosurg 1995;9(5):629–37.

24. Lamszus K. Meningioma pathology, genetics, and biology. J Neuropathol Exp Neurol 2004;63(4):275–86.

25. Shibuya M. Pathology and molecular genetics of meningioma: recent advances. Neurol Med Chir 2015;55(1):14–27.

26. Michael DB, Byers DM, Irwin LN. Gene expression following traumatic brain injury in humans: analysis by microarray. J Clin Neurosci 2005;12(3):284–90.

27. Monteiro GT, Pereira RA, Koifman RJ, et al. Head injury and brain tumours in adults: A case-control study in Rio de Janeiro, Brazil. Eur J Cancer 2006;42(7): 917–21.

28. Artico M, Cervoni L, Carloia S, et al. Development of intracranial meningiomas at the site of cranial fractures. Remarks on 15 cases. Acta Neurochir 1995;136(3–4): 132–4.

29. Caroli E, Salvati M, Rocchi G, et al. Post-traumatic intracranial meningiomas. Tumori 2003;89(1):6–8.

30. Annegers JF, Laws ER Jr, Kurland LT, et al. Head trauma and subsequent brain tumors. Neurosurgery 1979;4(3):203–6.

31. Kshettry VR, Ostrom QT, Kruchko C, et al. Descriptive epidemiology of World Health Organization grades II and III intracranial meningiomas in the United States. Neuro Oncol 2015;17(8):1166–73.

32. Cushing H. Meningiomas: their classification, regional behaviour, life history, and surgical end results. New York: Hafner Publisher Company; 1962.

33. Ashok R, Asthagiri RRL. Surgical management of parasagittal and convexity meningiomas. In: Quinones-Hinojosa A, editor. Schmidek & Sweet operative neurosurgical techniques: indications, methods, and results, vol. 1, 6th edition. Philadelphia: Elsevier; 2012. p. 399–408.

34. Mirimanoff RO, Dosoretz DE, Linggood RM, et al. Meningioma: analysis of recurrence and progression following neurosurgical resection. J Neurosurg 1985; 62(1):18–24.

35. Hentschel SJ, DeMonte F. Olfactory groove meningiomas. Neurosurg Focus 2003;14(6):e4.

36. McLendon RE, Russell DS. Russell and Rubinstein's pathology of tumors of the nervous system. 7th edition. London: Hodder Arnold; 2006.

37. McDermott MW, Rootman J, Durity FA. Subperiosteal, subperiorbital dissection and division of the anterior and posterior ethmoid arteries for meningiomas of the cribriform plate and planum sphenoidale: technical note. Neurosurgery 1995;36(6):1215–8 [discussion: 1218–9].

38. Komotar RJ, Starke RM, Raper DM, et al. Endoscopic endonasal versus open transcranial resection of anterior midline skull base meningiomas. World Neurosurg 2012;77(5–6):713–24.

39. Attia M, Kandasamy J, Jakimovski D, et al. The importance and timing of optic canal exploration and decompression during endoscopic endonasal resection of tuberculum sella and planum sphenoidale meningiomas. Neurosurgery 2012;71(1 Suppl Operative):58–67.

40. Kadis GN, Mount LA, Ganti SR. The importance of early diagnosis and treatment of the meningiomas of the planum sphenoidale and tuberculum sellae: a retrospective study of 105 cases. Surg Neurol 1979;12(5):367–71.

41. Liu Y, Chotai S, Ming C, et al. Characteristics of midline suprasellar meningiomas based on their origin and growth pattern. Clin Neurol Neurosurg 2014;125: 173–81.

42. Chi JH, McDermott MW. Tuberculum sellae meningiomas. Neurosurg Focus 2003;14(6):e6.

43. Clark AJ, Jahangiri A, Garcia RM, et al. Endoscopic surgery for tuberculum sellae meningiomas: a systematic review and meta-analysis. Neurosurg Rev 2013; 36(3):349–59.

44. Shimoji K, Yasuma Y, Mori K, et al. Unique radiological appearance of a microcystic meningioma. Acta Neurochir 1999;141(10):1119–21.

45. Katzman GL. Meningioma. In: Osborn AG, editor. Diagnostic imaging brain, vol. 2. Salt Lake city (UT): Amirsys; 2004. p. 56–64.

46. Goldsher D, Litt AW, Pinto RS, et al. Dural "tail" associated with meningiomas on Gd-DTPA-enhanced MR images: characteristics, differential diagnostic value, and possible implications for treatment. Radiology 1990;176(2): 447–50.

47. Wilms G, Lammens M, Marchal G, et al. Thickening of dura surrounding meningiomas: MR features. J Comput Assist Tomogr 1989;13(5):763–8.

48. Nakamura M, Roser F, Michel J, et al. Volumetric analysis of the growth rate of incompletely resected intracranial meningiomas. Zentralbl Neurochir 2005; 66(1):17–23.

49. Sankila R, Kallio M, Jaaskelainen J, et al. Long-term survival of 1986 patients with intracranial meningioma diagnosed from 1953 to 1984 in Finland. Comparison of the observed and expected survival rates in a population-based series. Cancer 1992;70(6):1568–76.
50. Simpson D. The recurrence of intracranial meningiomas after surgical treatment. J Neurol Neurosurg Psychiatry 1957;20(1):22–39.
51. Soni RS, Patel SK, Husain Q, et al. From above or below: the controversy and historical evolution of tuberculum sellae meningioma resection from open to endoscopic skull base approaches. J Clin Neurosci 2014;21(4):559–68.
52. Dehdashti AR, Ganna A, Witterick I, et al. Expanded endoscopic endonasal approach for anterior cranial base and suprasellar lesions: indications and limitations. Neurosurgery 2009;64(4):677–87 [discussion: 687–9].
53. Schroeder HW. Indications and limitations of the endoscopic endonasal approach for anterior cranial base meningiomas. World Neurosurg 2014;82(6 Suppl):S81–5.
54. de Divitiis E. Endoscopic endonasal transsphenoidal surgery: from the pituitary fossa to the midline cranial base. World Neurosurg 2013;80(5):e45–51.
55. Prosser JD, Vender JR, Alleyne CH, et al. Expanded endoscopic endonasal approaches to skull base meningiomas. J Neurol Surg B Skull Base 2012; 73(3):147–56.
56. Brunworth J, Padhye V, Bassiouni A, et al. Update on endoscopic endonasal resection of skull base meningiomas. Int Forum Allergy Rhinol 2015;5(4): 344–52.
57. Simal-Julian JA, Miranda-Lloret P, Botella-Asuncion C, et al. Full endoscopic endonasal expanded approach to the petroclival region: optimizing the carotid-clival window. Acta Neurochir 2014;156(8):1627–9.
58. Ceylan S, Koc K, Anik I. Extended endoscopic transphenoidal approach for tuberculum sellae meningiomas. Acta Neurochir 2011;153(1):1–9.
59. Gardner PA, Kassam AB, Thomas A, et al. Endoscopic endonasal resection of anterior cranial base meningiomas. Neurosurgery 2008;63(1):36–52 [discussion: 52–4].
60. Liu JK, Christiano LD, Patel SK, et al. Surgical nuances for removal of tuberculum sellae meningiomas with optic canal involvement using the endoscopic endonasal extended transsphenoidal transplanum transtuberculum approach. Neurosurg Focus 2011;30(5):E2.
61. de Divitiis E, Esposito F, Cappabianca P, et al. Tuberculum sellae meningiomas: high route or low route? A series of 51 consecutive cases. Neurosurgery 2008; 62(3):556–63 [discussion: 556–63].
62. Wang Q, Lu XJ, Ji WY, et al. Visual outcome after extended endoscopic endonasal transsphenoidal surgery for tuberculum sellae meningiomas. World Neurosurg 2010;73(6):694–700.
63. Rogers DA, Elstein AS, Bordage G. Improving continuing medical education for surgical techniques: applying the lessons learned in the first decade of minimal access surgery. Ann Surg 2001;233(2):159–66.
64. Leng LZ, Brown S, Anand VK, et al. "Gasket-seal" watertight closure in minimal-access endoscopic cranial base surgery. Neurosurgery 2008;62(5 Suppl 2): ONSE342–3 [discussion: ONSE343].
65. Hu F, Gu Y, Zhang X, et al. Combined use of a gasket seal closure and a vascularized pedicle nasoseptal flap multilayered reconstruction technique for high-flow cerebrospinal fluid leaks after endonasal endoscopic skull base surgery. World Neurosurg 2015;83(2):181–7.

66. Liu JK, Schmidt RF, Choudhry OJ, et al. Surgical nuances for nasoseptal flap reconstruction of cranial base defects with high-flow cerebrospinal fluid leaks after endoscopic skull base surgery. Neurosurg focus 2012;32(6):E7.
67. Zanation AM, Carrau RL, Snyderman CH, et al. Nasoseptal flap reconstruction of high flow intraoperative cerebral spinal fluid leaks during endoscopic skull base surgery. Am J Rhinol Allergy 2009;23(5):518–21.
68. Patel MR, Shah RN, Snyderman CH, et al. Pericranial flap for endoscopic anterior skull-base reconstruction: clinical outcomes and radioanatomic analysis of preoperative planning. Neurosurgery 2010;66(3):506–12 [discussion: 512].
69. Marosi C, Hassler M, Roessler K, et al. Meningioma. Crit Rev Oncol Hematol 2008;67(2):153–71.
70. Lomax NJ, Scheib SG. Quantifying the degree of conformity in radiosurgery treatment planning. Int J Radiat Oncol Biol Phys 2003;55(5):1409–19.
71. Flickinger JC, Kondziolka D, Maitz AH, et al. Gamma knife radiosurgery of imaging-diagnosed intracranial meningioma. Int J Radiat Oncol Biol Phys 2003; 56(3):801–6.
72. Pollock BE, Stafford SL, Utter A, et al. Stereotactic radiosurgery provides equivalent tumor control to Simpson Grade 1 resection for patients with small- to medium-size meningiomas. Int J Radiat Oncol Biol Phys 2003;55(4):1000–5.
73. Couldwell WT, Cole CD, Al-Mefty O. Patterns of skull base meningioma progression after failed radiosurgery. J Neurosurg 2007;106(1):30–5.

Endoscopic Management of Esthesioneuroblastoma

Christopher R. Roxbury, MD[a], Masaru Ishii, MD, PhD[a], Gary L. Gallia, MD, PhD[b], Douglas D. Reh, MD[a],*

KEYWORDS

- Esthesioneuroblastoma • Olfactory neuroblastoma • Endoscopic
- Expanded endonasal approach • Skull base

KEY POINTS

- Esthesioneuroblastoma is a rare sinonasal malignancy presenting with nonspecific sinonasal complaints.
- Diagnosis is confirmed histopathologically, with characteristic small, round, blue cells in a neurofibrillary stroma with prominent microvascularity and lobular architecture.
- Higher histologic grade (Hyams) portends worse prognosis.
- Preoperative assessment and imaging are essential to guide surgical approach.
- Endoscopic endonasal resection is feasible in select cases with the goal of obtaining negative margins.

INTRODUCTION

Esthesioneuroblastoma (ENB), also known as olfactory neuroblastoma, is a rare malignant tumor of the nasal cavity first described by Berger and colleagues[1] in 1924. These tumors have a propensity for local invasion into surrounding structures and distant metastases, most commonly to the neck, lungs, and bones.

Patients with ENB typically present with nonspecific chief complaints of nasal obstruction and epistaxis, and definitive diagnosis is made on biopsy. Histopathology is consistent with lobular architecture, small round blue cells in characteristic Homer-Wright pseudorosettes and Flexner-Wintersteiner rosettes, and prominent microvascularity (**Fig. 1**). Hyams[2] developed a histopathologic grading system classifying ENB

The authors have no relevant financial conflicts of interest to disclose.
[a] Department of Otolaryngology–Head and Neck Surgery, Johns Hopkins University School of Medicine, 601 North Caroline Street, 6th Floor, Baltimore, MD 21287, USA; [b] Department of Neurosurgery, Johns Hopkins University School of Medicine, 600 North Wolfe Street, Phipps Building, Room 101, Baltimore, MD 21287, USA
* Corresponding author. Department of Otolaryngology–Head and Neck Surgery, Johns Hopkins University, 601 North Caroline Street, 6th Floor, Baltimore, MD 21287.
E-mail address: dreh1@jhmi.edu

Otolaryngol Clin N Am 49 (2016) 153–165
http://dx.doi.org/10.1016/j.otc.2015.09.010
0030-6665/16/$ – see front matter © 2016 Elsevier Inc. All rights reserved.

oto.theclinics.com

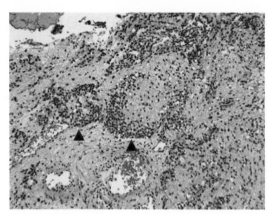

Fig. 1. Histopathologic sample of esthesioneuroblastoma. Note Homer-Wright rosettes (*arrowheads*) (H&E stain). (*Courtesy of* Dr James J. Sciubba, Lutherville-Timonium, MD.)

into four groups, with poorer prognosis occurring with increasing grade from I to IV (**Table 1**). Several attempts have been made to stage ENB based on imaging and surgical characteristics, with the most commonly used systems being developed by Kadish and coworkers,[3] Dulguerov and Calcaterra,[4] and Biller and coworkers,[5] with a more recent modification of the Kadish system by Morita and coworkers[6] (**Table 2**).

Management of ENB is generally surgical, with evidence suggesting that surgery with adjuvant radiation may provide the best prognosis.[7] Many surgical approaches have been described, including extracranial approaches,[8] craniofacial resection,[9,10] endoscopic-assisted craniofacial resection,[11,12] and most recently purely endoscopic expanded endonasal resection.[13,14] This article describes purely endoscopic surgical management of ENB and reviews outcomes of this approach described in the literature.

TREATMENT GOALS AND PLANNED OUTCOMES

Like other malignant sinonasal tumors, treatment goals and expected outcomes depend on extent of disease and tumor grade at presentation. Overall 5- and 10-year survival rates based on Surveillance, Epidemiology, and End Results tumor

Table 1
Hyams grading system

Microscopic Features	Grade I	Grade II	Grade III	Grade IV
Architecture	Lobular	Lobular	±Lobular	±Lobular
Pleomorphism	Absent/slight	Present	Prominent	Marked
Neurofibrillary matrix	Prominent	Present	May be present	Present
Rosettes	Homer-Wright	Homer-Wright	Flexner-Wintersteiner	Flexner-Wintersteiner
Mitoses	Absent	Present	Prominent	Marked
Necrosis	Absent	Absent	Present	Prominent
Glands	May be present	May be present	May be present	May be present
Calcification	Variable	Variable	Absent	Absent

Table 2
Summary of currently used staging systems

Modified Kadish		Biller		Dulguerov	
A	Tumor limited to nasal cavity	T1	Tumor of nasal cavity/ paranasal sinuses (excluding sphenoid) with or without erosion of anterior fossa bone	T1	Tumor of nasal cavity and/ or paranasal sinuses, sparing most superior ethmoid cells
B	Extension to paranasal sinuses	T2	Extension into orbit or protrusion into anterior fossa	T2	Tumor involving nasal cavity and/or paranasal sinuses (including sphenoid) with extension to or erosion of the cribriform plate
C	Extension beyond nasal cavity/paranasal sinuses	T3	Involvement of brain that is resectable with margins	T3	Tumor extending to orbit or protruding into anterior fossa
D	Metastatic disease	T4	Unresectable	T4	Tumor involving brain

registry data were 62.1% and 45.6%.[15] In the original report by Kadish and co-workers[3] of 17 patients with ENB, 100% of patients with group A disease (seven of seven), 80% (four of five) with group B disease, and 40% (two of five) with group C disease survived 3 or more years.[3] A more recent study showed 2-year survival of 75% (six of eight) in patients with group A or B disease versus 29% (5 of 17) in those with group C disease.[16] Another study showed high Hyams grade as a poor prognostic indicator with median survival of 9.8 years in low-grade tumors (grade I or II) and 6.9 years in high-grade tumors (III or IV).[17] The goal of treatment of ENB is complete surgical resection with negative margins. However, the treatment plan should be individualized for each patient. In cases where a negative margin is unattainable or returns positive postoperatively, or in those cases with positive nodal or distant metastases, adjuvant radiation and chemotherapy should be discussed. In advanced cases where cure is unlikely, the surgeon must have an honest discussion with the patient and his or her family regarding goals of care and palliative care.

PREOPERATIVE PLANNING AND PREPARATION

Preoperative planning begins with comprehensive history and physical by the neurosurgeon and the otolaryngologist–head and neck surgeon. Special emphasis must be placed on any factors that could increase the difficulty of the case, such as a history of chronic rhinosinusitis and previous functional endoscopic sinus surgery. As in all surgical patients, preoperative clearance must be performed by the appropriate internist and/or anesthesiologist to ensure that the patient can safely undergo general anesthesia.

A complete physical examination with special attention to the head and neck must also be performed. Findings of interest include signs of advanced disease, such as cranial nerve deficits or proptosis, and evidence of cervical lymphadenopathy. The examination should conclude with careful nasal endoscopy (**Fig. 2**) with particular attention to anatomic variants that could reduce endoscopic access, including septal deviation or spurs, turbinate hypertrophy, or conchae bullosa.

Preoperative imaging is essential to determining not only the extent of disease but also the ability to obtain a negative surgical margin. Imaging should also guide the

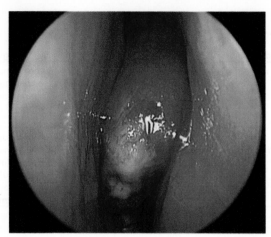

Fig. 2. Endoscopic appearance of left nasal cavity ENB.

surgeon's choice of open versus endoscopic approaches. In general, those patients with disease extent lateral to the meridian of the orbit, with significant intraorbital or intracranial involvement, and/or those with involvement of the facial soft tissues should be offered a traditional craniofacial resection rather than an expanded endonasal approach. Ultimately, careful preoperative evaluation and surgeon experience should guide the choice of surgical approach that is most likely to yield negative margins in the safest and least invasive manner possible. Complete preoperative imaging should include high-resolution computed tomography (CT) and MRI (**Fig. 3**) with intraoperative image guidance protocols. A PET scan should also be performed to assess for occult regional and metastatic disease.

PATIENT POSITIONING

The patient is placed in the supine position and the head secured using a Mayfield three-point head fixator. The neck is placed in extension with slight rotation toward the surgeons. The video monitor is placed on the patient's left, across from the surgeons and monitors for both intraoperative CT and MRI navigation are placed adjacent to

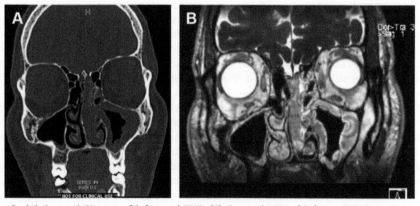

Fig. 3. (A) Coronal CT scan of left nasal ENB. (B) Coronal MRI of left nasal ENB.

the video monitor. Care is taken to secure essential equipment including the nasal endoscope, suction tubing, suction monopolar electrocautery, pistol-grip bipolar electrocautery, tissue shaver, and drill in a manner that it is easily accessible to the surgeons. Foot pedals are placed side by side at the surgeons' feet. Once proper set up and functioning of all instrumentation is confirmed, the patient is registered to the neuronavigation systems and the nasal cavity is irrigated with clindamycin solution. Perioperative antibiotics are administered and a time-out procedure is performed in anticipation of beginning the case. Surgical resection is performed with an endoscopic sinus and neurosurgeon team using a two-surgeon, three- to four-handed technique.

PROCEDURAL APPROACH

The nasal cavity is first examined with the 0-degree endoscope and the tumor is debulked using the microdebrider, taking care to avoid injury to native mucosa. Once adequate debulking is performed, the nasal septum is assessed and endoscopic septoplasty is performed for access if needed. If the posterior septum is limiting access, a back-biting forceps may be used to perform a posterior septectomy, taking care to preserve the mucosa unilaterally in the event that a nasoseptal flap is needed for skull base reconstruction at the end of the case. Middle turbinates are resected for access to the skull base.

Although a unilateral transcribriform transethmoid approach for preservation of olfaction in early stage tumors has been developed,[18] the more common bilateral approach is described here. This approach continues with bilateral maxillary antrostomies, total ethmoidectomies, sphenoidotomies, and frontal sinusotomies. Septal incisions are then planned anteriorly, posteriorly, and inferiorly to incorporate the tumor into the excised specimen. A nasoseptal flap may also be planned and raised at this time on the side of the septum opposite the tumor using a Colorado-tip Bovie electrocautery in anticipation of skull base reconstruction, as previously described by Hadad and coworkers.[19] A nasoseptal flap can only be used if all septal margins near the tumor are negative, so frozen sections should be obtained before this is undertaken. Next, the sphenoid rostrum, intersphenoid sinus septum, and posterior nasal septum are meticulously removed. A diamond drill or cutting instrumentation is used, taking care to avoid torque on the intersinus septum. This is especially important in cases where the intersinus septum attaches to the carotid canal to avoid inadvertent carotid injury. Care is taken to remove all posterior ethmoid cells that restrict access to the planum sphenoidale, which must be adequately exposed because this is the posterior limit of the skull base resection.

After appropriate access to the planum sphenoidale is achieved, attention is then turned back to the frontal sinuses. Using visualization with angled endoscopes, a modified Lothrop procedure is performed. At the end of this stage of the procedure, the surgeons have access to the entire anterior skull base from the sella turcica posteriorly to the posterior tables of the frontal sinuses anteriorly, extending laterally to the bilateral laminae papyraceae.

Before en bloc resection of the tumor involving the cribriform plate, circumferential margins are taken for frozen section analysis, taking care to maintain proper orientation of all specimens. Contiguous margins are generally taken from the sinonasal cavity and the extracranial surface of the skull base. Margins are taken until negative frozen section margins are achieved. Any bone involved with the tumor or adjacent to positive mucosal margins is also removed. Areas of bone that cannot be resected are aggressively drilled.

After negative circumferential margins are achieved, attention is then turned to en bloc resection of the tumor. At this time, control of the bilateral anterior and posterior ethmoid arteries is performed (**Fig. 4**). There is often bone overlying these structures that must be carefully drilled or removed with a curette. Once the arteries are exposed, they are coagulated using an endoscopic pistol grip bipolar electrocautery. Coagulation should be performed as medially as possible to avoid retraction into the orbit and retrobulbar hematoma. Lateral osteotomies are then performed and the dura is dissected away from the skull base. Using a Kerrison rongeur, the bone just medial to the orbit is removed. Next, an anterior osteotomy is created just posterior to the posterior table of the frontal sinuses (the anterior margin) and a posterior osteotomy is created at the level of the planum sphenoidale (the posterior margin). These osteotomies are subsequently connected to the lateral osteotomies. The crista galli is then dissected from the surrounding dura and excised by drilling its attachment to the posterior table and, once blue lined, carefully fracturing it, effectively separating the skull base from the cribriform plate (**Fig. 5**).

Next, attention is turned to dural resection. Incisions are planned anteriorly, posteriorly, and laterally to the dura involved by the tumor. The dura and the olfactory nerves are incised sharply, and the distal margins of the nerves sent for frozen section. The falx cerebri is then incised anteriorly to posteriorly, while applying gentle, inferior traction on the specimen. Arachnoid adhesions are dissected and cut sharply and the cribriform and tumor specimen is subsequently removed from the nasal cavity. After the specimen is resected, dural margins are taken and additional resection is performed, if needed, until margins are negative.

Skull base reconstruction is then performed using the previously harvested nasoseptal flap (**Fig. 6**). If a nasoseptal flap cannot be performed because of extent of tumor or if the harvested flap is of insufficient length, synthetic materials are used. Closure is typically performed in layers with a subdural inlay graft and an onlay graft over the skull base bony edges. The onlay grafts and/or nasoseptal flap are supported with intranasal packing of Gelfoam (Gelfoam Pfizer Inc, New York, NY) and Surgicel (Surgicel Ethicon Inc, Bridgewater, NJ). A Merocel sponge (Merocel Medtronic Inc, Minneapolis, MN), Nasopore (Nasopore Stryker Inc, Kalamazoo, MI), or Foley catheter is placed last as a buttress.

POSTOPERATIVE CARE

All patients are monitored postoperatively in the neurologic intensive care unit. A spiral head CT is performed to evaluate for any postoperative bleeding or pneumocephalus,

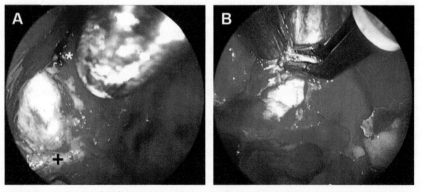

Fig. 4. (*A*) Exposure of left anterior ethmoid after cauterization (*asterisk*) and posterior ethmoid artery (*plus*) after lateral osteotomies. (*B*) Cauterization of left posterior ethmoid artery.

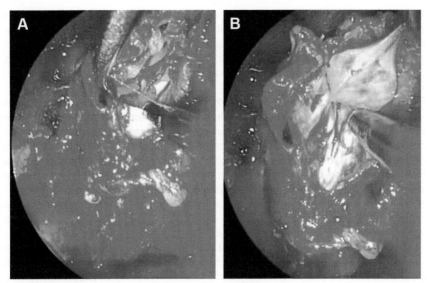

Fig. 5. Dissection (*A*) and removal (*B*) of the crista galli.

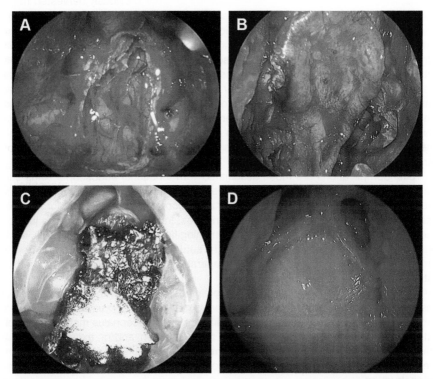

Fig. 6. (*A*) Skull base after ENB resection before reconstruction. (*B*) Skull base after nasoseptal flap rotated into position. (*C*) Postoperative appearance of nasoseptal flap at 3 months status post radiation. (*D*) Postoperative appearance of nasoseptal flap at 9 months status post radiation.

and to assess the positioning of nasal packing. Transfer to the surgical floor generally occurs on postoperative Day 1, and an MRI scan is performed within 2 days of the surgery to assess extent of resection. Lumbar drainage is routinely continued for 36 to 48 hours postoperatively. Intravenous antibiotics are continued throughout the hospital stay, and the patient is discharged on an oral antibiotic until the nasal packing is removed.

Routine postoperative nasal endoscopy is performed at 2-week intervals after discharge to assess for integrity of the skull base. Conservative nasal debridement may be performed during these visits, but any crusting along the skull base is not disturbed so as not to disrupt the graft reconstructions. Once endoscopic examination confirms an intact skull base, nasal saline irrigation can safely begin. Radiation therapy can be started at 3 weeks postoperatively, but is generally started at 6 to 8 weeks. In those patients with extensive mucosal spread or regional metastases to the neck, postoperative chemotherapy is added. Sinonasal irrigations and regular in-office debridements are conducted to limit the crusting in the area of the reconstruction that may occur during radiation (see **Fig. 6**).

Postoperative surveillance includes MRI at 3- to 4-month intervals for the first year postoperatively, 6-month intervals during the second postoperative year, and yearly thereafter. A PET/CT scan is generally performed at 1 year in our practice.

COMPLICATIONS

Complications of expanded endonasal resection of ENB are categorized into immediate and delayed postoperative complications. Immediate complications are vascular, orbital, intracranial, neurologic, or systemic. Vascular complications include epistaxis, intracranial hemorrhage, and cerebrovascular accident. Intracranial hemorrhage is extremely rare and most commonly associated with injury to the orbitofrontal branches of the anterior cerebral artery. Cerebrovascular accident is considered less common in purely endoscopic endonasal resection compared with traditional craniofacial resection, because the latter may require prolonged retraction on the frontal lobes. Catecholamine production should also be considered. Although this phenomenon is rare, hypertensive crisis could result from tumor manipulation intraoperatively.[20]

Orbital complications are those associated with functional endoscopic sinus surgery and include epiphora caused by nasolacrimal duct injury, retrobulbar hematoma caused by incomplete cauterization and/or retraction of anterior or posterior ethmoid arteries, ophthalmoplegia, diplopia, and blindness. Intracranial complications include pneumocephalus, cerebrospinal fluid leak, meningitis, and intracranial abscess. Meningitis and intracranial abscess are seen in the setting of inadequate dural closure with intracranial exposure to nasal flora. Perioperative antibiotics are administered to mitigate these potential complications.

A small amount of pneumocephalus is typical postoperatively, but a large degree of pneumocephalus or a tension pneumocephalus may lead to depressed mental status and, if extreme, cerebral herniation. The cause of pneumocephalus may be a combination of failure of adequate skull base reconstruction and/or excessive lumbar drainage. Management includes adjustment of lumbar drainage rate, needle decompression, or return to the operating room for revision endoscopic skull base reconstruction.

Rates of cerebrospinal fluid leak in expanded endonasal skull base tumor resection have decreased over time. An initial rate of 20% to 30%[21,22] was described in earlier papers, with more recent papers suggesting a rate closer to 10% or less.[23–25] We suggest a stepwise approach to repair of cerebrospinal fluid leak based on the size and location of the defect, with small defects repaired with layered free grafts and larger defects repaired with pedicled nasoseptal flaps or, in extreme cases, free tissue transfer.

Neurologic complications following endonasal endoscopic ENB resection include cranial nerve palsies, seizures, and dysosmia. All patients are given postoperative anticonvulsants to prevent seizures. All patients are counseled that they will be permanently anosmic following the surgery.

Delayed postoperative complications are those associated with the surgical approach and consist of persistent nasal crusting or iatrogenic chronic rhinosinusitis. Rarely, a mucocele may develop because of sinus outflow tract obstruction from scarring. As all patients are closely monitored for recurrence with imaging postoperatively and mucocele surveillance should also be routinely performed. Careful attention must also be paid to possible complications of postoperative radiation therapy including cataracts, epiphora, and osteoradionecrosis.

REHABILITATION AND RECOVERY

The endoscopic endonasal approach to ENB described here is generally well tolerated. Inpatient hospital recovery varies and is typically less than 1 week. There are no acute or subacute rehabilitation needs postoperatively. Early postoperative management typically requires strict cerebrospinal fluid leak precautions including no nose blowing, and no strenuous activity for 1 month after surgery. Patients are asked to sleep with the head of bed elevated at least 30° and are provided with stool softeners to prevent Valsalva while in the restroom during the first postoperative week. Late postoperative management focuses on nasal hygiene and includes careful debridement of nasal crusts and regular saline rinses after the integrity of the skull base has been confirmed.

OUTCOMES

Although ENB is a rare entity and data remain limited, there is growing evidence that expanded endoscopic approaches to resection of this tumor are feasible, effective, and safe. There have been several other small case series describing outcomes in treatment with expanded endonasal approaches. The largest series are described here. A comprehensive review of all studies evaluating endoscopic resection of ENB is provided in **Table 3**.

To date, the largest series of endoscopic ENB resection includes 23 patients, of which 19 were primary cases and 4 were recurrences. In this series, a negative margin was achieved in 17 of 19 primary cases with no evidence of disease in 22 of 23 cases at a mean follow-up of 45.2 months. There were no reported cases of meningitis and four cases of postoperative cerebrospinal fluid leak.[26] A series of 19 patients with ENB was described by Nicolai and colleagues[27] in which there was only one recurrence and a 5-year survival of 100%. This study included a total of 134 patients with sinonasal malignancies treated with endoscopic resection, and the overall complication rate was noted to be 8.7%.

In 2005, Unger and colleagues[28] updated their experience of 14 patients who underwent endoscopic resection of ENB with adjuvant radiosurgery. Of these, 12 were primary cases and 2 were revisions. A total of 5 of 14 (35.7%) showed disease progression and underwent repeat radiotherapy (four) or craniotomy (one). After a median follow-up of 58 months, 100% of patients were still living and at least 13 had no evidence of recurrence. A series of 11 patients described by Lund and colleagues[29]

Table 3
Summary of studies evaluating endoscopic resection of ENB

Series, Ref No, Year	N	Stage	Postoperative Therapy	Recurrence (mo)	Follow-up Range (Mean), Months	Status at Last Follow-up
Anderhuber et al,[31] 1999[a]	6	B5, C1	GKS (6)	1 (26)	DFS, 29.2	NED (5)
Stammberger et al,[32] 1999[a]	8	B7, C1	GKS (8)	1 (26)	DFS, 37.2	NED (7)
Walch et al,[33] 2000[a]	3	B2, C1	GKS (3)	None	39–71 (53.3)	NED (3)
Unger et al,[28] 2005[a]	14	B5, C9	GKS (14)	3 (18, 34, 79)	13–128 (59.8)	All pts alive, NED (likely 13)
Casiano, et al,[13] 2001[b]	5	A1, B2	XRT (3)	None	6–63 (30.8)	NED (4), AWD (1)
Poetker et al,[34] 2005	5	A1, B2, C1	XRT (3), chemo (1)	1 (3, 30)	38–95 (68)	NED (4)
Castelnuovo et al,[35] 2007[c]	10	A3, B4, C3	XRT (9), chemo (1)	None	15–79 (median 37)	NED (10)
Dave et al,[36] 2007[b]	10	A5, B2, C2	XRT (9)	None	3–105 (40.5)	NED (9)
Suriano et al,[37] 2007	9	A3, B6	XRT (9)	None	26–60 (42.8)	NED (9)
Lund et al,[29] 2007	11	NR	NR	NR	NR	5-y survival: 89% 5-y DFS: 56%
Zafereo et al,[38] 2008	3	A2, B1	XRT (1)	1 (38, 70)	21–147 (67.3)	NED (3)
Schwartz et al,[39] 2008	3	NR	XRT (2)	NR	NR	NR
Nicolai et al,[27] 2008[c]	19	A3, B11, C5	NR	1	NR	5-y survival: 100%
Dehdashti et al,[40] 2009	4	NR	NR	0 noted in 1 case	20 (1 case)	NED (1)
Folbe et al,[26] 2009[b]	23	A2, B11, C5, D1	XRT (16)	NR	11–152 (45.2)	NED (22)
Gallia et al,[30] 2012	11	A2, B2, C5, D2	XRT (11), XRT/chemo (3)	None	11–57 (28.5)	NED (11)
Song et al,[41] 2012	5	A2, B2, C1	XRT (4)	NR	Mean 88 mo	NED (5)
De Bonnecaze et al,[42] 2014	8	A1, B3, C4	XRT (4), XRT/chemo (4)	2 (22, 50)	24–198 (95)	NED (7), DOD (1)

Abbreviations: AWD, alive with disease; DFS, disease-free survival; DOD, died of disease; GKS, gamma knife radiosurgery; NED, no evidence of disease; NR, not reported; XRT, radiation therapy.
[a] There is an overlap between these series.
[b] There is an overlap between these series.
[c] There is an overlap between these series.
Data from Refs.[13,21,27–42]

showed a 5-year survival of 89% and a 5-year disease-free survival of 56%, with one case converted from an endoscopic approach to a craniofacial resection.

Finally, in the most recent update of the Johns Hopkins Hospital cohort of endoscopic ENB resection, Gallia and colleagues[30] were able to attain negative margins in 100% of patients (11 of 11) with no evidence of postoperative cerebrospinal fluid leak or meningitis. All patients underwent postoperative radiotherapy and three underwent chemotherapy in addition. Over a mean follow-up of 28.5 months (range, 10–57 months), 100% showed disease-free survival.

SUMMARY

ENB is an uncommon malignant tumor of the nasal cavity and paranasal sinuses, with frequent extension to the skull base and surrounding structures at presentation. Although the standard of care for these tumors was previously craniofacial resection, there is a growing body of evidence to suggest that an expanded endonasal approach to resection in selected cases may be a feasible alternative allowing for gross total resection with negative histopathologic margins and acceptable rates of postoperative complications.

REFERENCES

1. Berger L, Luc R, Richard D. L'esthesioneuroepitheliome olfactif. Bull Assoc Fr Etud Cancer 1924;13:410–21.
2. Hyams VJ. Tumors of the upper respiratory tract and ear. In: Hyams VJ, Batsakis JG, Michaels L, editors. Atlas of tumor pathology. Washington, DC: Armed Forces Institute of Pathology; 1988. p. 240–8, 2nd series, Fascile 25.
3. Kadish S, Goodman M, Wang CC. Olfactory neuroblastoma: a clinical analysis of 17 cases. Cancer 1976;37:1571–6.
4. Dulguerov P, Calcaterra T. Esthesioneuroblastoma: the UCLA experience 1970–1990. Laryngoscope 1992;102:843–9.
5. Biller HF, Lawson W, Sachdev VP, et al. Esthesioneuroblastoma: surgical treatment without radiation. Laryngoscope 1990;100:1199–201.
6. Morita A, Ebersold MJ, Olsen KD, et al. Esthesioneuroblastoma: prognosis and management. Neurosurgery 1993;32:706–14.
7. Dulguerov P, Allal AS, Calcaterra TC. Esthesioneuroblastoma: a meta-analysis and review. Lancet Oncol 2001;2(11):683–90.
8. Skolnik EM, Massari FS, Tenta LT. Olfactory neuroepithelioma. Review of world literature and presentation of two cases. Arch Otolaryngol 1966;84:644–53.
9. Doyle PJ, Paxton HD. Combined surgical approach to esthesioneuroepithelioma. Trans Am Acad Ophthalmol Otolaryngol 1971;75:526–31.
10. Sheehan JM, Jane JA. Esthesioneuroblastoma. In: Winn HR, editor. Youman's neurological surgery. Philadelphia: Elsevier; 2004. p. 1333–41.
11. Yuen AP, Fan YW, Fung CF, et al. Endoscopic-assisted crnaionasal resection of olfactory neuroblastoma. Head Neck 2005;27:488–93.
12. Thaler ER, Kotapka M, Lanza D, et al. Endoscopically assisted anterior cranial skull base resection of sinonasal tumors. Am J Rhinol 1999;13:303–10.
13. Casiano RR, Numa WA, Falquez AM. Endoscopic resection of esthesioneuroblastoma. Am J Rhinol 2001;15:271–9.
14. Gallia GG, Reh DD, Salmasi V, et al. Endonasal endoscopic resection of esthesioneuroblastoma: the Johns Hopkins Hospital experience and review of the literature. Neurosurg Rev 2011;34:465–75.

15. Jethanamest D, Morris LG, Sikora AG, et al. Esthesioneuroblastoma: a population-based analysis of survival and prognostic factors. Arch Otolaryngol Head Neck Surg 2007;133:276–80.

16. Miyamoto RC, Gleich LL, Biddinger PW, et al. Esthesioneuroblastoma and sinonasal undifferentiated carcinoma: impact of histological grading and clinical staging on survival and prognosis. Laryngoscope 2000;110:1262–5.

17. Van Gompel JJ, Giannini C, Olsen KD, et al. Long-term outcome of esthesioneuroblastoma: Hyams grade predicts patient survival. J Neurol Surg B Skull Base 2012;73:331–6.

18. Wessell A, Singh A, Litvack Z. Preservation of olfaction after unilateral endoscopic approach for resection of esthesioneuroblastoma. J Neurol Surg Rep 2014;75:e149–53.

19. Hadad G, Bassagasteguy L, Carrau RL, et al. A novel reconstructive technique after endoscopic expanded endonasal approaches: vascular pedicle nasoseptal flap. Laryngoscope 2006;116:1882–6.

20. Salmasi V, Schiavi A, Binder ZA, et al. Intraoperative hypertensive crisis due to a catecholamine-secreting esthesioneuroblastoma. Head Neck 2015;37:E74–80.

21. Frank G, Pasquini E, Doglietto F, et al. The endoscopic extended transsphenoidal approach for craniopharyngiomas. Neurosurgery 2006;59:ONS75–83.

22. Snyderman CH, Kassam AB, Carrau R, et al. Endoscopic reconstruction of cranial base defects following endonasal skull base surgery. Skull Base 2007;17:73–8.

23. Greenfield JP, Anand VK, Kacker A, et al. Endoscopic endonasal transethmoidal transcribriform transfovea ethmoidalis approach to the anterior cranial fossa and skull base. Neurosurgery 2010;66:883–92.

24. Kassam AB, Thomas A, Carrau RL, et al. Endoscopic reconstruction of the cranial base using a pedicled nasoseptal flap. Neurosurgery 2008;63:ONS44–52.

25. Hanna E, DeMonte F, Ibrahim S, et al. Endoscopic resection of sinonasal cancers with and without craniotomy: oncologic results. Arch Otolaryngol Head Neck Surg 2009;135:1219–24.

26. Folbe A, Herzallah I, Duvvuri U, et al. Endoscopic endonasal resection of esthesioneuroblastoma: a multicenter study. Am J Rhinol Allergy 2009;23:91–4.

27. Nicolai P, Battaglia P, Bignami M, et al. Endoscopic surgery for malignant tumors of the sinonasal tract and adjacent skull base: a 10-year experience. Am J Rhinol 2008;22:308–16.

28. Unger F, Walch C, Stammberger H, et al. Combined endoscopic surgery and radiosurgery as treatment modality for olfactory neuroblastoma (esthesioneuroblastoma). Acta Neurochir 2005;147:595–601.

29. Lund V, Howard DJ, Wei WI. Endoscopic resection of malignant tumors of the nose and sinuses. Am J Rhinol 2007;21:89–94.

30. Gallia GL, Reh DD, Lane AP, et al. Endoscopic resection of esthesioneuroblastoma. J Clin Neurosci 2012;19:1478–82.

31. Anderhuber W, Stammberger H, Walch C, et al. Rigid endoscopy in minimally invasive therapy of tumours of the paranasal sinuses and skull base. Minim Invasive Ther Allied Technol 1999;8:25–32.

32. Stammberger H, Anderhuber W, Walch C, et al. Possibilities and limitations of endoscopic management of nasal and paranasal sinus malignancies. Acta Otorhinolaryngol Belg 1999;53:199–205.

33. Walch C, Stammberger H, Anderhuber W, et al. The minimally invasive approach to olfactory neuroblastoma: combined endoscopic and stereotactic treatment. Laryngoscope 2000;110:635–40.

34. Poetker DM, Toohill RJ, Loehrl TA, et al. Endoscopic management of sinonasal tumors: a preliminary report. Am J Rhinol 2005;19:307–15.
35. Castelnuovo P, Bignami M, Delu G, et al. Endonasal endoscopic resection and radiotherapy in olfactory neuroblastoma: our experience. Head Neck 2007;29: 845–50.
36. Dave SP, Bared A, Casiano RR. Surgical outcomes and safety of transnasal endoscopic resection of anterior skull base tumors. Otolaryngol Head Neck Surg 2007;136:920–7.
37. Suriano M, De Vincentiis M, Colli A, et al. Endoscopic treatment of esthesioneuroblastoma: a minimally invasive approach combined with radiation therapy. Otolaryngol Head Neck Surg 2007;136:104–7.
38. Zafereo ME, Fakhri S, Prayson R, et al. Esthesioneuroblastoma: 25-year experience at a single institution. Otolaryngol Head Neck Surg 2008;138:452–8.
39. Schwartz TH, Fraser JF, Brown S, et al. Endoscopic cranial base surgery: classification of operative approaches. Neurosurgery 2008;62:991–1005.
40. Dehdashti AR, Ganna A, Witterick I, et al. Expanded endoscopic endonasal approach for anterior cranial base and suprasellar lesions: indications and limitations. Neurosurgery 2009;64:677–87.
41. Song CM, Won TB, Lee CH, et al. Treatment modalities and outcomes of olfactory neuroblastoma. Laryngoscope 2012;122:2389–95.
42. De Bonnecaze G, Chaput B, Al Hawat A, et al. Long-term oncological outcome after endoscopic surgery for olfactory esthesioneuroblastoma. Acta Otolaryngol 2014;134:1259–64.

Endoscopic Endonasal Management of Skull Base Chordomas

Surgical Technique, Nuances, and Pitfalls

João Mangussi-Gomes, MD[a,b], André Beer-Furlan, MD[a,c],
Leonardo Balsalobre, MD[a,b], Eduardo A.S. Vellutini, MD, PhD[a,c],
Aldo C. Stamm, MD, PhD[a,b,*]

KEYWORDS

- Endoscopic endonasal approach • Endoscopy • Chordoma • Skull base chordoma
- Clival chordoma

KEY POINTS

- The expanded endoscopic endonasal approach has revolutionized the management of ventral skull base tumors.
- Skull base chordomas are prone to endoscopic resection because of their midline location.
- Approach selection, technique, and nuances of the surgical management of skull base chordomas are discussed.

Videos of the transnasal/transseptal binostril approach to skull base lesions and the endoscopic endonasal approach to a skull base chordoma accompany this article at http://www.oto.theclinics.com/

INTRODUCTION

Chordoma is a rare primary bone tumor thought to arise from transformed notochord remnants[1] with an estimated incidence rate of 0.08 to 0.09 per 100,000.[2,3] It occurs

Financial Support, Industry Affiliations, Grants, and/or Financial Disclosures: A.C. Stamm receives book royalties from Thieme Medical Publishers. The other authors have nothing to disclose.
^a São Paulo Skull Base Center, Rua Afonso Brás, 525, cj. 13, São Paulo 04511-011, Brazil; ^b São Paulo ENT Center, Edmundo Vasconcelos Hospital, Rua Afonso Brás, 525, cj. 13, São Paulo 04511-011, Brazil; ^c DFVneuro Neurosurgical Group, Rua Dona Adma Jafet, 74, cj.121, São Paulo 01308-050, Brazil
* Corresponding author. Rua Afonso Brás, 525, Cj 13, São Paulo 04511-011, Brazil.
E-mail addresses: astamm@terra.com.br; cof@centrodeorl.com.br

most commonly in males with a peak incidence in their fourth to fifth decades of life and rarely affects children and adolescents.[2,4]

This type of tumor presents a predilection by the axial skeleton and may be encountered in the sacrum, mobile spine and skull base. Although it was historically assumed that chordomas were more common in the sacral region, data from the Surveillance, Epidemiology and End Results database show similar distribution among these three sites.[2] More recent analysis reports a slight predilection for the cranial region, where 42% of all chordomas might occur.[3]

Skull base chordomas (SBC) are essentially midline lesions that occur at the vicinity of the clivus (spheno-occipital bones) and represent only 0.15% of all intracranial tumors.[5] They are considered a low-malignancy neoplasm with slow growing pattern that rarely metastasizes. However, chordomas have a local aggressive behavior and high recurrence rates.[6–8] Treatment of SBC is complex and challenging and local control of the disease relies mainly on surgical excision of the tumor usually followed by high-dose radiation therapy for residual and/or recurrent lesions.[4,8–12]

The development of the expanded endoscopic endonasal approach (EEA) has improved surgical and prognostic results of SBC.[11,13,14] The EEA provides access to the entire ventral skull base from the frontal sinus to the second cervical vertebra in the sagittal plane and from the sella to the jugular foramen and occipital condyle in the coronal plane. This surgical technique has a particular importance in the management of ventral midline skull base tumors and it has definitely become a safe and reliable option on the armamentarium of skull base approaches.[15]

Defining the surgical approach to treat SBC depends basically on the patient's neurologic symptoms, location and extension of the tumor, and its relation to cranial nerves (CNs) and major vessels. Frequently, more than one surgical route may be necessary to achieve maximal tumor resection.[10,16,17]

Based on the clinical experience of our group and literature review, we highlight important aspects of approach selection, technique, and nuances of surgical management of SBC.

TREATMENT GOALS AND PLANNED OUTCOMES

Surgical treatment of SBC is challenging because of its location, local invasiveness, high recurrence rates, and proximity to critical neurovascular structures. Although gross total resection is one of the most important prognostic factors in cases of SBC, the benefits of total removal must always be balanced against the risks of an extensive and potentially morbid surgical dissection.[4,18,19] The two main goals of the treatment are to achieve gross total resection of the tumor, and to avoid surgical morbidity and mortality by minimizing manipulation and lesion of CNs, important arteries, and other vessels and by adequately closing the resulting skull base defect.[9,16,18–20]

SURGICAL TECHNIQUE AND PROCEDURE
Preoperative Planning

Radiologic evaluation
Radiologic investigation and preoperative planning for SBC has greatly improved because of rapidly evolving imaging methods. Computed tomography (CT) and magnetic resonance imaging (MRI) should always be performed in cases of suspected SBC for bone and soft tissue assessment, respectively. The combination of these two radiologic modalities permits the definition of important diagnostic and therapeutic characteristics of skull base tumors: radiologic appearance, location, extension, and relation to critical neurovascular structures.

SBCs typically present as midline extradural masses originating within bone and tend to expand posteriorly and laterally. They usually present as well-delineated soft tissue masses that may displace and compress adjacent structures. More advanced tumors show local invasiveness and characteristic bone destruction.

CT scans demonstrate best bone erosion, osteolysis, and intratumoral calcifications. There is typically no surrounding sclerosis. Moderate to marked heterogeneous enhancement following administration of iodinated contrast material can also be depicted (**Fig. 1**A).[21]

MRI is particularly reliable to evaluate tumor extension because it provides excellent tissue contrast and exquisite anatomic details. Most chordomas are hypointense or isointense on T1-weighted images. High signal correlates with hemorrhage or mucinous collection.[22] T2-weighted images characteristically demonstrate a high signal. Gadolinium enhancement is mostly heterogeneous and often presents a "honeycomb" appearance (**Fig. 1**B–D).[21,23]

Chondroid chordomas represent 5% to 15% of all chordomas and are characterized by the partial replacement of their gelatinous matrix by cartilaginous tissue.[9,24] Compared with typical chordomas, they normally present in a more lateral position

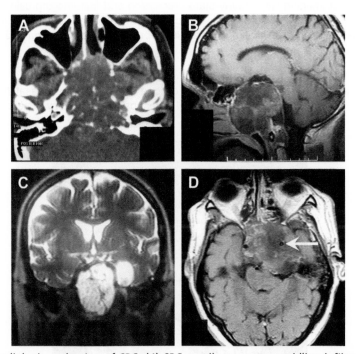

Fig. 1. Radiologic evaluation of SBC. (*A*) SBC usually presents as midline infiltrative and destructive lesions within the clival region on CT scans; osteolysis and intratumoral calcifications may also be evidenced. (*B*) Sagittal T1-weighted MRI depicts a large heterogeneous mass extending anteriorly to the nasal cavity and posteriorly to the posterior fossa, with low to iso signal intensity. (*C*) On coronal T2-weighted image this clival lesion presented high signal intensity and a bright appearance. (*D*) Axial T1-weighted image clearly shows the extension of the lesion and the complete encasement of internal carotid artery (ICA) on both sides (encased left ICA, *arrow*). This lesion was biopsied and histopathologic analysis confirmed the diagnosis of chordoma.

and intratumoral calcifications are more often evidenced on CT scans. Because of the differences in composition chondroid chordomas may not appear as bright as typical chordomas on T2-weighted MRIs. These findings are important prognostic factors because of significantly better survival rates of patients with chondroid chordomas.[8,21,25]

Tumor-vascular relationship

Angiographic studies (CT, MRI, or conventional) are also important whenever vascular compromise is suspected (**Fig. 2**). The presence of arterial displacement or encasement must be assessed before surgery so the dissection and debulking of the tumor can proceed safely. Arterial narrowing is highly suggestive of adventitia invasion, which hinders a total resection when the encased artery cannot be sacrificed. Despite not being routinely performed for SBC, conventional angiography studies may help to define whether sacrifice of an encased artery is possible or not by defining the patient's tolerance and collateral flow on balloon test occlusion.[20,21]

Tumor–cranial nerves relationship

The location and extension of the SBC determines the pattern of CN displacement and involvement, hence the surgical corridors available for tumor resection. New MRI technologies (fast imaging with steady-state precession and fast imaging using steady-state acquisition) now permit clear identification of the CN and its relationship to the skull base lesion, instead of simply assuming it based on the extension and position of the tumor.[26,27]

Approach selection

The main approaches to the skull base are divided into anterior (transbasal, transphenoidal, transoral, and EEA), anterolateral (pterional and orbitozygomatic), lateral

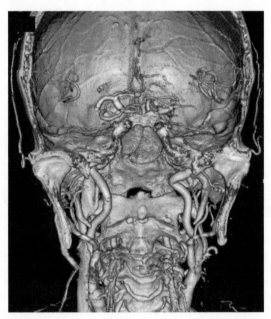

Fig. 2. Example of a CT-angiography scan. The anatomy, course, and caliber of major vessels are clearly depicted. Their relationship with skull base tumors and any other related lesions can also be evaluated.

(subtemporal and anterior petrosal), and posterolateral approaches (posterior petrosal, subocciptal retrosigmoid, and transcondylar). In the past decades, the microsurgical anterior approaches where gradually replaced by the expanded EEA. Because of the midline origin of the SBC, the endoscopic endonasal transclival approach (EETA) is frequently the first and best option when defining the surgical route. As a general rule, a second approach should always be considered in chordomas with lateral extension.[17,28,29]

Exceptions for not choosing the EETA as the first surgical route are inability to resolve the patient's main neurologic symptoms and complaints through the EETA, need for craniocervical junction stabilization/fusion, and impossibility to adequately reconstruct the resulting skull base defect.

Nasosinusal assessment

Once the EEA is included in the treatment plan of an SBC, the preoperative radiologic assessment of the nasosinusal region is imperative. A CT scan with thin slices (no more than 3 mm) with coronal, axial, and parasagittal images of the paranasal sinuses and skull base is crucial before surgery (**Box 1**).

Equipments and instrumentation

Adequate instrumentation is paramount for the EEA to the clivus and posterior fossa and its lack is considered a contraindication to performing the procedure (**Box 2**).

Patient Preparation and Positioning

The surgery is performed under hypotensive general anesthesia with total intravenous anesthetic agents, preferentially propofol and remifentanil. Routine prophylactic antibiotic is administered intravenously 30 to 60 minutes before surgery begins and an additional dose is administered if the procedure lasts more than 6 hours.[30]

Neuromuscular blockade must be avoided during the procedure when intraoperative neurophysiologic monitoring is anticipated. As a rule, CN VI, motor, and somatosensory evoked potentials must be monitored in all EEA to the posterior fossa. Monitoring the remaining CNs is performed according to the tumor size and location.

The patient is placed in a supine position on the operating table with dorsum elevated 30°, which might reduce bleeding during surgery and improve quality of the surgical field.[31,32] The neck is slightly flexed, and head extended 15° and turned toward the surgeon. Head must be secured in the anatomic position within a three-pin head holder if intraoperative neuronavigation is planned. Using magnetic material is prohibited in all cases if intraoperative MRI is to be performed.

Box 1
Evaluation of the nasosinusal region

- Nasal septum deviations
- Integrity and degree of aeration of the paranasal sinuses (particularly the sphenoid sinus)
- Location and presence of intersinus septae
- Presence of an Onodi cell
- Presence and extent of bone erosions, dehiscence, or hyperosteosis of the skull base
- Position of the internal carotid arteries (specially the paraclival segment)
- Thickness and incline of the clivus (basal angle)

> **Box 2**
> **Instrumentation for the EEA**
>
> *The equipment must include*
>
> - High-quality endoscopes: 0-, 45-, and 70-degree scopes; 5-mm 0-degree endoscope allows better visualization than the standard 4-mm scope
> - High-definition video equipment (camera and monitor)
> - Long and delicate drills with diamond burrs of various sizes
> - Long and delicate endoscopic bipolar forceps (**Fig. 3**)
> - Long and delicate dissection instruments
> - Adequate hemostatic material

Lateral aspect of the thigh and/or the inferior abdomen are prepared and draped for harvesting a fat and/or fascia lata graft for reconstruction of the skull base defect at the end of the procedure.

After adequately preparing and draping the patient, patties soaked in adrenaline 1:1000 are placed in the nasal cavity for 10 minutes before the surgical procedure begins.

Procedural Approach

Basic anatomic considerations: the clival region

The clivus (from the Latin, meaning "slope") separates the nasopharynx from the posterior cranial fossa. It is composed of the posterior portion of the sphenoid body (basisphenoid) and the basilar part of the occipital bone (basiocciput) and it is further subdivided into three parts: (1) the upper clivus is formed by the basisphenoid bone at the level of the sphenoid sinus and includes the dorsum sella, and the floor of the sella delineates its inferior limit; (2) the middle clivus corresponds to the rostral part of the basiocciput and it is located above a line connecting the caudal ends of the petroclival fissures, approximately at the level of the sphenoid sinus floor, and lateral limits are the internal carotid artery (ICA) protuberances; and (3) the lower clivus is formed by the caudal part of the basiocciput and is limited inferiorly by the foramen magnum.

Approaching the posterior fossa through the upper two-thirds of the clivus requires the opening of the sphenoid sinus. When the posterior fossa is approached through the lower clivus, bone removal may be done solely below the sphenoid floor.

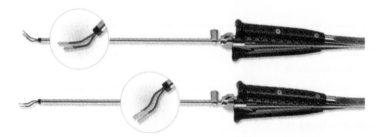

Fig. 3. Stamm skull base bipolar forceps. Example of long, delicate, and ergonomic bipolar forceps frequently used in skull base surgeries. Tips with varying angles facilitate their usage in different scenarios. (Permission granted by Integra LifeScience Corp., Plainsboro, NJ, USA.)

The intracranial surface of the upper two-thirds of the clivus faces the pons and is concave from side to side. The lower third lies in front of the medulla. There are two layers of dura overlying the inner surface of the clivus: the periosteal outer layer and the meningeal inner layer. The basilar venous plexus is located between these two layers at the level of the upper and middle clivus. It forms interconnecting venous channels between the inferior petrosal sinuses laterally, the cavernous sinuses superiorly, and the marginal sinus and epidural venous plexus inferiorly. The upper and middle clivus are separated from the petrous portion of the temporal bone on each side by the petroclival fissure. The abducens nerve (CN VI) arises from the pontomedullary junction and then runs superiorly over the petroclival fissure between the dural layers until it reaches and enters Dorello canal. Care must be taken not to injure this nerve when dissecting near the petroclival fissures (**Figs. 4–6**).[16,20]

Preparing the transnasal corridor

The surgical procedure is initiated with the combined transnasal/transseptal binostril approach (**Box 3**, Video 1).[16,20,33] Advantages of the transnasal/transseptal binostril access include that it allows two surgeons to simultaneously operate using both nostrils; it permits the harvesting of large mucosal flaps with robust pedicles, which aids the closure of skull base defects; and it permits the complete preservation of the nasosseptal mucosa on one side and thus avoids septal perforations.

Approaching the tumor

The clival bone is fully exposed and its removal is initiated with a high-speed drill with 5- to 6-mm diamond burrs and continued carefully with micro-Kerrison punches if

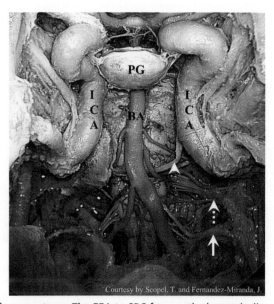

Courtesy by Scopel, T. and Fernandez-Miranda, J.

Fig. 4. Posterior fossa anatomy. The EEA to SBC frequently demands dissection of the clival region and posterior fossa. After extensively drilling bone, this beautiful anatomy is contemplated and important structures are pointed. Solid arrow indicates left hypoglossal nerve; dashed arrow points to the left lower cranial nerves (IX, X, and XI) reaching the jugular foramen; arrowhead indicates the left abducens (VI) nerve. BA, basilar artery; PG, pituitary gland. (*Courtesy of* Tiago Fernando Scopel, MD and Juan C. Fernandez-Miranda, MD, Pittsburgh, PA.)

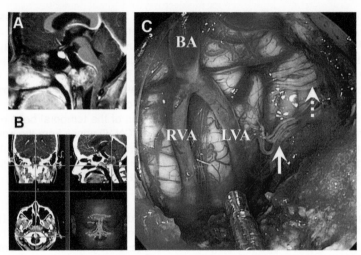

Fig. 5. A 15-year-old girl presented with a rounded and well-delimitated tumor within the lower clivus. The mass presented heterogeneous enhancement after contrast administration on T1-weighted MRI; it extended posteriorly, displacing the basilar artery and compressing the brainstem (*A*). Because of the midline location of the tumor, EEA was the best option. With the valuable aid of an intraoperative neuronavigation system inferior extension of the tumor and margins of surgical dissection could be clearly defined; the mass extended down to the level of the odontoid process (vertebra C2) (*B*). Intraoperative endoscopic view of the surgical field after gross total removal of the tumor (*C*). LVA, left vertebral artery; RVA, right vertebral artery; solid arrow, left hypoglossal nerve (XII) roots; dashed arrow, left lower cranial nerves (IX and X) roots; vertebrobasilar junction is lying immediately over pontomedullary sulcus. The patient did well after surgery and presented no neurologic deficits. Histopathologic and immunohistochemical analysis of the surgical specimen confirmed the diagnosis of skull base chordoma.

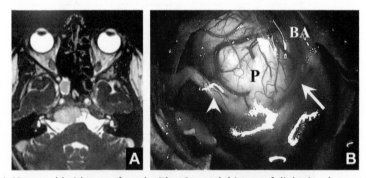

Fig. 6. A 13-year-old girl was referred with a 6-month history of diplopia when moving her gaze to the right. She had been submitted to a previous surgery for partial tumor removal and anatomopathologic analysis revealed a clivus chordoma. MRIs evidenced a well-delimitated mass in the middle clivus, extending laterally to the right petroclival fissure, where it stood posterior to the ipsilateral ICA (*A*). An EEA was then performed. The tumor was adherent to the right abducens (VI) nerve and dissection of its interdural segment was necessary. Intraoperative endoscopic view of the posterior fossa at the level of the middle clivus after partial removal of the tumor (*B*). P, pons; arrowhead, cisternal and interdural segments of the right VI nerve after dissection; arrow, right anterior inferior cerebellar artery. The patient's diplopia worsened discretely after surgery but no clinical abducens palsy/paresis was evident. Diplopia completely remitted 2 weeks after surgery.

Box 3
Combined transnasal/transseptal binostril approach

- Nasal septum is infiltrated with solution of ropivacaine 0.3% with adrenaline 1:100,000

- Septoplasty incision is made anteriorly and mucoperichondrial/mucoperiosteal flaps are elevated bilaterally

- Most of the septal cartilage and bone are removed and an L-shaped cartilaginous/bony strut must be preserved to support the nasal dorsum and tip

- The mucosal flaps are elevated posteriorly until both natural sphenoid ostia are completely exposed

- A large neurovascular pedicled nasoseptal flap is harvested with monopolar diathermy needle; the length and width of the flap must be generous and is defined according to the location, extension, and shape of the estimated skull base defect

- Nasoseptal flaps can be rotated posteriorly toward the rhinopharynx or safely placed into the maxillary sinus through a large maxillary antrostomy

- Turbinates are usually kept intact; middle and/or inferior turbinectomies might be necessary if the tumor extends too laterally and a transpterygoid approach is required

- A wide opening of the anterior sphenoid wall is created with micro-Kerrison rongeur and sphenoid rostrum can be drilled

- Delicate cutting forceps and 4- to 5-mm diamond burrs are used to carefully lower sinus septa and sphenoid floor

- The sinus mucosa that lies over the posterior sphenoid wall is reflected, exposing the clival bone

---

necessary (Video 2). Removing the involved clival bone not only permits access to the SBC itself, but also contributes to the complete resection and clearance of the tumor. The extent of bone removal must be tailored to the size and location of the lesion and, generally, bone removal and drilling must not be discontinued until healthy bone is reached.

The limits of a traditional transclival approach usually are superiorly (floor of the sella), inferiorly (craniocervical junction), and laterally (ICAs, hypoglossal canal, and occipital condyles). Micro-Doppler probes and/or an intraoperative navigation system are useful tools for the correct identification of the course of ICAs and other major arteries.

SBC that extends superiorly toward the interpeduncular cistern poses a greater challenge even for the more experienced skull base surgeons. Access to the retrosellar region might only be possible through pituitary transposition and posterior clinoidectomy, putting hypophyseal integrity and function at risk.[34] The transcavernous approach to the retrosellar region seems to be a good option for these cases.[35] Chordomas that extend inferiorly below the foramen magnum may still be treated through the endoscopic endonasal dissection down to the second cervical vertebral body. Nevertheless, a posterior occipital-cervical fusion may be necessary before the EEA if craniocervical junction instability is anticipated.

Adequate resection of SBC involves removal of the infiltrated bone, dura mater, and intradural component. Once the periosteal layer of the dura is incised, the basilar venous plexus and CN VI on each side are identified. Bleeding from the basilar plexus and venous sinuses cannot be cauterized safely but is usually controlled with packing with Spongostan Powder (Ethicon, Somerville, NJ). Large tumors often encroach on and obliterate much of the plexus, but if the lesion is not too large or if the plexus is not completely compressed, profuse and intense bleeding can occur. Judicious packing, time, patience, and experience are required to its adequate control.

The opening of the meningeal layer of the dura at the level of the middle and superior clivus must be accomplished with great care to avoid injury to the underlying basilar artery. Once the dura is opened, minor bleeding is stopped with bipolar cautery. It is finally possible to carefully introduce the zero-degree and angled endoscopes into the intradural space. Depending on the extent of the necessary surgical dissection it is then possible to identify the following posterior fossa structures (see **Figs. 4–6**): arteries (vertebral arteries, basilar artery and its perforating pontine branches, anteroinferior cerebellar arteries, superior cerebellar arteries, posterior cerebral arteries), brainstem and cerebellopontine angle, retrosellar region and mammillary bodies, and CNs II to XII.

Once the anatomy is appreciated, meticulous dissection is required to remove the tumor. To optimize the surgeon's view, persistent hemostasis of the tissues of the nasal cavity and sphenoid sinus needs to be maintained to minimize soiling of the endoscopes. Frequent irrigation and controlled suction with tip-protected cannulas are used to maintain the quality of the surgical field.

A four-handed microsurgical technique is used to resect the tumor. The limits of the tumor and normal anatomy must be identified. Because of the gelatinous nature of chordomas controlled suction is often sufficient for the debulking of the tumor. Microsurgical dissection around the tumor must be performed whenever possible to preserve the related structures.

Intraoperative MRI can be performed once the chordoma resection is thought to be complete. The patient is rescanned while still under general anesthesia and any residual tumor can be evidenced. Updated images can also be used for image guidance and intraoperative neuronavigation.[17]

Reconstruction

Repair of the skull base defect in the region of the clivus is challenging not only because of the size of the defect but also because of the high flow of cerebrospinal fluid (CSF), lack of supporting structures, and the effects of gravity. The main objective of the reconstruction is to provide complete separation between cranial and sinonasal cavities. When adequately performed, this prevents postoperative CSF leakage, pneumocephalus formation, and the occurrence of intracranial infection.[36] Skull base reconstruction is usually performed in a multilayer fashion and should always include a neurovascular pedicled mucosal flap (**Box 4**).[37,38]

Nuances and Pitfalls of the Technique

Major principles of the EEA to SBC include the following:

- The vidian nerves are important landmarks to the identification of the lacerum segment of the ICA
- Neuronavigation tools are helpful in defining the limits of bone removal, especially in cases where the pneumatization of the sphenoid sinus is not favorable or in reoperations
- Parapharyngeal ICA must be evaluated when approaching the inferior clival region
- It is recommend to leave a thin bone overlying the paraclival ICA as a protection during deep clival bone drilling
- The required bone drilling to create an adequate intradural exposure must be completely finished before opening the dura

---

Box 4
Skull base reconstruction performed in a multilayer fashion and including a neurovascular pedicled mucosal flap

- If the defect is too large, it must first be filled with abdominal fat and then covered with free grafts of fascia lata or a synthetic dural substitute

- Edges from the remaining dura should ideally overlap the graft to prevent displacement of the graft

- Over these grafts more fat grafts might be placed to regularize and to anteriorize the reconstruction plane

- Sphenopalatine artery pedicled mucosal flaps are then rotated and placed over the grafts securing them in place; nasoseptal flaps are often sufficient to completely close the skull base defect; situations where it is unavailable or insufficient require secondary pedicled flaps, such as the lateral nasal wall flap

- Mucosal edges of the flap should be in direct contact with denuded bone so that adherence and healing may occur more easily

- Fibrin glue and Surgicel patties (Johnson & Johnson, New Brunswick, NJ) are not typically necessary but may be used to help to hold the grafts and flaps in position

- Spongostan powder (Ethicon, Somerville, NJ) and Gelfoam (Pfizer, New York, NY) are layered directly over the flap, followed by packing with gauze soaked in antibiotic ointment

- The packing is then supported by a nasal tampon, such as RapidRhino 900 (Arthrocare, Austin, TX)

- Lumbar drainage is not routinely used; nevertheless, it must always be considered when high-flow CSF leak is identified intraoperatively; lumbar drain is usually kept in place for 3 to 5 days

- Broad-spectrum antibiotics are used for 10 days or as long as necessary

---

- Early VI CN identification is important for the complete dural opening and safe resection of the tumor (see **Fig. 6**)
- The inclination of the clivus (basal angle) must be considered when planning the skull base reconstruction; if the basal angle is obtuse, the nasosseptal flap may be short to cover the inferior region of the skull base defect
- Multilayer reconstruction of the posterior fossa is always imperative

COMPLICATIONS AND MANAGEMENT

The EEA to SBC carries potential risks of complications. CNs and blood vessels are especially at risk. Adoption of neurosurgical principles, detailed anatomic knowledge, and meticulous dissection of important structures are all required to avoid injuries.[39]

Generically, the complications are classified according to time of appearance as immediate or delayed and according to severity as minor and major. Immediate complications occur during surgery. The most frequent of these are intraoperative bleeding and injuries to the brain and CNs. Delayed complications include CSF leakage, meningitis, epistaxis, nasal synechiae, and infection.[40]

Minor complications present little morbidity and do not compromise the patient's life, although they may be annoying and troublesome. Most of the minor complications resolve with time and only conservative treatment is warranted. Major complications might represent significant morbidity and the possibility of mortality. Intracranial complications can result from direct injury to the brain, CNs, meninges, blood vessels, or venous sinuses. The resulting deficits are loss of function of the damaged structures (brain and/or CNs), loss of vascular supply to critical neurologic areas, and mass compressive effects (hematoma, others).

Through the EETA the following blood vessels are visualized and put at risk of damage and intraoperative bleeding:

- Maxillary, sphenopalatine arteries and their branches
- ICAs
- Basilar, vertebral arteries and their branches
- Small brainstem perforating arteries
- Venous sinuses of the skull base (basilar venous plexus and cavernous sinus)

CSF leakage can cause symptoms directly and predispose to meningitis and pneumocephalus. Pneumocephalus without evidence of CSF leaks are normal findings after EEA to skull base lesions and demand only careful observation.[41] The best management of postoperative CSF leaks depends on the severity of the leak. For minimum leaks, repeated lumbar punctures should relieve intracranial pressure and facilitate the healing of small skull base defects. However, for moderate to severe leaks nasal endoscopy and careful evaluation of the reconstructed skull base area is paramount. Surgical re-exploration is advised when large dehiscence areas are identified or suspected or the pedicled flap is irreversibly compromised (eg, a necrotic flap). Placement of a lumbar drain or a ventricular derivation should always be considered when there is evidence of high intracranial pressure.[40]

POSTPROCEDURAL CARE

A satisfactory postoperative result depends on appropriate operative technique and meticulous postoperative care. Wide-spectrum antibiotics are given during the operation and for 10 days postoperatively or until the nasal packing is removed. Adequate postoperative care of the surgical site requires appropriate instrumentation, including 4-mm, zero-degree, and 45-degree endoscopes; straight and curved atraumatic aspirators; and microforceps for outpatient debridement and follow-up.

- The anterior packing is removed within 5 to 7 days
- The ribbon gauze is removed after 10 to 14 days
- Vigilance is required in the postoperative period for CSF leaks and infections
- After the removing the packing the nasal cavity is carefully suctioned and any residual bony fragments are removed
- The patient is instructed to perform frequent nasal irrigations with buffered 0.9% saline solution

EXPECTED OUTCOMES AND CLINICAL RESULTS IN THE LITERATURE

Surgical outcomes and clinical results depend greatly on the experience of the involved surgical team.[28] Most of the available studies regarding the validity of EEA in the context of SBC are small and have short follow-up periods. They are also extremely heterogeneous in respect to patient inclusion criteria, treatment protocols, and methods of data collection, analysis and report. **Table 1** summarizes the findings of the most relevant studies to date. The results of our group are also shown.

SUMMARY

The EEA is the main surgical route used to resect SBC. Because of its midline origin, the EETA is frequently the first and best option. As a general rule, a second transcranial approach should always be considered in chordomas with lateral extension.

Table 1
Results of the most relevant studies to date on the validity of EEA for the treatment of SBC: surgical outcomes and clinical results

Author, Year	No. of Patients	Mean Age (y)	Male Gender (%)	Recurrent Lesions (%)	GTR Rate (%)	Postoperative Complications CSF Leak (%)	Meningitis (%)	New Neuropathy (%)	Mean F-U (mo)	Recurrence Rates (%)
Frank et al,[42] 2006	9	62	33	44	33	0	0	0	24	11
Zhang et al,[43] 2008	7	39	29	43	86	—[a]	—[a]	—[a]	20	14
Carrabba et al,[44] 2008	12	48	59	18	59	24	0	6	16	0
Hong Jiang et al,[45] 2009	12	39	33	—[a]	58	0	0	0	21	17
Solares et al,[46] 2010	4	43	—[a]	25	75	—[a]	—[a]	—[a]	15	25
Fraser et al,[47] 2010	7	52	71	14	71	0	0	0	18	14
Koutourousiou et al,[28] 2012	60	41	70	42	General: 67 Primary tumors: 83 Recurrent tumors: 44; 2003–2007, 36; 2008–2001, 89	27 → 16[b]	3	7	18	33
Tan et al,[48] 2012	14	48	57	50	General: 50 Primary tumors: 71 Recurrent tumors: 29	21 → 0[b]	0	0	42	15
Saito et al,[49] 2012	6	59	50	83	50	0	17	0	—[a]	—[a]
Chibbaro et al,[50] 2014	54	49	61	40	General: 65 Primary tumors: 88 Recurrent tumors: 30	8	14	0	34	11
Shidoh et al,[51] 2014	9	56	44	—[a]	33	11	22	0	—[a]	—[a]
Present group's experience 32 (updated data from Vellutini et al,[17] 2014)	32	43	66	44	47	22 → 9[b]	12	0	F-U range: 6 mo–12 y	—[a]

Abbreviations: F-U, follow-up; GTR, gross total removal.
[a] Data not available.
[b] Data before and after (→) introduction of the nasoseptal flap into skull base surgery.
Data from Refs.[17,28,42–51]

Endoscopic management of SBC requires anatomic knowledge, appropriate case selection, surgeon's experience, available resources, and surgical equipment.

SUPPLEMENTARY DATA

Supplementary data related to this article is found online at http://dx.doi.org/10.1016/j.otc.2015.09.011.

REFERENCES

1. Bouropoulou V, Bosse A, Roessner A, et al. Immunohistochemical investigation of chordomas: histogenetic and differential diagnostic aspects. Curr Top Pathol 1989;80:183–203.
2. McMaster ML, Goldstein AM, Bromley CM, et al. Chordoma: incidence and survival patterns in the United States, 1973-1995. Cancer Causes Control 2001;12(1):1–11.
3. Chambers KJ, Lin DT, Meier J, et al. Incidence and survival patterns of cranial chordoma in the United States. Laryngoscope 2014;124(5):1097–102.
4. Di Maio S, Temkin N, Ramanathan D, et al. Current comprehensive management of cranial base chordomas: 10-year meta-analysis of observational studies. J Neurosurg 2011;115(6):1094–105.
5. Sen C, Triana A. Cranial chordomas: results of radical excision. Neurosurg Focus 2001;10(3):E3.
6. Stüer C, Schramm J, Schaller C. Skull base chordomas: management and results. Neurol Med Chir (Tokyo) 2006;46(3):118–24.
7. Jones PS, Aghi MK, Muzikansky A, et al. Outcomes and patterns of care in adult skull base chordomas from the Surveillance, Epidemiology, and End Results (SEER) database. J Clin Neurosci 2014;21(9):1490–6.
8. Walcott BP, Nahed BV, Mohyeldin A, et al. Chordoma: current concepts, management, and future directions. Lancet Oncol 2012;13(2):e69–76.
9. Jahangiri A, Jian B, Miller L, et al. Skull base chordomas: clinical features, prognostic factors, and therapeutics. Neurosurg Clin N Am 2013;24(1):79–88.
10. Fernandez-Miranda JC, Gardner PA, Snyderman CH, et al. Clival chordomas: a pathological, surgical, and radiotherapeutic review. Head Neck 2014;36(6):892–906.
11. Koutourousiou M, Snyderman CH, Fernandez-Miranda J, et al. Skull base chordomas. Otolaryngol Clin North Am 2011;44(5):1155–71.
12. Amit M, Na'ara S, Binenbaum Y, et al. Treatment and outcome of patients with skull base chordoma: a meta-analysis. J Neurol Surg B Skull Base 2014;75(6):383–90.
13. Komotar RJ, Starke RM, Raper DMS, et al. The endoscope-assisted ventral approach compared with open microscope-assisted surgery for clival chordomas. World Neurosurg 2011;76(3–4):318–27.
14. Graffeo CS, Dietrich AR, Grobelny B, et al. A panoramic view of the skull base: systematic review of open and endoscopic endonasal approaches to four tumors. Pituitary 2014;17(4):349–56.
15. Prevedello DM, Doglietto F, Jane JA, et al. History of endoscopic skull base surgery: its evolution and current reality. J Neurosurg 2007;107(1):206–13.
16. Stamm AC, Balsalobre L, Hermann D, et al. Endonasal endoscopic approach to clival and posterior fossa chordomas. Oper Tech Otolaryngol Head Neck Surg 2011;22(4):274–80.

17. Vellutini Ede AS, Balsalobre L, Hermann DR, et al. The endoscopic endonasal approach for extradural and intradural clivus lesions. World Neurosurg 2014; 82(6 Suppl):S106–15.

18. Lanzino G, Dumont AS, Lopes MB, et al. Skull base chordomas: overview of disease, management options, and outcome. Neurosurg Focus 2001;10(3):E12.

19. Tzortzidis F, Elahi F, Wright D, et al. Patient outcome at long-term follow-up after aggressive microsurgical resection of cranial base chordomas. Neurosurgery 2006;59(2):230–7.

20. Stamm AC, Pignatari SSN, Vellutini E. Transnasal endoscopic surgical approaches to the clivus. Otolaryngol Clin North Am 2006;39(3):639–56.

21. Erdem E, Angtuaco EC, Van Hemert R, et al. Comprehensive review of intracranial chordoma. Radiographics 2003;23(4):995–1009.

22. Meyers SP, Hirsch WL, Curtin HD, et al. Chordomas of the skull base: MR features. AJNR Am J Neuroradiol 1992;13(6):1627–36.

23. Mohyeldin A, Prevedello DM, Jamshidi AO, et al. Nuances in the treatment of malignant tumors of the clival and petroclival region. Int Arch Otorhinolaryngol 2014; 18:157–72.

24. Chugh R, Tawbi H, Lucas DR, et al. Chordoma: the nonsarcoma primary bone tumor. Oncologist 2007;12(11):1344–50.

25. Stark AM, Mehdorn HM. Chondroid clival chordoma. N Engl J Med 2003; 349(10):e10.

26. Schmitz B, Hagen T, Reith W. Three-dimensional true FISP for high-resolution imaging of the whole brain. Eur Radiol 2003;13(7):1577–82.

27. Mikami T, Minamida Y, Yamaki T, et al. Cranial nerve assessment in posterior fossa tumors with fast imaging employing steady-state acquisition (FIESTA). Neurosurg Rev 2005;28(4):261–6.

28. Koutourousiou M, Gardner PA, Tormenti MJ, et al. Endoscopic endonasal approach for resection of cranial base chordomas: outcomes and learning curve. Neurosurgery 2012;71(3):614–24.

29. Benet A, Prevedello DM, Carrau RL, et al. Comparative analysis of the transcranial "far lateral" and endoscopic endonasal "far medial" approaches: surgical anatomy and clinical illustration. World Neurosurg 2014;81(2):385–96.

30. Holloway KL, Smith KW, Wilberger JE, et al. Antibiotic prophylaxis during clean neurosurgery: a large, multicenter study using cefuroxime. Clin Ther 1996; 18(1):84–94.

31. Thongrong C, Kasemsiri P, Carrau RL, et al. Control of bleeding in endoscopic skull base surgery: current concepts to improve hemostasis. ISRN Surg 2013; 2013:e191543.

32. Ko M-T, Chuang K-C, Su C-Y. Multiple analyses of factors related to intraoperative blood loss and the role of reverse Trendelenburg position in endoscopic sinus surgery. Laryngoscope 2008;118(9):1687–91.

33. Stamm AC, Pignatari S, Vellutini E, et al. A novel approach allowing binostril work to the sphenoid sinus. Otolaryngol-Head Neck Surg 2008;138(4):531–2.

34. Kassam AB, Prevedello DM, Thomas A, et al. Endoscopic endonasal pituitary transposition for a transdorsum sellae approach to the interpeduncular cistern. Neurosurgery 2008;62(3 Suppl 1):57–72.

35. Fernandez-Miranda JC, Gardner PA, Rastelli MM, et al. Endoscopic endonasal transcavernous posterior clinoidectomy with interdural pituitary transposition. J Neurosurg 2014;121(1):91–9.

36. Snyderman CH, Kassam AB, Carrau R, et al. Endoscopic reconstruction of cranial base defects following endonasal skull base surgery. Skull Base 2007;17(1):73–8.

37. Hadad G, Bassagasteguy L, Carrau RL, et al. A novel reconstructive technique after endoscopic expanded endonasal approaches: vascular pedicle nasoseptal flap. Laryngoscope 2006;116(10):1882–6.
38. Patel MR, Taylor RJ, Hackman TG, et al. Beyond the nasoseptal flap: outcomes and pearls with secondary flaps in endoscopic endonasal skull base reconstruction. Laryngoscope 2014;124(4):846–52.
39. Prevedello DM, Ditzel Filho LFS, Solari D, et al. Expanded endonasal approaches to middle cranial fossa and posterior fossa tumors. Neurosurg Clin N Am 2010; 21(4):621–35.
40. Ransom ER, Chiu AG. Prevention and management of complications in intracranial endoscopic skull base surgery. Otolaryngol Clin North Am 2010;43(4): 875–95.
41. Banu MA, Szentirmai O, Mascarenhas L, et al. Pneumocephalus patterns following endonasal endoscopic skull base surgery as predictors of postoperative CSF leaks. J Neurosurg 2014;121(4):961–75.
42. Frank G, Sciarretta V, Calbucci F, et al. The endoscopic transnasal transsphenoidal approach for the treatment of cranial base chordomas and chondrosarcomas. Neurosurgery 2006;59(1 Suppl 1):ONS50–7.
43. Zhang Q, Kong F, Yan B, et al. Endoscopic endonasal surgery for clival chordoma and chondrosarcoma. ORL J Otorhinolaryngol Relat Spec 2008;70(2):124–9.
44. Carrabba G, Dehdashti AR, Gentili F. Surgery for clival lesions: open resection versus the expanded endoscopic endonasal approach. Neurosurg Focus 2008;25(6):E7.
45. Hong Jiang W, Ping Zhao S, Hai Xie Z, et al. Endoscopic resection of chordomas in different clival regions. Acta Otolaryngol 2009;129(1):71–83.
46. Solares CA, Grindler D, Luong A, et al. Endoscopic management of sphenoclival neoplasms: anatomical correlates and patient outcomes. Otolaryngol-Head Neck Surg 2010;142(3):315–21.
47. Fraser JF, Nyquist GG, Moore N, et al. Endoscopic endonasal minimal access approach to the clivus: case series and technical nuances. Neurosurgery 2010;67(3 Suppl Operative):ons150–8.
48. Tan NC-W, Naidoo Y, Oue S, et al. Endoscopic surgery of skull base chordomas. J Neurol Surg B Skull Base 2012;73(6):379–86.
49. Saito K, Toda M, Tomita T, et al. Surgical results of an endoscopic endonasal approach for clival chordomas. Acta Neurochir (Wien) 2012;154(5):879–86.
50. Chibbaro S, Cornelius JF, Froelich S, et al. Endoscopic endonasal approach in the management of skull base chordomas: clinical experience on a large series, technique, outcome, and pitfalls. Neurosurg Rev 2014;37(2):217–24.
51. Shidoh S, Toda M, Kawase T, et al. Transoral vs. endoscopic endonasal approach for clival/upper cervical chordoma. Neurol Med Chir (Tokyo) 2014;54(12):991–8.

Sinonasal Malignancies of Anterior Skull Base

Histology-driven Treatment Strategies

Paolo Castelnuovo, MD[a,b], Mario Turri-Zanoni, MD[a,b,*],
Paolo Battaglia, MD[a,b], Paolo Antognoni, MD[c], Paolo Bossi, MD[d],
Davide Locatelli, MD[b,e]

KEYWORDS

- Radiotherapy • Chemotherapy • Endoscopic endonasal • Paranasal sinuses
- Skull base cancer • Olfactory neuroblastoma • Adenocarcinoma
- Mucosal melanoma

KEY POINTS

- Endoscopic endonasal surgery represents an oncologically sound alternative to open surgery in selected patients with sinonasal malignancies with lower morbidity, faster recovery, and better quality-of-life outcomes.
- A correct diagnosis by means of histology, immunohistochemistry, or molecular biology represents the key factor for initiating an appropriate treatment strategy.
- Integration of multimodal treatment strategies, including different regimens of chemotherapy, photon, and heavy-ion radiotherapy, is able to improve survival rates, especially for high-grade and advanced-stage tumors.
- Cooperation in a multidisciplinary oncologic skull base team is mandatory to offer patients the best treatment options, and to minimize complications and failures.

Conflicts of interest: The authors certify that they have no conflict of interest or financial relationship with any entity mentioned in this article. No sponsorships or grants were received.
[a] Unit of Otorhinolaryngology, Department of Biotechnology and Life Sciences (DBSV), Ospedale di Circolo e Fondazione Macchi, University of Insubria, via Guicciardini 9, Varese 21100, Italy; [b] Department of Biotechnology and Life Sciences (DBSV), Head and Neck Surgery & Forensic Dissection Research Center (HNS&FDRc), University of Insubria, via Guicciardini 9, Varese 21100, Italy; [c] Division of Radiation Oncology, University of Insubria, viale Borri 57, Varese 21100, Italy; [d] Head and Neck Cancer Medical Oncology Unit, Fondazione IRCCS Istituto Nazionale dei Tumori, via Venezian 1, Milano 20133, Italy; [e] Unit of Neurosurgery, University of Insubria, via Guicciardini 9, Varese 21100, Italy
* Corresponding author. Unit of Otorhinolaryngology, Ospedale di Circolo e Fondazione Macchi, University of Insubria, via Guicciardini 9, Varese 21100, Italy.
E-mail address: tzmario@inwind.it

Otolaryngol Clin N Am 49 (2016) 183–200
http://dx.doi.org/10.1016/j.otc.2015.09.012
0030-6665/16/$ – see front matter © 2016 Elsevier Inc. All rights reserved.

oto.theclinics.com

INTRODUCTION

Sinonasal tumors are rare diseases, accounting for 3% to 5% of head and neck malignant neoplasms and the 0.2% to 0.8% of all tumors.[1] There are several histologic subtypes with different natural histories. The most frequent tumors of this region have epithelial origin and poor prognosis, such as squamous cell carcinoma, intestinal-type adenocarcinoma (ITAC), undifferentiated carcinoma, and neuroendocrine carcinoma (NEC). Although there are several staging systems, none are ideal or universally used. However, stage at presentation is generally highly predictive of survival and, despite a maximum treatment of the primary tumor, local, regional, or distant recurrences can occur even after many years.[2] From a surgical standpoint, the introduction of craniofacial resection (CFR) in the 1960s represented a significant advance in the care of these patients and has served as the mainstay for their treatment for the past 50 years.[3] However, this approach has been associated with perioperative mortality and major complications in 0% to 13% and 35% to 63% of patients, respectively.[4] The advances in endoscopy have revolutionized the management of sinonasal and skull base lesions. Many complex cancers that traditionally required open approaches are now amenable to purely endoscopic endonasal resection, providing less invasive surgery with lower morbidity but with comparable oncologic outcomes in terms of survival rates.[5] The endoscopic endonasal approach has become accepted with precise indications for the treatment of selected skull base cancers. Therefore, at present, external traditional and endoscopic approaches should not be considered as two competing techniques, but rather as different approaches useful for suitable cases, performed in centers with extensive experience, according to the oncologic principle of radicality. At present, the surgical strategy has to be driven by the cancer histology and its extension rather than the available surgical expertise and equipment, and therefore surgeons have to be equally comfortable in managing patients by open craniofacial as well as endoscopic approaches.[6] So far, no standard and uniform protocols of treatment of such aggressive tumors have been reported, given their rarity, heterogeneity in histology and stages of diseases, and in the absence of prospective studies. Surgery followed by radiotherapy (RT) has been generally adopted as the usual treatment strategy. However, some studies also explored the role and feasibility of induction chemotherapy and the prognostic value of the response to it in several histotypes.[7,8] Recently, heavy-ion therapy using proton or carbon ion beams has been introduced in the treatment of these tumors as exclusive therapy or in the postoperative setting with encouraging outcomes.[9] Proton/carbon ion beam therapy, compared with conventional photon therapy, provides a more accurate and intense dose to the tumor area, with potentially greater control of disease.[10] Moreover, this therapy may produce less toxic side effects in particularly critical areas exposed to late RT toxicities and potentially can help in organ preservation strategies for locally advanced cases, especially to avoid orbital exenteration.[11] In this scenario, even in the absence of prospective data, the integration of multiple modalities of treatment tailored to the histology; molecular profile; and, in selected cases, to the response to induction chemotherapy seems to be the best approach for these rare and aggressive cancers.[12] This article discusses the current evidence for the multimodal management of sinonasal and anterior skull base (ASB) cancers, focusing on the different treatment protocols driven by histologic subtypes. Preoperative work-up, indications and exclusion criteria, surgical techniques, and postoperative management are analyzed. Oncologic outcomes stratified according to histology are presented and future directions for the management of these cancers are discussed.

DIAGNOSTIC WORK-UP

Diagnosis is often made late because these tumors are asymptomatic or produce nonspecific symptoms in their early stages. Nasal endoscopy under local anesthesia can help to determine the site and extent of the tumor. Computed tomography (CT) and contrast-enhanced MRI can provide information on the exact location and the extent of the disease. In many cases, both imaging modalities are necessary for an accurate treatment plan. After imaging, an endoscopic-assisted biopsy of the sinonasal lesion is mandatory in order to clearly identify the specific histotype of cancer. What seems to be crucial is reaching the correct histologic diagnosis considering that histology and molecular pattern of the tumor can guide the type of treatment to be administered. For this reason, when dealing with rare and particularly aggressive histotypes, a second histopathologic opinion is mandatory for confirming or reaching the correct diagnosis. Before planning the treatment, complete staging of the patient is advisable. To this end, ultrasonography examination of the neck and contrast-enhanced CT scan of the chest and abdomen are performed to rule out regional or systemic dissemination of the disease. In contrast, a total body PET-CT scan is preferred in cases of aggressive histotypes (ie, sarcoma, malignant melanoma, undifferentiated and NEC) and for advanced-stage lesions.

MULTIDISCIPLINARY TREATMENT PROTOCOLS

The multimodal treatment protocols currently available are tailored for specific histologic subtypes.

Squamous Cell Carcinoma

This is the most common tumor of the sinonasal tract in the United States, originating in approximately 60% of cases from the maxillary sinus. The standard treatment of this tumor is radical surgery followed by adjuvant intensity-modulated radiotherapy (IMRT).[12–14] Elective irradiation of the neck should be considered for locally advanced lesion (T3–T4) because of the frequency of cervical lymph node metastases (23%).[1] Platinum-based adjuvant chemoradiotherapy is generally used only in cases of positive margins after surgery and for pathologic evidence of neural or lymphovascular invasion.[1] When dealing with poorly differentiated squamous cell carcinoma in advanced stages (T3–T4), induction chemotherapy regimens including mainly a combination of a taxane and platinum followed by surgery and adjuvant (chemo)radiation or by definitive (chemo)radiation showed promising results. In the MD Anderson Cancer Center experience with 46 consecutive cases, a partial or complete response to this induction chemotherapy protocol was observed in 67% of patients and it was predictive of treatment outcome and prognosis.[7]

Adenocarcinoma

This is the most common mucosal epithelial malignancy in Europe, occurring predominantly in the ethmoid sinuses (85%) and olfactory region (13%). Men develop adenocarcinoma 4 times more frequently than women, implying an occupational hazard related to wood and leather dusts exposure.[15] This finding also explains the multifocality of tumors observed in different mucosal area of the nasal cavities, even distant to each other, especially for ITAC. For this reason, a bilateral ethmoid labyrinth resection is always recommended, because the contralateral ethmoid may be exposed to the same carcinogenic risk factors as the neoplastic nasal fossa (**Fig. 1**).[15,16] Surgery is the mainstay for the treatment of such cancers. Endoscopic endonasal surgery is effective as a single treatment modality for early-stage (T1–T2) low-grade lesions,

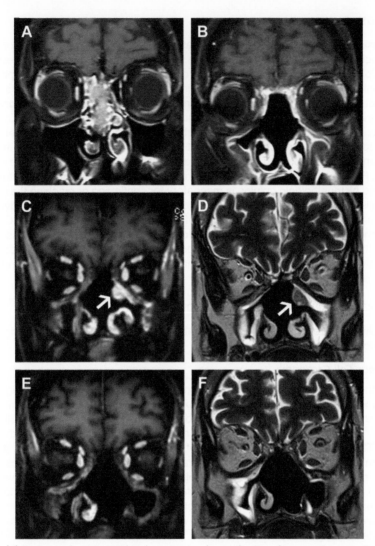

Fig. 1. (*A*) Preoperative T1-weighted contrast-enhanced coronal magnetic resonance (MR) scan showing right ethmoid ITAC. The patient underwent an endoscopic resection with transnasal craniectomy followed by adjuvant IMRT (70 Gy). The lesion was staged pT3N0M0. Two-year postoperative contrast-enhanced MR scan was free of disease (*B*). Four-year postoperative contrast-enhanced coronal MR scan T1 (*C*) and T2 (*D*) weighted showed a local recurrence of disease (*white arrows*) localized on the left papyracea (contralateral to the primary tumor). The recurrence was treated surgically through an endoscopic endonasal approach. Six-year postoperative contrast-enhanced coronal MR scan T1 (*E*) and T2 (*F*) weighted was clear, without evidence of recurrences.

radically resected with negative margins. In contrast, postoperative IMRT improves survival rates for high-grade sinonasal adenocarcinomas (G3, signet-ring variant, solid type) regardless of the stage of disease at presentation. The role of adjuvant IMRT is also widely accepted for advanced-stage lesions (T3–T4) and in the presence of positive surgical margins.[17] Given the possibility of tumor spread to leptomeninges at diagnosis or late during the follow-up, a prophylactic brain irradiation could be considered in high-grade lesions with intracranial invasion.[18] Elective treatment of the neck lymph nodes is not routinely performed in sinonasal adenocarcinoma because the risk of regional metastases is low (7%).[1] Moreover, in the presence of advanced-stage ITAC (T3–T4), a chemotherapy regimen based on cisplatin, fluorouracil, and leucovorin followed by surgery and radiation has been proposed for tumors with functional p53 protein, being highly effective with promising results in terms of disease-free survival.[8]

Olfactory Neuroblastoma

Olfactory neuroblastoma (ONB) arises from the neural-epithelial olfactory mucosa. The mainstay treatment of ONB generally comprises radical surgical resection.[19] In our experience, surgical excision should include the dura of the ASB together with the ipsilateral olfactory bulb in every case, not only to obtain a free-margins resection of the disease but also for staging purposes.[19] The removal of both olfactory bulbs is performed only for bilaterally extended cancers. Postoperative irradiation has been shown to reduce local recurrence rates and improve survival, so it is recommended in all cases, irrespective of extent of disease at diagnosis.[19–21] Radiation treatment is typically delivered using IMRT, which provides optimal sparing of radiation dose to sensitive normal structures, such as the optic nerve or brain. The recent introduction of intensity-modulated proton beam radiation therapy (IMPBRT) deserves particular mention, showing promising results for the management of ONB both as exclusive primary therapy and in the postoperative setting.[22] Cervical lymph node metastases are infrequent at presentation for patients diagnosed with ONB, with reported rates between 5% and 12%. However, given the high reported rates of late regional failures and limited morbidity-associated IMRT, elective neck radiation may warrant consideration in patients with intracranial disease at presentation (Kadish C).[20,21] Particular attention should be paid to Hyams grading, which accurately characterizes tumor biology and represents an independent predictor of locoregionally recurrence of disease and overall survival (OS).[20] For this reason, it is a valuable asset to consider when contemplating adjuvant or neoadjuvant therapies. In detail, poorly differentiated ONB, namely Hyams grade IV lesions, presenting in locally advanced stages (T3–T4), could benefit from different regimens of induction chemotherapy (etoposide/cisplatin[23] or cyclophosphamide/vincristine[24]) to improve both disease control and survival rates; however, the existing data do not provide any definitive indication in this field.

Neuroendocrine Carcinoma: Small Cell and Large Cell Types

Sinonasal NEC is a highly aggressive tumor, usually presenting at advanced stages, developing a broad range of systemic metastases (47.6% of patients) in a short interval of time, without significant possibilities for cure and a dismal prognosis. For such cancer, aggressive multimodal therapy seems to be the most effective approach, although survival remains poor. Recent data reported that neoadjuvant chemotherapy mainly consisting of etoposide and cisplatin followed by surgical resection and adjuvant IMRT or IMPBRT could be effective, improving survival outcomes and reducing recurrence rates, therefore its standard use was recommended for these patients.[25,26] Moreover, the response to such induction chemotherapy can also represent a strong prognostic factor.[26]

Sinonasal Undifferentiated Carcinoma

This is a highly aggressive carcinoma of uncertain histogenesis, with or without neuroendocrine differentiation, typically presenting with locally extensive disease and showing a greater tendency to metastasize compared with conventional squamous cell carcinoma. From a histopathologic viewpoint, sinonasal undifferentiated carcinoma (SNUC) may be difficult to distinguish from high-grade ONB and sinonasal NEC.[27] The nuances of differentiating these neoplasms are not merely academic because there are significant differences in prognosis and treatment strategies. Given the advanced stage of disease at presentation, high incidence of distant failure, and its chemosensitivity, neoadjuvant chemotherapy followed by either chemoradiation or surgery followed by postoperative IMRT shows promise for ideal management of SNUC.[28,29]

Hemangiopericytoma

This is a rare tumor of vascular origin with low risk of malignancy and distant metastasis but with a strong tendency to recur locally. The mainstay of treatment is wide surgical excision with clear resection margins as a single treatment modality, because the tumors are fairly radioresistant and chemoresistant.[30]

Adenoid Cystic Carcinoma

Sinonasal adenoid cystic carcinoma (ACC) is salivary gland tumor with high propensity for perineural spread (eg, trigeminal branches) and bony invasion, which can lead to significant skull base involvement and intracranial extension, including cavernous sinus and middle cranial fossa. Surgery combined with postoperative radiation provides the best OS in such patients.[31] The goal of surgery is to radically resect the lesion whenever feasible; however, also the debulking of the gross volume of the tumor mass may make sense when dealing with this kind of cancer. The rationale for adjuvant irradiation may be to clear positive margins (microscopic or macroscopic) that are left after surgery. Postoperative radiation may be delivered using conventional photon radiotherapy (eg, IMRT) or taking advantage of recently introduced particle therapy, especially carbon ion therapy, which showed promising rates of local control of the disease not only in the postoperative setting but also for inoperable cases.[32] Pretreatment methionine-PET can be useful for predicting the therapeutic efficacy of heavy-particle therapy for these patients.[33] Globally, although local recurrences develop in a significant percentage of patients (65%), survival from ACC exceeds that of the other sinonasal cancers.[31]

Mesenchymal Tumors: Soft Tissue Sarcomas and Ewing Sarcoma

In these patients the first treatment strategy is generally chemotherapy, with or without radiotherapy, leaving the surgical option only for nonresponders or in case of recurrence of disease.[34] Specific treatment strategies can be adopted for Ewing sarcoma, particularly affecting children between 7 and 15 years of age. At present, neoadjuvant chemotherapy followed by radical surgery and adjuvant irradiation (brachytherapy or conventional IMRT) seems to be the best treatment option for this subset of young patients.[35] In this regard, a treatment regimen including vincristine, ifosfamide, doxorubicin, and etoposide followed by complete endoscopic resection and brachytherapy was described with promising results (AMORE framework: Ablative surgery, MOulage brachytherapy and REconstruction).[36]

Hematolymphoid Tumors

The role of surgery for such tumors is only to obtain a proper histologic diagnosis in order to guide the appropriate regimen of chemotherapy and/or radiation therapy.[37] For this reason, a minimally invasive endoscopic endonasal approach is paramount in order to minimize the surgical morbidity for the patients. Surgery may also be useful in the posttreatment setting to exclude persistence of disease whenever a radiological suspect needs to be proved.

Mucosal Melanoma

Surgery with curative or palliative intent is considered the primary treatment of choice for sinonasal mucosal melanoma (MM).[38,39] Minimally invasive endoscopic approaches are generally associated with better survival rates than those obtained with mutilating external surgeries. In this regard, Lund and colleagues[38] hypothesized that aggressive surgery might cause severe disturbances in immunobalance and, consequently, may promote dramatic recurrence and/or explain cases with rapid systemic dissemination.

The indication for adjuvant IMRT is debated, with several studies reporting that postoperative IMRT improves only local control of disease without affecting survival.[38,39] For this reason, at present, adjuvant IMRT is generally delivered only in the presence of involved surgical margins. Particle therapies such as carbon ion irradiation have emerged in the last few years as effective options, improving survival outcomes of this serious disease. However, future large-scale studies are necessary to validate these preliminary results.[40] In addition, in the presence of metastatic spread of disease, selected cancer-specific molecular abnormalities might lead to the development of tailored targeted therapies; for example, by using inhibitors of KIT and mitogen-activated protein kinase pathways, which are currently under intense investigation.[39]

SURGICAL APPROACHES
Indications and Contraindications

From a surgical perspective, the degree of intracranial extension and orbital involvement have been shown to be independent prognostic factors and are also the determinants of whether an entirely endoscopic endonasal approach is possible.[41,42] However, a combination of endoscopic endonasal technique with subfrontal craniotomy is an effective option for extensive tumors with anterior or lateral involvement of the frontal sinus, infiltration of the dura far over the orbital roof, or with extensive infiltration of the brain.[43] For this reason, all patients scheduled for a purely endoscopic endonasal approach must be informed about the possibility of switching to a combined cranioendoscopic resection (CER), even intraoperatively, if deemed necessary. The currently indications and contraindications for these minimally invasive approaches are detailed in **Table 1**. Patients were considered inoperable in the presence of massive infiltration of the orbital apex, cavernous sinus involvement, and internal carotid artery encasement.

Preparation and Patient Positioning

The endoscopic transnasal approaches require adequate instrumentation for a correct procedure. The surgical set should include several dissectors of different sizes, and delicate scissors of different angles. Delicate bipolar forceps with straight and angled tips can be very useful. Moreover, an intraoperative magnetic navigation system is strongly advisable. Patients are placed in anti-Trendelenburg position, under general anesthesia. A perioperative prophylactic antibiotic regimen including third-generation cephalosporin is used. Some minutes before surgery, the nasal cavities are packed with cottonoids soaked in 2% oxymetazoline, 1% oxybuprocaine, and adrenaline (1:100,000) solution to reduce bleeding and improve transnasal operative spaces.

Surgical Techniques

According to the site of origin, extension, and tumor histology, the endoscopic resection can be performed unilaterally (resection extended anteroposteriorly from the

Table 1
Indications and contraindications for the endoscopic endonasal management of sinonasal and ASB malignancies

Indications	Contraindications
Ethmoid cancer involving lamina papyracea, cribriform plate, or roof of the ethmoid	Infiltration in nasal bones, palate, skin, and subcutaneous tissue
Lesions involving the medial portion of the frontal sinus	Massive involvement of the frontal sinus
Lesions vegetating in the sphenoid or involving maxillary sinus (medial, superior, and posterior walls)	Erosion of lateral, anterior, or inferior bony walls of the maxillary sinus
Involvement of nasolacrimal duct or medial wall of the lacrimal sac	Massive involvement of the lacrimal pathway
Pterygopalatine fossa invasion and limited infratemporal fossa extension	Massive infratemporal fossa extension
Periorbital layer invasion	Orbit content infiltration
Infiltration of ASB dura or olfactory bulbs	Massive infiltration of the dura over the orbital roof or brain parenchyma infiltration

posterior wall of the frontal sinus to the planum sphenoidale and laterolaterally from the nasal septum to the lamina papyracea) or bilaterally (resection extended from one lamina papyracea to the opposite one).[44] The previous focus of oncologic surgery on en-bloc resection to avoid the risk of tumor spilling is now debated, gradually being replaced by the concept of disassembling the lesion, having under view the limits between normal and diseased mucosa. The step-by-step technique of endoscopic endonasal resection (EER) is summarized later.

Tumor origin identification
The lesion is gradually debulked starting from the core, in order to identify its site of origin. In this phase, it is crucial to preserve the surrounding anatomic structures, because these are useful landmarks for orientating the subsequent surgical steps.

Exposure of the surgical field
Removal of the posterior two-thirds of the nasal septum is performed to gain better exposure of the surgical field and to optimize the endonasal maneuverability of dedicated instruments, using the 2-nostrils 4-hands technique. In this step, a wide sphenoidotomy with removal of intersinus septum and sphenoid rostrum is crucial to expose the posteroinferior margin of the dissection. The frontal sinus is approached by Draf type IIb sinusotomy in the case of monolateral EER, whereas Draf type III median sinusotomy is performed if the EER involves both sides. The frontal sinusotomy represents the anterosuperior margin of the dissection, allowing precise identification of the beginning of the anterior cranial fossa.

Centripetal removal
Once the posteroinferior and anterosuperior margins of the resection are exposed, a subperiosteal dissection of the nasoethmoidal-sphenoidal complex is performed unilaterally or bilaterally (according to the extension of disease), to expose the lateral margins.[44] The lamina papyracea is included in the dissection when the tumor is in close proximity to or frankly involved in it. When required by the extension of disease, an endoscopic medial maxillectomy can be performed, to achieve good control of the

whole maxillary sinus. This surgical phase has to be associated with nasolacrimal duct exposure and resection, just below the lacrimal sac. Superiorly, the dissection is continued in the anteroposterior direction, by resecting the olfactory fibers and the basal lamella of the ethmoidal turbinate, to mobilize the monoblock. The entire nasoethmoidal-sphenoidal complex is then isolated and pushed toward the central part of the nasal fossa (centripetal technique) to extract it transorally or through the nasal vestibule.[44] The surgical margins are checked by frozen section and, if necessary, the dissection is continued until free margins are obtained.

Skull base removal
According to the extension of the disease, the EER can be extended to include the ASB as well (endoscopic resection with transnasal craniectomy).[45] The ethmoid roof is exposed using a drill with a diamond burr (**Fig. 2**A). The anterior and posterior ethmoidal arteries are identified, cauterized, and divided. The crista galli is carefully detached from the dura and removed with blunt instruments, preserving the integrity of the dural layer (**Fig. 2**B).

Intracranial work
The key point for subsequently performing an optimal skull base reconstruction is to properly dissect the epidural space over the orbital roofs laterally, the planum

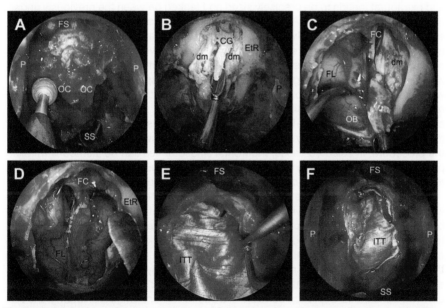

Fig. 2. Step-by-step endoscopic resection with transnasal craniectomy of a sinonasal malignancy encroaching on the ASB. (*A*) After removing the ethmoidal box bilaterally, the ethmoid roof is exposed using a drill with a diamond burr; (*B*) crista galli removal, preserving the integrity of the dural layer; (*C*) transnasal resection of the dural layer together with the right olfactory bulb affected by the tumor; (*D*) bilateral resection of the ASB dura from the frontal sinuses back to the sphenoid and from one papyracea to the other; (*E*) skull base reconstruction using a free graft of iliotibial tract placed intradurally (first layer); (*F*) the second layer of iliotibial tract was placed in the epidural gap. CG, crista galli; dm, dura mater; EtR, ethmoidal roof; FC, falx cerebri; FL, frontal lobe; FS, frontal sinus; ITT, free graft of autologous iliotibial tract; OB, olfactory bulb; OC, olfactory cleft; P, papyracea; SS, sphenoid sinuses.

sphenoidale posteriorly, and the posterior wall of the frontal sinus anteriorly before starting the resection of the dura. The dura is then incised and circumferentially cut with angled scissors or a dedicated scalpel, far enough away from the suspected area of tumor spread (**Fig. 2**C, D). The falx cerebri is clipped in the anterior portion before its resection, to avoid sagittal sinus bleeding; then its posterior portion at the level of the sphenoethmoidal planum is resected. The arachnoid plane over the intracranial portion of the tumor is then dissected and separated from the brain parenchyma. The specimen, including the residual tumor, the ASB, and the overlying dura, together with 1 or both of the olfactory bulbs, is removed transnasally. The dural margins are sent for frozen sections. With small tumors, the dural resection can be performed by leaving the ethmoidal complex attached to the skull base at the level of the olfactory grooves in a monoblock fashion.

Skull Base Reconstruction

The resulting skull base defect is reconstructed by the endoscopic endonasal multi-layer technique, performed preferably using autologous materials. In our experience, the fascia lata and/or the iliotibial tract possess the best characteristics in terms of thickness, pliability, and strength.[45] For the first intradural layer of duraplasty, the graft has to be at least 30% larger than the dural defect and split anteriorly on the midline to adjust to the falx cerebri in case of bilateral resection.[45] The second layer, intracranial and extradural, needs to be precisely sized and tacked between the previously under-mined dura and the residual ASB bone (**Fig. 2**E, F). Pieces of fatty tissue are placed to eliminate the dead space between the second and third layers and to flatten the residual denuded ASB. The third extracranial layer has to cover all the exposed ASB, but must not overlap the frontal sinusotomies. The borders of the second and third layers are properly fixed with fibrin glue. In the case of a tumor sparing the nasal septum and without multifocal localizations (eg, not ITAC), for the third layer of the skull base reconstruction it is also possible to use a mucoperiosteum/mucoperichondrium pedicled nasoseptal flap (Hadad-Bassagasteguy flap).[46] Its use facilitates rapid healing of the surgical cavity, especially in patients who require adjuvant irradiation. At the end of the procedure, in selected cases, the frontal sinusotomies can be stented with rolled polymeric silicone sheaths to allow subsequent frontal sinus debridement with no risks for the duraplasty. The surgical cavity is packed for about 48 hours.

For lesions filling the frontal sinus or encroaching on the ASB with intradural extension over the orbital roof or with brain parenchyma infiltration, the EER has to be combined with an external approach (CER).[43] The procedure is performed by 2 surgical teams (neurosurgeons and otorhinolaryngologists), working simultaneously through a transnasal and transcranial corridor, respectively. The endonasal approach allows the ethmoidal labyrinth to be mobilized in a monoblock, by removing the nasal septum and rostrum and dissecting the sphenoid posteriorly and the lamina papyracea later-ally. The transcranial approach consists of a subfrontal (or frontal) craniotomy, the size and shape of which depends on the surgical requirements. The craniotomy is performed a few millimeters above the orbital upper arches in order to obtain an approach to the frontal skull base as broad and tangential as possible, to reduce as much as possible any excessive retraction of the cerebral parenchyma and thus avoid excessive kinking of the pericranium flap during the ASB reconstruction. A bony flap including the anterior and posterior wall of the frontal sinus is harvested. After detaching the bony flap from the dural layer and clipping the sagittal sinus emissaries to control the bleeding, the exposed dura is incised, the cerebral falx is dissected, and the intracranial portion of the tumor is carefully resected from the brain parenchyma. The intracranial dissected lesion, together with the ethmoidal box, are extracted transcranially by the two surgical teams cooperating through the different approaches. The dural defect is rebuilt by suturing the dura mater to the temporal fascia or fascia lata. The ASB defect is reconstructed using a galeoperiosteum flap that is folded over and fixed with sutures to the remaining sphenoidal border and to the orbital process of the frontal bone (medial edge). The bony flap is put back into place and fixed with titanium plaques and screws. The galeal skin flap is then relocated and sutured. At the end of the procedure, the endoscopic endonasal approach is useful to verify the watertight closure and to apply connective tissue in overlay fashion (temporal fascia or fascia lata), for reinforcing the ASB reconstruction.

Complications

In general, the complication rate and overall morbidity of endoscopic procedures compares favorably with those of external procedures such as CFR, even though the extent of surgery is comparable with that of open procedures.[2,5,41,42] The absence of facial incisions and osteotomies, improved visualization of tumor borders, less postoperative pain, shorter hospitalization time, and the reduced intraoperative mortality are the major advantages promoting the EER as a good alternative to traditional external procedures whenever feasible, despite the longer surgical training and extensive experience required.[41] The 2 largest endoscopic series of recent years reported an overall complication rate of 9% to 11% and a mortality of 0% to 1%,[41,42] compared with an overall complication rate of 36.3% and mortality of 4.5% for CFR.[4] As expected, the most frequent major complication in endoscopic series was cerebrospinal fluid (CSF) leak, with a prevalence of 3% to 4.3%.[41,42] A recent analysis performed by the Italian group on a subset of 62 patients who underwent endoscopic removal of tumor with dural resection showed that the occurrence of CSF leak is related to the learning curve of the surgical team and to the refinement of surgical technique.[45] Other possible complications observed were infections (local or systemic), epiphora, mucocele formation, and epistaxis. The overall complication rates increased with T4 lesions and larger tumors and if an endoscopic craniectomy was added.[47]

Postoperative Care

All patients undergoing skull base reconstruction require a brain CT scan on the first postoperative day to rule out complications and to evaluate the extent of pneumocephalus, and they must observe complete bed rest keeping the head in a 20° upright position until the third postoperative day. Nasal packing is gradually removed under endoscopic vision within 48 hours. Intravenous third-generation cephalosporin therapy is started the day before surgery and continued for at least 5 days. During the early postoperative period, stool softeners are suggested and the patient is recommended to avoid blowing the nose or exerting physical effort for some weeks. Nasal irrigation with saline solution and application of mupirocin ointment twice daily is recommended for at least 2 months.

Follow-up

All patients are followed according to a protocol that includes monthly endoscopic examinations and MRI every 4 months during the first year; endoscopic examination and MRI every 2 and 6 months, respectively, during the second year; and thereafter both examinations at 6-month intervals until the fifth year. Thereafter, patients are followed with endoscopy and MRI every 12 months until the 10th year. During this period, attention should be given also to potential metastatic dissemination of disease. Our protocol includes a whole-body staging of the disease performed once per year using chest radiograph and neck ultrasonography for low-grade tumors and PET-CT for aggressive histologies (eg, MM, NEC, SNUC, sarcoma).[2,5] For specific histotypes showing a late recurrence pattern (eg, ONB), a long-term close follow-up for more than 10 years or, whenever possible, extended for an individual's lifetime is recommended.[12]

OUTCOMES

Because endoscopic techniques have been applied with curative intent, there have been many publications reported in literature, although most of them have been characterized by small numbers, mixed histologies, and short follow-up.[41,42] Data emerging from these studies underline that the endoscopic approach is safe and effective and it can be undertaken in cases of appropriate histology and extent of disease, with the expectation of equivalent results to CFR and in many cases with reduced morbidity and hospital stay. However, at present, it is mandatory to perform analysis of survival outcomes in relation to specific histologies, in order to clarify the role of endoscopic surgery in the multidisciplinary management of such cancers and, possibly, to refine it based on available data.

Olfactory Neuroblastoma

Endoscopic surgery has an accepted role for the resection of this tumor, showing encouraging outcomes that are higher than for other sinonasal cancers (**Fig. 3**). In a

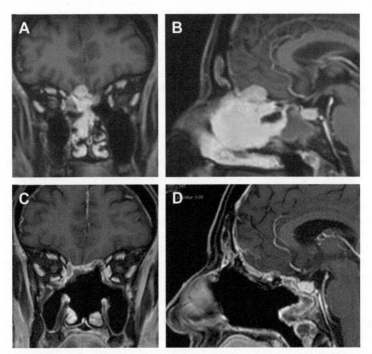

Fig. 3. Preoperative T1-weighted contrast-enhanced MR scan in coronal (*A*) and sagittal (*B*) views showing an olfactory neuroblastoma with intracranial extension and right olfactory bulb involvement (Kadish C). The tumor was excised through an endoscopic resection with transnasal craniectomy followed by adjuvant IMRT (68 Gy on the surgical area and 54 Gy on the neck with retropharyngeal nodes). Postoperative MR scan obtained 5 years after surgery (*C, D*) excluded local recurrence of disease.

meta-analysis of 23 publications comparing endoscopic with open surgery, endoscopic surgery was associated with better survival (10-year OS of 90% compared with 65% for open resection).[48] Hyams grading represents an independent prognostic factor, as shown by the Gustave Roussy experience on 44 cases published in 2013, in which 5-year OS of patients with Hyams grade IV was 14.8% versus 100%, 90.9%, and 86.2% respectively for patients with Hyams grade I, II, and III. The University of Virginia reported 15-year and 20-year disease-free survival (DFS) of 82.6% and 81.2%, respectively,[49] and the MD Anderson Cancer Center found a median time to recurrence of 6.9 years and incidences of overall recurrence and distant metastasis of 46% and 15%, respectively.[20] These data suggest that recurrences may occur late, even beyond 10 years after the initial diagnosis, confirming that lifelong follow-up is required irrespective of the treatment.

Neuroendocrine Carcinoma

The limited number of cases published, difficulties of diagnosis, and heterogeneity of treatment approaches has hampered meaningful evaluations.

The largest series (28 patients) was reported by Mitchell and colleagues[25] with 5-year OS, disease-specific survival (DSS), and DFS of 66.9%, 78.5%, and 43.8%, respectively. The incidences of local, regional, and distant failure were 21%, 25%, and 18%, respectively.[25] Other studies reported local recurrence rates of 45% to 50% and distant metastasis rates of 35% to 42%, which shows the aggressive biological behavior of this cancer.[25–27]

Sinonasal Undifferentiated Carcinoma

The prognosis of SNUC is generally dismal with patients presenting with locally advanced disease in 67% to 81% of cases and nodal or distant metastasis in 13% to 21% of cases.[50] Al-Mamgani and colleagues[51] published a series of 21 patients divided between chemoradiation therapy, neoadjuvant chemotherapy, or surgery as primary modes of treatment. Predictors of local control on multivariate analysis were T staging and treatment with 3 treatment modalities compared with 2 modalities (**Fig. 4**). This series reported the best survival outcomes published to date (OS of 74%), suggesting that a tailored treatment approach is better than any 1 strategy.[51]

Squamous Cell Carcinoma

Published studies on endoscopic resection of squamous cell carcinoma consist of small series, the largest of which reported a 5-year DSS rate of 61%.[1,41,42,52] The University of Pittsburgh Medical Center recently presented its experience of 34 patients treated with endoscopic surgery.[13] The cohort consisted mostly (85%) of stage T3 to T4 tumors. Seventy-four percent of patients were treated with the purely endoscopic endonasal approach and 26% were treated with combined transcranial/transfacial and endoscopic endonasal approaches. Twenty-seven patients had definitive resection and 7 had debulking surgery. The definitive resection group had 5-year DFS and OS rates of 62% and 78%, respectively. The positive margin rate was 19% in the definitive resection group. Survival was comparable with that for open surgery.[13]

Adenocarcinoma

Preliminary experiences published more than 10 years ago suggested that the endoscopic technique is safe and effective in sinonasal adenocarcinoma resection, obtaining acceptable oncologic outcomes and minimizing morbidity and hospitalization time for the patients.[41,42] Thereafter, Antognoni and colleagues[16] reported a series of

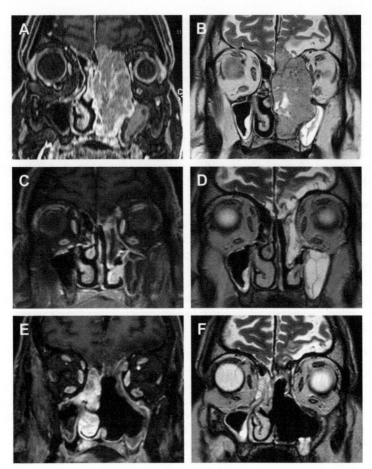

Fig. 4. Contrast-enhanced T1-weighted (*A*) and T2-weighted (*B*) MR scan showing a sino-nasal undifferentiated carcinoma involving the left ethmoid with intracranial extension, staged cT4bN0M0. The patient was initially treated with chemotherapy (carboplatin and taxol), obtaining a partial response (postchemotherapy MR scan is shown in *C, D*). The remaining lesion was surgically removed through an endoscopic endonasal approach, followed by adjuvant IMRT (62 Gy). The 2-year posttreatment MR scan (*E, F*) was clear, without evidence of recurrence.

30 consecutive patients with 5-year OS, DSS, and Recurrence-free survival of 72.7%, 78%, and 69.2%, respectively, outlining the efficacy of a treatment regimen based on endoscopic resection followed by adjuvant irradiation. The largest series reported to date was recently described by Nicolai and colleagues[18] analyzing 169 consecutive patients affected by ITAC and obtaining 5-year OS and event-free survival of 68.9% and 63.6%, respectively. Advanced pT stage, high grade, and positive surgical margins were independently predictive of poor survival. Comparable rates of 5-year OS were also observed by Camp and colleagues[53] (68% from a series of 123 patients) and Vergez and colleagues[54] (62% from a series of 159 patients). These data strongly support a definitive paradigm shift in the management of ITAC toward a schedule including endoscopic surgery with or without adjuvant IMRT in place of external surgical techniques, which have a role only in a minority of patients.

Mucosal Melanoma

Sinonasal MM is one of the most aggressive tumors of the head and neck region, with a very high propensity to recur and metastasize, regardless of the radicality of resection and adjuvant treatments administered.[1] In this regard, the seventh edition of the American Joint Commission for Cancer staging system (2010) omitted the T1 and T2 stages for upper aerodigestive tract MM, allowing the staging of lesions only as T3 or T4a-T4b.[55] Such dismal prognosis is supported by Lund and colleagues'[38] analysis of a series of 115 surgically treated patients, with 5-year OS of 28% and DFS of 23.7%. Adjuvant radiotherapy did not improve local control or survival. As expected, cervical metastases conferred a dramatically worse outcome.[38] Other studies found that OS was not superior to 50% at 3 years and between 26.9% and 38.7% at 5 years, confirming the aggressive behavior of the disease.[39,56] Moreover, there was no statistically significant association between T and N stage and the risk of death.[39,56] This observation confirms the high risk of failure for sinonasal MM even in apparently less aggressive lesions.

OPEN ISSUES

The role of endoscopic surgery in the multidisciplinary management of sinonasal malignancies is continually being refined. In this regard, prospective analysis of data focusing on specific histologies will be paramount to understanding the natural history of, and the development of the best treatment options for, each tumor.

Recent advances in irradiation modalities, such as particle therapy with carbon ion or proton beam, need future studies to understand the potential to improve oncologic outcomes. Induction chemotherapy in specific histologies has to be further investigated to select patients who could benefit from this treatment in terms of survival rates, organ preservation, or better definition of the subsequent treatments according to response to the chemotherapy.

The possibilities to stratify tumors based on new molecular biology techniques and the tailoring of the treatment based on behavior of the tumor will further refine decision making in the future. Constant training of the multidisciplinary oncologic skull base team should help to reach these goals, minimizing the rate of complications and failures.

SUMMARY

Endoscopic surgery offers an oncologically sound alternative to open surgery in selected patients with sinonasal malignancies. It offers the advantages of lower morbidity, faster recovery, and better quality-of-life outcomes. Globally, a correct classification by means of histology, immunohistochemistry, or molecular biology represents the key factor for initiating an appropriate treatment strategy. Recent data emphasized the role of appropriate histology-driven and patient-tailored adjuvant or neoadjuvant treatments by expert multidisciplinary teams in the management of sinonasal malignancies, including otolaryngologists, neurosurgeons, ophthalmologists, radiation oncologists, medical oncologists, occupational doctors, and pathologists. Although the optimal strategy is yet to be determined, individualized treatment that takes into account the stage of tumor, patient comorbidities, and histologic characteristics can achieve better survival. Pathology-specific and long-term follow-up survival data are required to further define the role of endoscopic surgery in the setting of multidisciplinary care.

REFERENCES

1. Lund VJ, Stammberger H, Nicolai P, et al. European position paper on endoscopic management of tumours of the nose, paranasal sinuses and skull base. Rhinology Suppl 2010;22:1–143.
2. Castelnuovo P, Battaglia P, Turri-Zanoni M, et al. Endoscopic endonasal surgery for malignancies of the anterior cranial base. World Neurosurg 2014;82:22–31.
3. Ketcham AS, Wilkins RH, Vanburen JM, et al. A combined intracranial facial approach to the paranasal sinuses. Am J Surg 1963;106:698–703.
4. Patel SG, Singh B, Polluri A, et al. Craniofacial surgery for malignant skull base tumors: report of an international collaborative study. Cancer 2003;98:1179–87.
5. Castelnuovo P, Lepera D, Turri-Zanoni M, et al. Quality of life following endoscopic endonasal resection of anterior skull base cancers. J Neurosurg 2013;119(6):1401–9.
6. Harvey RJ, Winder M, Parmar P, et al. Endoscopic skull base surgery for sinonasal malignancy. Otolaryngol Clin North Am 2011;44(5):1081–140.
7. Hanna EY, Cardenas AD, DeMonte F, et al. Induction chemotherapy for advanced squamous cell carcinoma of the paranasal sinuses. Arch Otolaryngol Head Neck Surg 2011;137(1):78–81.
8. Licitra L, Suardi S, Bossi P, et al. Prediction of TP53 status for primary cisplatin, fluorouracil, and leucovorin chemotherapy in ethmoid sinus intestinal-type adenocarcinoma. J Clin Oncol 2004;22:4901–6.
9. Ramaekers BL, Pijls-Johannesma M, Joore MA, et al. Systematic review and meta-analysis of radiotherapy in various head and neck cancers: comparing photons, carbon-ions and protons. Cancer Treat Rev 2011;37:185–201.
10. Patel SH, Wang Z, Wong WW, et al. Charged particle therapy versus photon therapy for paranasal sinus and nasal cavity malignant diseases: a systematic review and meta-analysis. Lancet Oncol 2014;15(9):1027–38.
11. Reyes C, Mason E, Solares CA, et al. To preserve or not to preserve the orbit in paranasal sinus neoplasms: a meta-analysis. J Neurol Surg B Skull Base 2015;76(2):122–8.
12. Su SY, Kupferman ME, DeMonte F, et al. Endoscopic resection of sinonasal cancers. Curr Oncol Rep 2014;16(2):369.
13. de Almeida JR, Su SY, Koutourousiou M, et al. Endonasal endoscopic surgery for squamous cell carcinoma of the sinonasal cavities and skull base: oncologic outcomes based on treatment strategy and tumor etiology. Head Neck 2014;37(8):1163–9.
14. Bhattacharyya N. Cancer of the nasal cavity: survival and factors influencing prognosis. Arch Otolaryngol Head Neck Surg 2002;128:1079–83.
15. Cantù G, Solero CL, Mariani L, et al. Intestinal type adenocarcinoma of the ethmoid sinus in wood and leather workers: a retrospective study of 153 cases. Head Neck 2011;33:535–42.
16. Antognoni P, Turri-Zanoni M, Gottardo S, et al. Endoscopic resection followed by adjuvant radiotherapy for sinonasal intestinal-type adenocarcinoma: retrospective analysis of 30 consecutive patients. Head Neck 2014;37(5):677–84.
17. Bhayani MK, Yilmaz T, Sweeney A, et al. Sinonasal adenocarcinoma: a 16-year experience at a single institution. Head Neck 2013;36(10):1490–6.
18. Nicolai P, Schreiber A, Villaret AB, et al. Intestinal type adenocarcinoma of the ethmoid: outcomes of a treatment regimen based on endoscopic surgery with or without radiotherapy. Head Neck 2015. http://dx.doi.org/10.1002/hed.24144.
19. Castelnuovo P, Bignami M, Delù G, et al. Endonasal endoscopic resection and radiotherapy in olfactory neuroblastoma: our experience. Head Neck 2007;29(9):845–50.

20. Ow TJ, Hanna EY, Roberts DB, et al. Optimization of long-term outcomes for patients with esthesioneuroblastoma. Head Neck 2014;36(4):524–30.
21. Dulguerov P, Allal AS, Calcaterra TC. Esthesioneuroblastoma: a metaanalysis and review. Lancet Oncol 2001;2(11):683–90.
22. Nishimura H, Ogino T, Kawashima M, et al. Proton-beam therapy for olfactory neuroblastoma. Int J Radiat Oncol Biol Phys 2007;68(3):758–62.
23. Van Gompel JJ, Giannini C, Olsen KD, et al. Long-term outcome of esthesioneuroblastoma: Hyams grade predicts patient survival. J Neurol Surg B Skull Base 2012;73(5):331–6.
24. Chao KS, Kaplan C, Simpson JR, et al. Esthesioneuroblastoma: the impact of treatment modality. Head Neck 2001;23(9):749–57.
25. Mitchell EH, Diaz A, Yilmaz T, et al. Multimodality treatment for sinonasal neuroendocrine carcinoma. Head Neck 2012;34(10):1372–6.
26. Bell D, Hanna EY, Weber RS, et al. Neuroendocrine neoplasms of the sinonasal region. Head Neck 2015. http://dx.doi.org/10.1002/hed.24152.
27. Su SY, Bell D, Hanna EY. Esthesioneuroblastoma, neuroendocrine carcinoma, and sinonasal undifferentiated carcinoma: differentiation in diagnosis and treatment. Int Arch Otorhinolaryngol 2014;18(Suppl 2):S149–56.
28. Bell D, Hanna EY. Sinonasal undifferentiated carcinoma: morphological heterogeneity, diagnosis, management and biological markers. Expert Rev Anticancer Ther 2013;13(3):285–96.
29. Fouad Mourad W, Hauerstock D, Shourbaji RA, et al. Trimodality management of sinonasal undifferentiated carcinoma and review of the literature. Am J Clin Oncol 2013;36(6):584–8.
30. Bignami M, Dallan I, Battaglia P, et al. Endoscopic, endonasal management of sinonasal haemangiopericytoma: 12-year experience. J Laryngol Otol 2010; 124(11):1178–82.
31. Lupinetti AD, Roberts DB, Williams MD, et al. Sinonasal adenoid cystic carcinoma: the M. D. Anderson Cancer Center experience. Cancer 2007;110(12):2726–31.
32. Takagi M, Demizu Y, Hashimoto N, et al. Treatment outcomes of particle radiotherapy using protons or carbon ions as a single-modality therapy for adenoid cystic carcinoma of the head and neck. Radiother Oncol 2014;113(3):364–70.
33. Toubaru S, Yoshikawa K, Ohashi S, et al. Accuracy of methionine-PET in predicting the efficacy of heavy-particle therapy on primary adenoid cystic carcinomas of the head and neck. Radiat Oncol 2013;8:143.
34. Szablewski V, Neuville A, Terrier P, et al. Adult sinonasal soft tissue sarcoma: analysis of 48 cases from the French Sarcoma Group database. Laryngoscope 2015; 125(3):615–23.
35. Potratz J, Dirksen U, Jürgens H, et al. Ewing sarcoma: clinical state-of-the-art. Pediatr Hematol Oncol 2012;29(1):1–11.
36. Meccariello G, Merks JH, Pieters BR, et al. Endoscopic management of Ewing's sarcoma of ethmoid sinus within the AMORE framework: a new paradigm. Int J Pediatr Otorhinolaryngol 2013;77(1):139–43.
37. Peng KA, Kita AE, Suh JD, et al. Sinonasal lymphoma: case series and review of the literature. Int Forum Allergy Rhinol 2014;4(8):670–4.
38. Lund VJ, Chisholm EJ, Howard DJ, et al. Sinonasal malignant melanoma: an analysis of 115 cases assessing outcomes of surgery, postoperative radiotherapy and endoscopic resection. Rhinology 2012;50(2):203–10.
39. Turri-Zanoni M, Medicina D, Lombardi D, et al. Sinonasal mucosal melanoma: molecular profile and therapeutic implications from a series of 32 cases. Head Neck 2013;35:1066–77.

40. Yanagi T, Mizoe JE, Hasegawa A, et al. Mucosal malignant melanoma of the head and neck treated by carbon ion radiotherapy. Int J Radiat Oncol Biol Phys 2009; 74(1):15–20.
41. Nicolai P, Battaglia P, Bignami M, et al. Endoscopic surgery for malignant tumours of the sinonasal tract and adjacent skull base: a 10-year experience. Am J Rhinol 2008;22:308–16.
42. Hanna E, DeMonte F, Ibrahim S, et al. Endoscopic resection of sinonasal cancers with and without craniotomy: oncologic results. Arch Otolaryngol Head Neck Surg 2009;135:1219–24.
43. Castelnuovo PG, Belli E, Bignami M, et al. Endoscopic nasal and anterior craniotomy resection for malignant nasoethmoid tumors involving the anterior skull base. Skull Base 2006;16:15–8.
44. Castelnuovo P, Battaglia P, Locatelli D, et al. Endonasal micro-endoscopic treatment of the malignant tumours of paranasal sinuses and anterior skull base. Oper Tech Otolaryngol Head Neck Surg 2006;17(3):152–67.
45. Villaret AB, Yakirevitch A, Bizzoni A, et al. Endoscopic transnasal craniectomy in the management of selected sinonasal malignancies. Am J Rhinol Allergy 2010; 24:60–5.
46. Hadad G, Bassagasteguy L, Carrau RL, et al. A novel reconstructive technique after endoscopic expanded endonasal approaches: vascular pedicle nasoseptal flap. Laryngoscope 2006;116(10):1882–6.
47. Nicolai P, Castelnuovo P, Bolzoni Villaret A. Endoscopic resection of sinonasal malignancies. Curr Oncol Rep 2011;13:138–44.
48. Devaiah AK, Andreoli MT. Treatment of esthesioneuroblastoma: a 16-year meta-analysis of 361 patients. Laryngoscope 2009;119(7):1412–6.
49. Levine PA. Would Dr. Ogura approve of endoscopic resection of esthesioneuro-blastomas? An analysis of endoscopic resection data versus that of craniofacial resection. Laryngoscope 2009;119(1):3–7.
50. Reiersen DA, Pahilan ME, Devaiah AK. Meta-analysis of treatment outcomes for sinonasal undifferentiated carcinoma. Otolaryngol Head Neck Surg 2012;147: 7–14.
51. Al-Mamgani A, van Rooij P, Mehilal R, et al. Combined-modality treatment improved outcome in sinonasal undifferentiated carcinoma: single-institutional experience of 21 patients and review of the literature. Eur Arch Otorhinolaryngol 2013;270(1):293–9.
52. Shipchandler TZ, Batra PS, Citardi MJ, et al. Outcomes for endoscopic resection of sinonasal squamous cell carcinoma. Laryngoscope 2005;115:1983–7.
53. Camp S, Van Gerven L, Vander Poorten V, et al. Long-term follow-up of 123 patients with adenocarcinoma of the sinonasal tract treated with endoscopic resection and postoperative radiation therapy. Head Neck 2014. http://dx.doi.org/10. 1002/hed.23900.
54. Vergez S, du Mayne MD, Coste A, et al. Multicenter study to assess endoscopic resection of 159 sinonasal adenocarcinomas. Ann Surg Oncol 2014;21(4): 1384–90.
55. Edge SB, Byrd DR, Compton CC, et al, editors. AJCC cancer staging manual. 7th edition. New York: Springer; 2010. p. 97–8.
56. Sun CZ, Li QL, Hu ZD, et al. Treatment and prognosis in sinonasal mucosal melanoma: a retrospective analysis of 65 patients from a single cancer center. Head Neck 2014;36:675–81.

Endoscopic Endonasal Management of Craniopharyngioma

Brad E. Zacharia, MD, MS[a], Muhamad Amine, MD[b],
Vijay Anand, MD[b], Theodore H. Schwartz, MD[b,c,d],*

KEYWORDS

- Craniopharyngioma • Endonasal • Endoscopic • Transsphenoidal • Suprasellar
- Transtuberculum • Transplanum

KEY POINTS

- Gross total resection of craniopharyngioma reduces the likelihood of recurrence.
- Planned subtotal resection +/− adjuvant radiation therapy may be a reasonable treatment approach in selected cases.
- The transsphenoidal corridor and endoscopic, endonasal technique are used to resect not only sellar and sellar-suprasellar but also purely suprasellar intraventricular craniopharyngioma.
- A key aspect of this technique is the expansion of the operative field by incorporation of the transtuberculum and transplanum approaches.
- The primary limitation of the transsphenoidal approach is its lateral reach, and as a general rule, this approach should not be applied to tumors extending more than a centimeter beyond the lateral limits of the exposure.

 A video of endoscopic endonasal resection of a supra sellar craniopharyngioma accompanies this article at www.oto.theclinics.com/

Disclosures: The authors have no relevant financial disclosures.
[a] Department of Neurosurgery, Penn State Hershey Medical Center, 30 Hope Drive, Hershey, PA 17033, USA; [b] Department of Otolaryngology–Head and Neck Surgery, New York Presbyterian Hospital, Weill Medical College of Cornell University, 525 E 68th Street, New York, NY 10065, USA; [c] Department of Neurosurgery, New York Presbyterian Hospital, Weill Medical College of Cornell University, 525 E 68th Street, New York, NY 10065, USA; [d] Department of Neuroscience, New York Presbyterian Hospital, Weill Medical College of Cornell University, 525 E 68th Street, New York, NY 10065, USA
* Corresponding author. Department of Neurosurgery, Weill Cornell Medical College, 525 East 68th Street, Box 99, New York, NY 10065.
E-mail address: schwarh@med.cornell.edu

Otolaryngol Clin N Am 49 (2016) 201–212
http://dx.doi.org/10.1016/j.otc.2015.09.013
0030-6665/16/$ – see front matter © 2016 Elsevier Inc. All rights reserved.

oto.theclinics.com

INTRODUCTION

Craniopharynigoma are rare, benign tumors of the central nervous system. Thought to arise from remnants of Rathke pouch in the sellar region, they represent less than 1% of all primary central nervous system tumors. Despite their benign histology, these tumors have posed a significant treatment challenge. Their central location in the sellar and suprasellar region and frequent invasion into critical neurovascular structures, such as the pituitary gland, hypothalamus, and optic apparatus, makes gross total resection (GTR) challenging. Although tumors may still recur after GTR the likelihood increases dramatically with subtotal resection.[1–6] Nevertheless, significant controversy exists regarding the optimal treatment strategy, with some groups pursuing conservative subtotal resection with either upfront or salvage radiotherapy or radiosurgery to lessen the risks of aggressive surgical resection.[1–18]

As these treatment paradigms have evolved, so too have the surgical techniques and approaches to craniopharyngioma, with the goal of maximizing resection and minimizing collateral damage. Traditional transcranial approaches require some degree of brain retraction and manipulation of cerebrovascular structures that lay between the surgeon and the pathology.[8,19] The transsphenoidal approach offers a more direct route to the sellar/suprasellar region and if performed with the operating microscope provides only a limited field of view, which often precludes safe and complete resection of these lesions.[19–23] The use of the transsphenoidal corridor was broadened with the development of expanded approaches, which offered a safe alternative method for reaching suprasellar craniopharyngioma.[24–32] The incorporation of the endoscope was the next step on the evolutionary ladder. By virtue of an improved field of view and superb illumination, this allowed for further expansion of the endonasal corridor. Finally, the development of a variety of complementary multilayer techniques to repair the skull base minimized the risk of postoperative cerebrospinal fluid (CSF) leak.[8,19] Several groups have now published their series incorporating these innovations into a fully endoscopic, endonasal, extended transsphenoidal approach for sellar and suprasellar craniopharyngioma.[2,8,33–42]

Epidemiology and Clinical Characteristics

Craniopharyngioma is a histologically benign, but locally aggressive sellar/suprasellar tumor characterized by a propensity to involve surrounding neurovascular structures. The overall incidence rate is between 1.3 and 1.7 cases per 1,000,000 person-years.[1,5,6,9,13] As is often noted in the literature, there is a bimodal age distribution with an incidence of 1.9 cases per 1,000,000 person-years in children ages 0 to 19 and an incidence of 2.1 cases per 1,000,000 person-years in adults aged 40 to 79.[1,7,10,12,14] The population-adjusted incidence rates suggest that craniopharyngioma has a slightly higher incidence in black persons. There is an even distribution between genders.[1,8,9]

Most craniopharyngiomas are located in the parasellar region. Most involve the suprasellar cistern to some degree. Occasionally the tumor can extend into neighboring cranial fossae and rarely is found in ectopic locations.[19,43] The most common presenting symptoms are related to increased intracranial pressure secondary to obstructive hydrocephalus (eg, headaches, nausea, and vomiting); visual dysfunction from direct compression of the optic chiasm, nerve, or tract; hormonal imbalance from pituitary stalk infiltration; and behavioral/developmental abnormality from hypothalamic injury (occurring primarily in children).[19,43]

Radiologic and Pathologic Characteristics

There are two major subtypes of craniopharyngioma. The adamantinomatous subtype is more prevalent in children and is thought to arise from neoplastic transformation of epithelial rests within the craniopharyngeal duct. The papillary subtype is almost exclusively found in adults and is thought to derive from metaplastic changes of epithelial cells within the pituitary stalk. Craniopharyngioma are characterized as a World Health Organization grade I neoplasm (**Fig. 1**).[2,24,26]

Most craniopharyngioma range in size from 2 to 4 cm, but can be significantly larger. They often have irregular borders and cystic components (46%–64%). The cystic components tend to be hyperintense on T2-weighted MRI. Enhancement of the cyst wall and heterogeneous enhancement of the solid portions is common. The adamantinomatous variant is frequently calcified. Close review of preoperative imaging is crucial to identify the relationships between the lesion and the chiasm, adjacent vasculature, pituitary stalk, and third ventricle (**Fig. 2**).[19,37,43]

TREATMENT GOALS AND PLANNED OUTCOMES

Although histologically benign, these lesions are locally aggressive and mandate intervention for the prevention and/or amelioration of neurologic symptoms. Surgical resection is a critical component of the treatment algorithm for craniopharyngioma. For many years attempted GTR was believed to be paramount to successful management of these lesions, and evidence suggests that recurrence rates are significantly improved when GTR is obtained.[5,6,13,44] With the advent of modern microsurgical techniques, imaging modalities, and improved endocrine management, GTR became feasible with reasonably low morbidity and mortality. Nevertheless, some groups contend that a conservative surgical approach, achieving subtotal resection, followed by radiation therapy should be considered the preferred treatment strategy.[2,7,10,12,14] The rationale is to avoid potential surgical morbidity that would adversely affect quality of life. This is especially true in children, in whom endocrinologic and hypothalamic injury can be devastating. There is no level 1 or level 2 evidence that supports one management paradigm over the other. Our general philosophy is one that aims to maximize tumor resection while minimizing postoperative complications. In most cases this means an attempt at complete resection with an endoscopic, endonasal approach followed by observation if successful or adjuvant therapy, such as radiation, if residual tumor remains.[2–4,8,11,15,17,18]

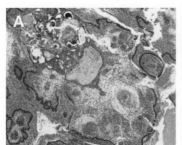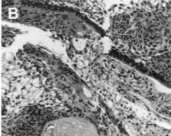

Fig. 1. Resection from a 63-year-old woman with a sellar/suprasellar mass. Hematoxylin and eosin stained sections at low (*A*) and high (*B*) power reveal classic adamantinomatous histology with squamous epithelium, palisaded columnar cells, islands of wet keratin, stellate reticulum, and calcifications.

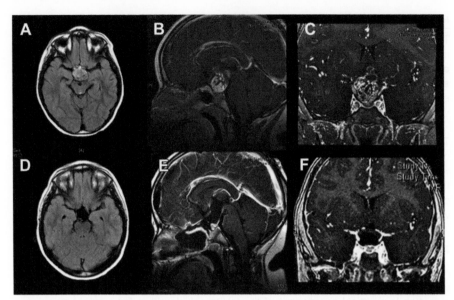

Fig. 2. MRI of craniopharyngioma. (*A*) Preoperative axial FLAIR. (*B*) Preoperative sagittal with gadolinium contrast. (*C*) Preoperative coronal with gadolinium contrast. (*D*) Postoperative axial FLAIR, note the absence of fluid attenuated inversion recovery (FLAIR) signal normally associated with retraction injury. (*E*) Postoperative sagittal with gadolinium contrast. (*F*) Postoperative coronal with gadolinium contrast.

The transsphenoidal corridor and endoscopic, endonasal technique can be used to resect sellar and suprasellar craniopharyngioma. A key aspect of this technique is the expansion of the operative field by incorporation of the transtuberculum and transplanum approaches.[1,6,13,43] This approach is adapted for use in tumors extending into the third ventricle, and those extending into the prepontine cistern. The primary limitation of the transsphenoidal approach is its lateral reach, and as a general rule, this approach should not be applied to tumors extending more than a centimeter beyond the lateral limits of the exposure.[1,7,9,10,12,43]

PREOPERATIVE PLANNING AND PREPARATION

Relevant anatomy from preoperative MRI should be reviewed in detail. Particular attention should be paid to the location of the optic nerves/chiasm, internal carotid, anterior cerebral, and middle cerebral arteries, and the pituitary gland/stalk. In addition, a detailed neurologic examination should be performed before any intended surgical intervention. Patients with optic chiasm compression should undergo comprehensive neuro-ophthalmologic evaluation, including formal visual field testing. All patients should undergo neuroendocrine assessment, including measurement of pituitary hormones.[2,45,46]

PATIENT POSITIONING

Patients are positioned supine on a standard operating table. Patients are then placed in pin fixation to allow for neuronavigation with preoperative MRI or computed tomography. The head is turned toward the surgeon about 30-degrees with slight neck extension. The abdomen and/or lateral thigh are prepared for a fat graft and/or fascia lata harvest.

PROCEDURAL APPROACH
Nasal and Sinus Stage

The surgical approach has been previously described in great detail (Video 1).[19–23,37,43] At the start of each case, 0.25 mL of 10% fluorescein (AK-FLUOR, Akorn, Lake Forest, IL) is injected in 10 mL of CSF via lumbar puncture to aid in visualization of intraoperative CSF leaks and closure of the skull base, which is an off-label use of fluorescein.[24–30,45,46] We often place a lumbar drain at the start of the operation because these intradural tumors generally have significant postresection CSF leaks, which benefit from transient CSF diversion. Before injection of fluorescein, the patient is pretreated with dexamethasone and diphenhydramine to minimize the risk of seizure or radiculopathy.

Following the placement of an arterial line, we place 4% cocaine pledgets into the nose to maximize decongestion. The table is placed in reverse Trendelenburg to improve venous outflow and minimize bleeding. The patient is then draped in a routine fashion. Our standard approach is a binostril, two-surgeon, four-handed technique. We start with a 0-degree, 18-cm long, 4-mm endoscope (Karl Storz, Tuttlingen, Germany). The nasal septum and rostrum are injected with 1% lidocaine with 1:100,000 epinephrine. Following adequate vasoconstriction, we find that by lateralizing the middle and superior turbinates one can achieve sufficient working room.[47] If the middle or superior turbinates limit visualization they can be resected, generally on one side, the left side to accommodate the endoscope, with a small risk of postoperative hyposmia. Because of the anticipated CSF leak, a vascularized nasoseptal flap is harvested based on the posterior nasoseptal artery (a branch of the sphenopalatine artery). This is set aside by tucking it into the nasopharynx being careful not to twist and strangulate the pedicle. We then proceed with a posterior septectomy by removing the exposed septal cartilage and vomer. If a large defect is anticipated, a Janus flap[48] can be created by harvesting the contralateral nasoseptal flap and creating a double flap. The remaining tissue edges of the nasal septum and maxillary crest are debrided with a tissue shaver. It is at this stage that a 0-degree, 30-cm long, 4-mm diameter endoscope is brought into the field and held in place with a scope holder. A wide sphenoidotomy and posterior ethmoidectomy are performed. To maximize exposure and prevent the nasoseptal flap from tenting, the "keel" (ie, the posterior inferior vomer), which articulates with the sphenoid floor, is removed. The choanal architecture remains intact following this step. The sphenoid intersinus septum must be removed to visualize the entire posterior wall of the sphenoid sinus. Important landmarks to expose are the lateral opticocarotid recess laterally, the planum sphenoidale superiorly, and the floor of the sphenoid and the clival recess inferiorly (**Fig. 3**). All of the mucosa from the posterior sphenoid wall is stripped. This serves two purposes: first, it decreases bleeding from the mucosa itself; and second, it prevents the development of a postoperative mucocele underneath the nasoseptal flap. The location of the internal carotid artery and the tumor are confirmed with neuronavigation.

Sellar/Suprasellar Stage

A high-speed drill and bone rongeurs are used to remove bone from the top of the sella, tuberculum, and variable portions of the planum sphenoidale depending on the size and location of the tumor (see **Fig. 3**). In the sagittal plane, bone is removed from cavernous sinus to cavernous sinus. The opening can also be enlarged inferiorly

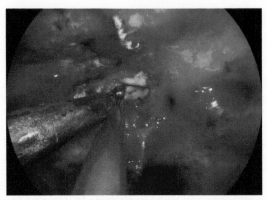

Fig. 3. Bone removal (intraoperative view, 0-degree endoscope). Thinned out planum being removed with up-going curette.

to include the upper portion of the clivus if there is extension of the tumor ventral to the brainstem. The dura above and below the superior intercavernous sinus is opened, and the sinus is cauterized and divided. The tumor is carefully dissected off any adjacent critical neurovascular structures, internally decompressed, and removed (**Fig. 4**). Given the ability to use bimanual techniques and the growing array of specialized endonasal, endoscopic instruments, we adhere to standard microsurgical principles. Every effort is made to preserve the stalk, superior hypophyseal arteries, and floor of the third ventricle (**Fig. 5**). In many cases, however, because of tumor extension into the third ventricle, the foramen of Monro and aqueduct of Sylvius can be clearly visualized at the end of the resection. This can often be best visualized with the use of an angled endoscope (see **Fig. 5**).

Closure Stage

The closure technique has evolved over time. Early in our experience, we placed fat grafts intracranially to eliminate large dead spaces. This was abandoned as unnecessary, a possible source of intracranial infection, and an obfuscation of postoperative

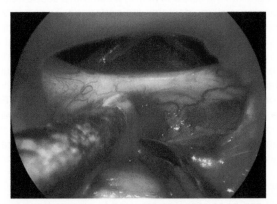

Fig. 4. Optic chiasm (intraoperative view, 0-degree endoscope). Tumor capsule is seen adherent to the undersurface of the optic chiasm. Care is taken to sharply dissect these attachments and not sacrifice blood supply to the optic apparatus. The bilateral A1 segments of the anterior cerebral artery are seen superior to the optic chiasm.

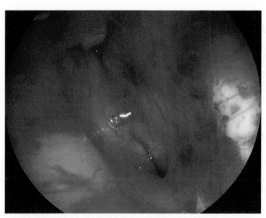

Fig. 5. Third ventricle (intraoperative view, 30-degree endoscope). Following complete resection of the craniopharyngioma a clear view is obtained into the third ventricle. The foramen of Monro and aqueduct of Sylvius are noted.

imaging. When there is a large defect in the skull base we use a "gasket seal" closure, which we have previously described.[2,8,33–42,44] Briefly, a piece of autologous fascia lata (1 cm larger than the skull base defect in every direction) is countersunk with a rigid Porex buttress (Porex Corp, Newman, GA). A vascularized nasoseptal flap is then placed over the gasket closure (**Fig. 6**). This is followed by DuraSeal (Covidien, Waltham, MA), a tissue adhesive/sealant, to hold the construct in place. FloSeal (Baxter, Deerfield, IL) is used to fill the remainder of the cavity, which aids in hemostasis. Lastly, Telfa (Kendall, Mansfield, MA) splints are inserted into the nasal passage to assist with hemostasis and are removed the following day. This technique has resulted in a near 0% risk of postoperative CSF leak.[49–51] Importantly, gentle emergence from anesthesia and extubation is desired to prevent disruption of the closure by way of increased intracranial pressure. However, this must be balanced with the risk of hypoventilation, which may necessitate supporting the airway. In this case, positive pressure should not be used for fear of creating pneumocephalus; rather, the patient may be reintubated.

POTENTIAL COMPLICATIONS

Given the proximity of craniopharyngioma to critical neurovascular structures there is always the potential for surgical complications. Manipulation of the optic nerves

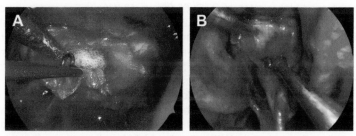

Fig. 6. Cranial base reconstruction (intraoperative view, 30-degree endoscope). (*A*) Gasket seal performed with inlay of undersized Medpor and oversized autologous fascia lata. (*B*) Previously harvested nasal septal flap being rotated into place over gasket seal.

and/or chiasm or disruption of the delicate vascular supply to these structures can lead to postoperative deterioration in vision. Direct injury to a major vascular structure is rare, but devastating. Prompt hemostasis via coagulation or clip ligation is critical. In the event of significant injury the surgical procedure is often aborted and the patient is taken for digital subtraction angiogram to assess the extent of vascular injury, extent of collateral circulation, and evaluate for development of dissections or pseudoaneurysm formation.

POSTPROCEDURAL CARE, REHABILITATION, AND RECOVERY

When placed, the lumbar drain is drained at 5 mL per hour for 24 hours and removed on postoperative Day 1 in the evening so the patient lays flat overnight and then can be ambulated on the second postoperative day with less risk of spinal headache. The drain is occasionally left longer if the gasket seal closure is not believed to be optimally situated. A postoperative contrast-enhanced MRI is obtained to rule out residual tumor, delineate the location of the fat graft, and observe for any significant hemorrhage. This also serves as a baseline scan to which follow-up imaging is later compared. Follow-up imaging is obtained at approximately 3 months after resolution of postoperative changes. A full endocrine panel is obtained immediately following surgery and then repeated in 4 to 6 weeks. In the immediate postoperative period the patient is monitored closely for the development of diabetes insipidus. Importantly, postoperative instructions should include CSF leak precautions, such as no straining, no nose blowing, and no bending at the waist. In addition, nasal sprays are avoided to monitor for the development of a CSF leak. After discharge the patient is seen by the otolaryngologist initially at 1 week for debridement and thereafter until healed. Continued follow-up is also important to rule out the development of a mucocele underneath the nasoseptal flap.[2,6,9]

OUTCOMES AND LITERATURE REVIEW

To accurately assess the endoscopic, endonasal approach one must consider the safety and efficacy relative to open approaches for craniopharyngioma. In regards to the extent of resection, GTR in transcranial series ranges from 9% to 90%[2–4,11,15,17,18] and in fully endoscopic, endonasal series rates are between 29% and 70%.[8,33–36,41,52] In our initial series we were able to achieve an 86% rate of GTR in surgeries in which it was intended.[8] There have been no prospective, randomized clinical trials addressing this question, and it is unlikely that one will ever be conducted. To this end, we completed a systematic review of the literature and found that relative to an open transcranial approach, patients undergoing endoscopic endonasal resection achieved higher rates of GTR (66.9% vs 48.3%).[53] The endoscopic cohort also had improved visual outcomes (56.2% vs 33.1%). We have found that extent of resection and visual outcomes are significantly associated with quality of life in patients undergoing endoscopic, endonasal resection of craniopharyngioma. Permanent diabetes insipidus developed in 42% and panhypopituitarism in 38%. These rates are consistent with the endoscopic and transcranial literature.[8,26,33–36,41,52] Not surprisingly the postoperative rate of CSF leakage is greater in the endoscopic (18.4%) than in the transcranial group (2.6%), although these rates have improved over time as closure techniques continue to be refined.[19,37,43,53] With our evolving skull base closure paradigm we achieved a CSF leak rate of 3.8% and even lower[49] in this patient cohort.[2,8,45,46] However, postoperative seizures occurred in 8.5% of transcranial cases, but never occurred when the endoscopic approach was used.[5,6,13,44,53] We also found that 69% of patients successfully returned to their preoperative profession or grade of educations, which is in line with other reports from the literature.

SUMMARY

Although benign in histology, craniopharyngioma results in significant morbidity and lost quality of life from visual loss, hypothalamic dysfunction, and endocrine dysregulation. The potential morbidity of GTR has led some to consider alternative treatment paradigms aimed at minimizing surgical insults. Parallel shifts in neurosurgical technique and minimal access endoscopic approaches have led to a marriage of treatment philosophy and technique.[2,7,8,10,12,14] The expanded endonasal approach affords a directed ventral, midline corridor to craniopharyngioma, which provides an unprecedented view and obviates brain retraction. As part of a minimally disruptive treatment paradigm, the expanded endonasal approach has the potential to improve rates of resection, improve postoperative visual recovery, and minimize surgical morbidity.

SUPPLEMENTARY DATA

Supplementary data related to this article is found online at 10.1016/j.otc.2015.09.013.

REFERENCES

1. Zacharia BE, Bruce SS, Goldstein H, et al. Incidence, treatment and survival of patients with craniopharyngioma in the Surveillance, Epidemiology and End Results program. Neuro Oncol 2012;14:1070–8.
2. Leng LZ, Anand VK, Lad SP, et al. Endoscopic management of craniopharyngiomas. Operat Tech Otolaryngol Head Neck Surg 2011;22(3):215–22.
3. Fahlbusch R, Honegger J, Paulus W, et al. Surgical treatment of craniopharyngiomas: experience with 168 patients. J Neurosurg 1999;90:237–50.
4. Van Effenterre R, Boch AL. Craniopharyngioma in adults and children: a study of 122 surgical cases. J Neurosurg 2002;97:3–11.
5. Weiner HL, Wisoff JH, Rosenberg ME, et al. Craniopharyngiomas: a clinicopathological analysis of factors predictive of recurrence and functional outcome. Neurosurgery 1994;35:1001–10 [discussion: 1010–1].
6. Tuniz F, Soltys SG, Choi CY, et al. Multisession cyberknife stereotactic radiosurgery of large, benign cranial base tumors: preliminary study. Neurosurgery 2009;65:898–907 [discussion: 907].
7. Tomita T, Bowman RM. Craniopharyngiomas in children: surgical experience at Children's Memorial Hospital. Childs Nerv Syst 2005;21:729–46.
8. Leng LZ, Greenfield JP, Souweidane MM, et al. Endoscopic, endonasal resection of craniopharyngiomas: analysis of outcome including extent of resection, cerebrospinal fluid leak, return to preoperative productivity, and body mass index. Neurosurgery 2012;70:110–24.
9. Bunin GR, Surawicz TS, Witman PA, et al. The descriptive epidemiology of craniopharyngioma. J Neurosurg 1998;89:547–51.
10. Stripp DCH, Maity A, Janss AJ, et al. Surgery with or without radiation therapy in the management of craniopharyngiomas in children and young adults. Int J Radiat Oncol Biol Phys 2004;58:714–20.
11. Baskin DS, Wilson CB. Surgical management of craniopharyngiomas. A review of 74 cases. J Neurosurg 1986;65:22–7.

12. Chiou SM, Lunsford LD, Niranjan A, et al. Stereotactic radiosurgery of residual or recurrent craniopharyngioma, after surgery, with or without radiation therapy. Neuro Oncol 2001;3:159–66.
13. Chakrabarti I, Amar AP, Couldwell W, et al. Long-term neurological, visual, and endocrine outcomes following transnasal resection of craniopharyngioma. J Neurosurg 2005;102:650–7.
14. Jeon C, Kim S, Shin HJ, et al. The therapeutic efficacy of fractionated radiotherapy and gamma-knife radiosurgery for craniopharyngiomas. J Clin Neurosci 2011;18:1621–5.
15. De Vile CJ, Grant DB, Kendall BE, et al. Management of childhood craniopharyngioma: can the morbidity of radical surgery be predicted? J Neurosurg 1996;85:73–81.
16. Crotty TB, Scheithauer BW, Young WF Jr, et al. Papillary craniopharyngioma: a clinicopathological study of 48 cases. J Neurosurg 1995;83:206–14.
17. Hoffman HJ, De Silva M, Humphreys RP, et al. Aggressive surgical management of craniopharyngiomas in children. J Neurosurg 1992;76:47–52.
18. Yaşargil MG, Curcic M, Kis M, et al. Total removal of craniopharyngiomas. Approaches and long-term results in 144 patients. J Neurosurg 1990;73:3–11.
19. Karavitaki N, Cudlip S, Adams CBT, et al. Craniopharyngiomas. Endocr Rev 2006;27:371–97.
20. Laws ER. Transsphenoidal microsurgery in the management of craniopharyngioma. J Neurosurg 1980;52:661–6.
21. Honegger J, Buchfelder M, Fahlbusch R, et al. Transsphenoidal microsurgery for craniopharyngioma. Surg Neurol 1992;37:189–96.
22. König A, Lüdecke DK, Herrmann HD. Transnasal surgery in the treatment of craniopharyngiomas. Acta Neurochir (Wien) 1986;83:1–7.
23. Maira G, Anile C, Rossi GF, et al. Surgical treatment of craniopharyngiomas: an evaluation of the transsphenoidal and pterional approaches. Neurosurgery 1995;36:715–24.
24. Prabhu VC, Brown HG. The pathogenesis of craniopharyngiomas. Childs Nerv Syst 2005;21:622–7.
25. Kato T, Sawamura Y, Abe H, et al. Transsphenoidal-transtuberculum sellae approach for supradiaphragmatic tumours: technical note. Acta Neurochir (Wien) 1998;140:715–8 [discussion: 719].
26. Karavitaki N, Wass JAH. Craniopharyngiomas. Endocrinol Metab Clin North Am 2008;37:173–93, ix–x.
27. Dusick JR, Esposito F, Kelly DF, et al. The extended direct endonasal transsphenoidal approach for nonadenomatous suprasellar tumors. J Neurosurg 2005;102: 832–41.
28. Maira G, Anile C, Albanese A, et al. The role of transsphenoidal surgery in the treatment of craniopharyngiomas. J Neurosurg 2004;100:445–51.
29. Couldwell WT, Weiss MH, Rabb C, et al. Variations on the standard transsphenoidal approach to the sellar region, with emphasis on the extended approaches and parasellar approaches: surgical experience in 105 cases. Neurosurgery 2004;55:539–47 [discussion: 547–50].
30. Kouri JG, Chen MY, Watson JC, et al. Resection of suprasellar tumors by using a modified transsphenoidal approach. Report of four cases. J Neurosurg 2000;92: 1028–35.
31. Kaptain GJ, Vincent DA, Sheehan JP, et al. Transsphenoidal approaches for the extracapsular resection of midline suprasellar and anterior cranial base lesions. Neurosurgery 2001;49:94–100 [discussion: 100–1].

32. Anand VK, Schwartz TH. Practical endoscopic skull base surgery. San Diego (CA): Plural Publishing; 2007.
33. Jane JA, Kiehna E, Payne SC, et al. Early outcomes of endoscopic transsphenoidal surgery for adult craniopharyngiomas. Neurosurg Focus 2010; 28(4):E9.
34. Campbell PG, McGettigan B, Luginbuhl A, et al. Endocrinological and ophthalmological consequences of an initial endonasal endoscopic approach for resection of craniopharyngiomas. Neurosurg Focus 2010;28(4):E8.
35. Frank G, Pasquini E, Doglietto F, et al. The endoscopic extended transsphenoidal approach for craniopharyngiomas. Neurosurgery 2006;59:ONS75–83 [discussion: ONS75–83].
36. Cavallo LM, Prevedello DM, Solari D, et al. Extended endoscopic endonasal transsphenoidal approach for residual or recurrent craniopharyngiomas. J Neurosurg 2009;111:578–89.
37. Laufer I, Anand VK, Schwartz TH. Endoscopic, endonasal extended transsphenoidal, transplanum transtuberculum approach for resection of suprasellar lesions. J Neurosurg 2007;106:400–6.
38. Scarone P, Klap P, Héran F, et al. Supradiaphragmatic retrochiasmatic craniopharyngioma in an 80-year-old patient operated by extended endoscopic endonasal approach: case report. Minim Invasive Neurosurg 2008;51:178–82.
39. Dehdashti AR, Ganna A, Witterick I, et al. Expanded endoscopic endonasal approach for anterior cranial base and suprasellar lesions: indications and limitations. Neurosurgery 2009;64:677–87 [discussion: 687–9].
40. Ceylan S, Koc K, Anik I. Extended endoscopic approaches for midline skull-base lesions. Neurosurg Rev 2009;32:309–19 [discussion: 318–9].
41. Gardner PA, Kassam AB, Snyderman CH, et al. Outcomes following endoscopic, expanded endonasal resection of suprasellar craniopharyngiomas: a case series. J Neurosurg 2008;109:6–16.
42. Fatemi N, Dusick JR, de Paiva Neto MA, et al. Endonasal versus supraorbital keyhole removal of craniopharyngiomas and tuberculum sellae meningiomas. Neurosurgery 2009;64:269–84 [discussion: 284–6].
43. Schwartz TH, Fraser JF, Brown S, et al. Endoscopic cranial base surgery: classification of operative approaches. Neurosurgery 2008;62:991–1002 [discussion: 1002–5].
44. Leng LZ, Brown S, Anand VK, et al. Gasket-seal watertight closure in minimal-access endoscopic cranial base surgery. Neurosurgery 2008;62:ONSE342–3 [discussion: ONSE343].
45. Tabaee A, Placantonakis DG, Schwartz TH, et al. Intrathecal fluorescein in endoscopic skull base surgery. Otolaryngol Head Neck Surg 2007;137:316–20.
46. Placantonakis DG, Tabaee A, Anand VK, et al. Safety of low-dose intrathecal fluorescein in endoscopic cranial base surgery. Neurosurgery 2007;61:161–5 [discussion: 165–6].
47. Nyquist GG, Anand VK, Brown S, et al. Middle turbinate preservation in endoscopic transsphenoidal surgery of the anterior skull base. Skull Base 2010;20: 343–7.
48. Nyquist GG, Anand VK, Singh A, et al. Janus flap: bilateral nasoseptal flaps for anterior skull base reconstruction. Otolaryngol Head Neck Surg 2010;142: 327–31.
49. Patel KS, Komotar RJ, Szentirmai O, et al. Case-specific protocol to reduce cerebrospinal fluid leakage after endonasal endoscopic surgery. J Neurosurg 2013;119:661–8.

50. Garcia-Navarro V, Anand VK, Schwartz TH. Gasket seal closure for extended endonasal endoscopic skull base surgery: efficacy in a large case series. World Neurosurg 2013;80:563–8.
51. Mascarenhas L, Moshel YA, Bayad F, et al. The transplanum transtuberculum approaches for suprasellar and sellar-suprasellar lesions: avoidance of cerebrospinal fluid leak and lessons learned. World Neurosurg 2014;82:186–95.
52. de Divitiis E, Cavallo LM, Cappabianca P, et al. Extended endoscopic endonasal transsphenoidal approach for the removal of suprasellar tumors: part 2. Neurosurgery 2007;60:46–58 [discussion: 58–9].
53. Komotar RJ, Starke RM, Raper DMS, et al. Endoscopic endonasal compared with microscopic transsphenoidal and open transcranial resection of craniopharyngiomas. World Neurosurg 2012;77:329–41.

Endoscopic Approaches to the Craniovertebral Junction

Varun R. Kshettry, MD[a], Brian D. Thorp, MD[b], Michael F. Shriver, BS[c],
Adam M. Zanation, MD[b,d], Troy D. Woodard, MD[e,f],
Raj Sindwani, MD[e,f], Pablo F. Recinos, MD[e,f,*]

KEYWORDS

- Endoscopic • Endonasal • Transnasal • Transclival • Craniovertebral
- Craniocervical • Odontoidectomy • Foramen magnum

KEY POINTS

- The endoscopic endonasal approach provides a direct surgical trajectory to anteriorly located lesions at the craniovertebral junction.
- Endoscopic endonasal odontoidectomy allows preservation of the soft palate, and patients can restart an oral diet on the first postoperative day.
- Lesions extending lateral to the lower cranial nerves cannot fully be treated via an endonasal approach.
- The use of vascularized pedicled flaps, such as the nasoseptal flap, has dramatically reduced the incidence of postoperative cerebrospinal fluid leak.
- A 2-surgeon 4-hand approach is recommended with collaborative expertise in rhinology and neurosurgery.

Disclosures: None.
[a] Rosa Ella Burkhardt Brain Tumor and Neuro-Oncology Center, Cleveland Clinic, 9500 Euclid Avenue, S73, Cleveland, OH 44195, USA; [b] Department of Otolaryngology—Head and Neck Surgery, University of North Carolina at Chapel Hill, 170 Manning Drive #7070, Chapel Hill, NC 27599-7070, USA; [c] Case Western Reserve University School of Medicine, 11100 Euclid Avenue, Cleveland, OH 44106, USA; [d] Department of Neurosurgery, University of North Carolina at Chapel Hill, 170 Manning Drive #7060, Chapel Hill, NC 27599-7060, USA; [e] Section of Rhinology, Sinus and Skull Base Surgery, Head and Neck Institute, Cleveland Clinic, 9500 Euclid Avenue, A71, Cleveland, OH 44195, USA; [f] Skull Base Surgery, Minimally Invasive Cranial Base and Pituitary Surgery Program, CCLCM, CWRU, 9500 Euclid Avenue, S-73, Cleveland, OH 44195, USA
* Corresponding author. Skull Base Surgery, Minimally Invasive Cranial Base and Pituitary Surgery Program, CCLCM, CWRU, 9500 Euclid Avenue, S-73, Cleveland, OH 44195.
E-mail address: recinop@ccf.org

Otolaryngol Clin N Am 49 (2016) 213–226
http://dx.doi.org/10.1016/j.otc.2015.08.003
0030-6665/16/$ – see front matter © 2016 Elsevier Inc. All rights reserved.

INTRODUCTION

Pathologic lesions located anterior or anterolateral at the craniovertebral (CVJ) pose a surgical challenge given their deep location and proximity to critical neurovascular structures. Historically, surgical treatment of these lesions using a standard midline suboccipital approach resulted in significant morbidity and mortality.[1,2] Over the last several decades, numerous alternative approaches have been described to treat these lesions more effectively. These include the far lateral, extreme lateral, direct lateral, transcervical, transoral, and transnasal approaches.[3–17]

The endonasal approach to the CVJ was originally described by Kassam and colleagues.[9,18] The advantage of the endonasal approach is that it provides direct surgical access to anterior and anterolateral CVJ lesions without the need to mobilize or retract cranial nerves, the lower brainstem, or upper cervical spinal cord. In addition, the endoscope can provide high illumination with a wide field of view.[19,20] However, the endoscopic endonasal approach to the CVJ requires substantial experience to overcome the learning curve associated with the technique and to minimize the risk of potential complications. In this article, the authors outline the surgical technique for the endoscopic endonasal approach to the CVJ, present illustrative cases, review outcomes, and discuss complication avoidance.

TREATMENT GOALS

The goals of surgery and the anticipated outcomes are discussed with the patient preoperatively. Goals may include obtaining a diagnosis (if not already known), decompression of neural structures, and maximizing survival and quality of life. The latter requires minimizing collateral damage to both nasal and neural structures and lessening the risk of complications.

PREOPERATIVE PLANNING

Preoperative evaluation begins with thorough radiographic assessment of pathologic and anatomic variations. Thin-slice (1.0 mm) computed tomography (CT) scan of the sinuses, CVJ, and upper cervical spine and volumetric MRI are performed. In addition to the volumetric T1 sequence with gadolinium, a high-resolution constructive interference in steady state sequence can be invaluable in showing the relationship of cranial nerves to the condition and the competency of dural membranes.[21] A preoperative CT angiogram may be performed in certain cases to further evaluate any anatomic variations in the paraclival carotid arteries (the segment of the carotid artery between the foramen lacerum and the cavernous sinus) and to assess intracranial collateralization patterns. These images may be fused and uploaded into a frameless stereotaxy image-guidance unit, which is used on all endoscopic endonasal cases.

In addition to radiographic evaluation, preoperative direct bilateral sinonasal evaluation is imperative. This evaluation is usually performed in the office by the participating otolaryngologist. Anatomic variations, such as septal deviation, spur formation, or perforation, may directly impact the operative approach or reconstruction technique. In addition, screening for concurrent paranasal sinus disease is necessary to determine the need for preoperative antibiotic treatment. If preoperative voice or swallowing symptoms exist, a preoperative swallow evaluation or direct laryngoscopy may be performed to provide baseline function and to appropriately counsel the patients on potential risks of exacerbation after surgery.

PATIENT POSITIONING

The patient is placed in supine position toward the right edge of the surgical bed. The arms are tucked to the side allowing sufficient access to the abdomen and right thigh should fat or fascia lata harvest be necessary. Accordingly, the monopolar electrocautery grounding pad is placed on the left thigh. For transclival approaches, the head may be placed on a donut or in a 3-point fixation device and secured to the bed. For cases of odontoidectomy before a posterior cervical fusion, placing the patient in a 3-point fixation device is imperative given that significant spinal instability will be present after odontoidectomy. The head may be placed in a neutral position for transclival cases, but gentle neck flexion is beneficial for odontoidectomy cases to align the approach trajectory with the surgeon.

The endotracheal tube is placed along the left side of the mouth. A throat pack or nasogastric tube is placed to avoid the collection of blood in the stomach, which may provoke postoperative emesis and affect the reconstruction. Neurophysiology monitoring may also prove helpful in select cases. Somatosensory and motor-evoked potentials may be used as well as monitoring of lower cranial nerves if affected by the condition. A neural integrity monitor electromyogram endotracheal tube (NIM 3.0; Medtronic, Minneapolis, MN) allows one to stimulate the vagus nerve and assess for motor response within the vocal cords.[22] Local anesthetic gels must be avoided with this endotracheal tube. In addition, it cannot be used in cases of intraoperative MRI, as it is MRI incompatible. Electrodes may also be placed in the trapezius muscle and tongue to monitor the accessory and hypoglossal nerves, respectively.

PROCEDURAL APPROACH
Nasal Approach

The nasal mucosa is injected with local vasoconstrictors. Using a 0° endoscope, the inferior turbinates are out-fractured. Resection of one or both of the middle turbinates can be performed to provide a wider corridor for passage of instruments. However, middle turbinectomy is typically not necessary when the approach is limited to the CVJ, unless there is significant platybasia. The choanae can then be visualized by following the nasal cavity floor back to the nasopharynx. The natural ostium of the sphenoid sinus is identified medial to the superior turbinate. In cases requiring vascularized reconstruction, a nasoseptal flap is harvested by first identifying the pedicle of the flap, which contains the posterior septal artery. Using needle-tip bovie electrocautery, the inferior cut is made from the posterior choana extending inferior and anterior along the floor of the nasal cavity. The superior cut is then made starting at the natural sphenoid ostium and extending superior and anterior along the nasal septum. During most endoscopic endonasal cases, the nasoseptal flap is tucked into the nasopharynx. However, when approaching the CVJ, the flap must be placed into the maxillary sinus to maximize visualization and avoid damaging the flap. Therefore, a maxillary antrostomy is performed on the side of the nasoseptal flap harvest by removing the uncinate process, and the nasoseptal flap is tucked into the maxillary sinus until needed for the reconstruction. Again, it should be noted that approaches for pathologic conditions limited to the CVJ might not require initial nasoseptal flap harvest. Rather, an inferior posterior septectomy that spares the pedicle to the nasoseptal flap can be used, which allows subsequent harvest if needed.

Wide sphenoidotomies can then be performed if warranted by the pathologic findings or at the discretion of the surgeon. The posterior nasal septum is disarticulated from the rostrum of the sphenoid sinus, and the rostrum is removed with a 4-mm coarse diamond burr or Kerrison rongeurs. Roughly 1 to 2 cm of the posterior septum is removed as well.

Wide bilateral sphenoidotomies creates a large, singular surgical cavity with adequate room for the passage of the endoscope and surgical instruments without conflict.

For access to the lower clivus and upper cervical spine, additional nasal exposure is performed. The floor of the sphenoid sinus is drilled down to create a wide communication between the sphenoid sinus and the nasopharynx. The nasopharyngeal mucosal and muscular layers along the midline are cauterized and lateralized. This process exposes the nasopharyngeal fascia, which is also elevated off the clivus and lateralized. The longus capitus (lower clivus), longus coli (upper cervical spine), and anterior atlanto-occipital membranes are also cauterized at the midline and lateralized to provide access to the lower clivus, anterior ring of C1, and the odontoid process.[23]

Endoscopic Endonasal Transclival Approach

For the purpose of this article, the discussion focuses on the transclival approach for access to the lower clivus and CVJ. Common conditions treated with these approaches include clival chordomas and ventrally located foramen magnum meningiomas. The relationship between the tumor, the lower cranial nerves, and carotid arteries should be carefully studied on preoperative imaging. Lesions extending lateral to the lower cranial nerves cannot fully be treated via an endonasal approach. During a midclival approach, the paraclival carotid arteries are at risk. An important anatomic landmark is the lacerum segment of the internal carotid artery (ICA), which roughly corresponds to the pontomesencephalic junction. In lower clival and foramen magnum approaches, which take place below the lacerum segment of the ICA, the risk of carotid artery injury is lower. In general, the ICA is lateral to the superior pharyngeal constrictor muscle and occipital condyle. However, major anatomic variations of the ICA can occur, particularly in elderly patients and in patients with significant congenital bony deformity of the craniocervical junction, and should be accounted for when planning the operation.[23–25]

After the nasal corridor has been accessed as previously described, the clivus is drilled with a 4-mm coarse diamond burr between the lacerum segments of the ICA superiorly and the occipital condyles inferiorly. The basilar plexus, which lies between the 2 layers of clival dura and communicates with the inferior petrosal sinus and cavernous sinus on each side, can often result in brisk bleeding when encountered. This bleeding is controlled with injectable hemostatic agents and gentle pressure with cotton patties. When this region has already been invaded by tumor, the basilar plexus is often already thrombosed.

For lesions that lie lateral to the occipital condyle, the anteromedial portion of the occipital condyles may be removed to gain additional lateral access. First, the rectus capitus anterior and the atlanto-occipital joint capsule are removed to expose the atlanto-occipital joint. A small groove is found on the superior aspect of the condyle, which estimates the level of the hypoglossal canal.[23] Above this groove is bone of the jugular tubercle, and below this groove is bone of the occipital condyle. The condyle can be removed up to the level of the hypoglossal canal. The inferior portion of the condyle that contains the alar ligament insertion is left intact as removal of this portion results in very little additional exposure but can increase risk of craniocervical instability.[26,27] In addition, the lateral extent of surgical exposure can be better visualized using angled endoscopes.[28,29] Inferior clivectomy, transection of the tectorial membrane, and resection of less than 75% of the anteromedial condyle for exposure of the anterior foramen magnum does not result in significant craniocervical instability enough to warrant fusion.[29]

Case Illustration

A 60-year-old man with a history of smoking and diabetes presented with headaches and double vision. His examination was remarkable for left abducens nerve palsy. MRI of the brain found a 3.0- × 2.5- × 3.8-cm enhancing clival mass extending laterally along bilateral petrous apices behind the horizontal petrous carotid arteries (**Fig. 1**). CT scan found destruction of the clival bone in the location of the mass (**Fig. 2**). An endoscopic endonasal resection was planned.

The patient was positioned supine with the head positioned neutral in a donut. Stereotactic image guidance was used. Nasal cavities were prepared with topical vasoconstrictor. The inferior turbinates were outfractured and the right middle turbinate was resected. A right nasoseptal flap was harvested using needle-tip electrocautery. A right maxillary antrostomy was performed, and the nasoseptal flap was tucked into the maxillary sinus to allow unimpeded access to the clivus. Wide bilateral sphenoidotomies, in addition to a posterior septectomy, was performed. The mucosa of the sphenoid sinus was stripped.

The sella and clinoidal ICAs were identified (**Fig. 3**), and the tumor, which had invaded much of the clival bone, was resected. The paraclival arteries were dissected out bilaterally. Angled endoscopes and instruments were used to remove the tumor extending posterolateral to the paraclival ICAs on both sides. The paraclival arteries and clivus were covered with the nasoseptal flap. Postoperative imaging confirmed gross total resection (**Fig. 4**). The patient did well after surgery and in follow-up had improvement in his abducens palsy.

Endoscopic Endonasal Odontoidectomy Approach

Although the transoral corridor has been used primarily for odontoidectomies, the transnasal approach affords the advantage of preserving the soft palate and retropharyngeal soft tissues, allowing patients to resume a normal diet on the first postoperative day.[12,18,30] In the transoral approach, the soft palate is typically retracted for a prolonged period. This approach can result in paresis of muscle movements, loss of retropharyngeal soft tissue volume, and scarring of the palate, which may lead to

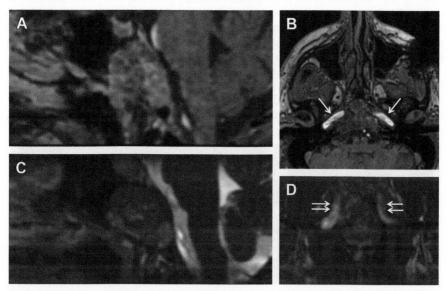

Fig. 1. Preoperative sagittal (*A*) and axial (*B*) postcontrast T1 MRI and sagittal (*C*) and coronal (*D*) constructive interference in steady state showing enhancing mass within clivus extending behind bilateral horizontal petrous carotid arteries (*white arrow*) and between bilateral paraclival ICAs (*double white arrow*).

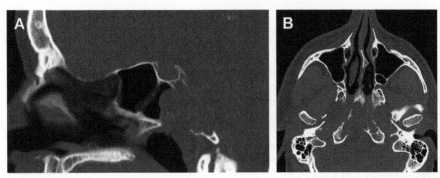

Fig. 2. Preoperative sagittal (*A*) and axial (*B*) CT scan shows an infiltrative mass involving the entire clivus.

velopalatine insufficiency. Preoperative radiographic evaluation is performed by obtaining a thin-cut CT scan and MRI, which include the nasal sinuses and CVJ. A line is draw from the anterior inferior nasal bone through the posterior aspect of the hard palate on sagittal imaging to delineate the nasopalatine line. The nasopalatine line is used to predict the caudal limit of exposure of the upper cervical spine (**Fig. 5**).[31]

Case Illustration

A 67-year-old woman with a remote history of an upper aerodigestive tract squamous cell carcinoma treated with primary radiotherapy presented with progressive upper extremity weakness, muscular wasting, fatigue, and cervical pain. Given these progressive symptoms, she was extremely deconditioned and wheelchair bound. Examination at the time of presentation found upper extremity weakness and muscle wasting, with sequelae of her prior radiation therapy including 1 cm trismus and xerostomia. Radiographic studies were done, which found basilar impression with severe narrowing of the spinal canal (**Fig. 6**). An endoscopic endonasal odontoidectomy was planned because it was the most direct surgical approach, and the patient's trismus made her a poor candidate for a transoral approach.

After appropriately positioning the patient and set up of stereotactic image guidance and neurophysiology monitoring as previously described, the nasal cavities were prepared with pledgets soaked with a topical vasoconstrictor. The inferior and middle turbinates were then lateralized bilaterally allowing easy visualization of the nasopharynx.

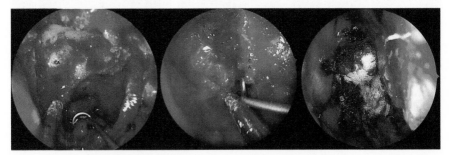

Fig. 3. (*Left*) Exposure of the sella and right clinoidal segment of the ICA and tumor resection from the clival region. (*Middle*) Use of angled endoscope and angled curettes to remove tumor behind the left paraclival ICA. (*Right*) Reconstruction with nasoseptal flap, hydrogel glue, and oxidized cellulose. SF, sellar floor; T, tumor.

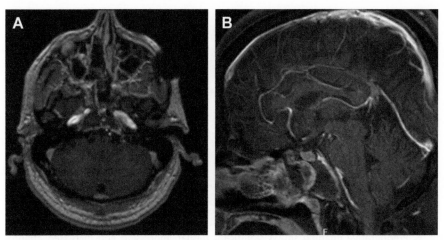

Fig. 4. Postoperative axial (*A*) and sagittal (*B*) postcontrast MRI shows complete resection.

To facilitate a 2-surgeon, 4-handed approach, an inferior posterior septectomy was performed preserving the posterior septal artery pedicle. This expanded the surgical working space and allowed clear visualization of the nasopharynx.

After obtaining the initial exposure, the nasopharyngeal mucosa and underlying paraspinal muscles were incised in the midline and lateralized, allowing visualization of

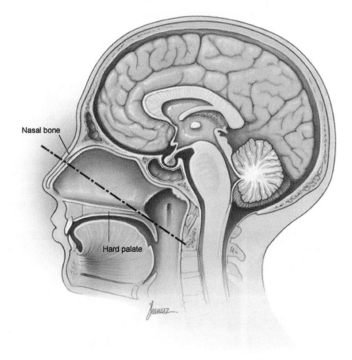

Fig. 5. The nasopalatine line, drawn from the inferior nasal bone to the posterior aspect of the hard palate and extended to the cervical spine, predicts the caudal extent of exposure. (*Courtesy of* Cleveland Clinic, Cleveland, OH; with permission.)

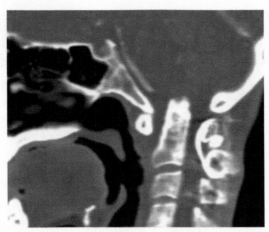

Fig. 6. Preoperative imaging shows significant basilar impression and increased atlanto-dens interval with resultant severe narrowing of the spinal canal.

the inferior clivus, atlanto-occipital membrane, and anterior arch of C1. A high-speed drill with a 4-mm coarse diamond burr was then used to drill the inferior clivus. Given the anatomic changes secondary to basilar impression, the dens was located just posterior to the inferior clivus that had been removed. The anterior arch of C1 was then progressively drilled to allow access to the dens (**Fig. 7**). Once the anterior arch of C1 was removed, visualized preodontoid fibrosis was removed allowing view of the dens. The dens was then progressively cored with maintenance of the outer cortex of the cap. The cap was then thinned and removed, resulting in excellent decompression as confirmed by pulsations of the thecal sac (**Fig. 8**). No cerebrospinal fluid (CSF) leak was encountered during this dissection, and the wound was then left to heal by secondary intention. Given that the anterior decompression resulted in expected instability, a posterior fusion was sequentially performed in the same operative setting. Postoperative imaging confirmed excellent decompression (**Fig. 9**).

Reconstruction

Postoperative CSF leak is the main limitation of endoscopic endonasal approaches. However, with the introduction and use of the nasoseptal flap and other vascularized reconstructive options, the incidence of postoperative CSF leak has dramatically decreased.[32,33] When approaching lesions at the level of the CVJ, it is essential to

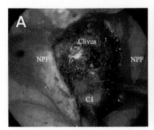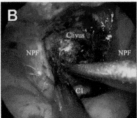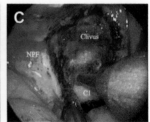

Fig. 7. (*A*) Visualization of the inferior clivus and anterior arch of C1 with lateralization of the nasopharyngeal mucosa and paraspinal musculature, or nasopharyngeal flap (NPF). (*B*) Further view of the inferior clivus and anterior arch of C1 with instruments placed on the atlanto-occipital membrane. (*C*) Initial drilling of the inferior clivus and anterior arch of C1.

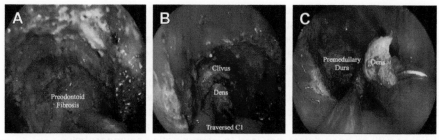

Fig. 8. (*A*) Visualization of preodontoid fibrosis after transgression of the anterior arch of C1. (*B*) Progressive coring of the dens with maintenance of the dens cap. (*C*) Removal of the thinned dens cap and visualization of decompressed premedullary dura.

make the nasoseptal flap large enough to reach the caudal limit of the defect. To have a nasoseptal flap of adequate dimensions, the inferior cut of the flap can be extended onto the nasal floor or even inferolaterally to incorporate the mucosa of the inferior turbinate.[34]

Several reconstructive techniques have been described. In cases in which a CSF leak has been noted, the dural defect is generally first covered with an inlay dural substitute or autologous free graft (eg, fascia lata). Then, the vascularized flap is placed for onlay coverage. It is of particular importance that the flap lays on bony edges of the defect that have been fully cleared of mucosa. Oxidized cellulose (Surgicel; Ethicon, Somerville, NJ) or dural sealant can be placed at the edges of the bone–flap interface to augment the repair. In cases in which there is a large clival bony defect, this dead space can be obliterated with autologous fat graft. Finally, the nasal cavity is filled with absorbable or nonabsorbable packing. In cases in which a CSF leak was not noted, the wound can be left to heal by secondary attention.

POTENTIAL COMPLICATIONS AND MANAGEMENT

One potential concern with endonasal approaches is the ability to obtain hemostasis. Adapted techniques, hemostatic agents, and specialized instrumentation designed for endoscopic endonasal procedures including the use of diamond burrs, injectable hemostatic agents, warm irrigation, and pistol grip bipolar devices have all made

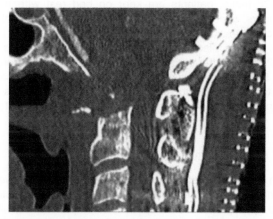

Fig. 9. Postoperative imaging shows odontoidectomy and complete decompression.

hemostasis feasible.[35–37] Arterial hypotension, which is often used to help control nasal mucosal bleeding, is strictly avoided when entering the intracranial space or when brainstem or upper cervical spinal cord compression is present to maintain adequate perfusion of the brain, brainstem, and spinal cord.

Postoperative CSF leak may occur despite meticulous reconstruction. The authors favor early surgical re-exploration for patients with postoperative CSF leak to identify the site of leak. Intrathecal fluorescein injection may be used to facilitate identification of the CSF fistula site in cases of low-flow leaks. CSF drainage through a lumbar sub-arachnoid drain is only used as an adjunctive measure after surgical repair, as CSF drainage with an open defect may lead to symptomatic pneumocephalus.

Carotid artery injury is a major known complication of the endoscopic endonasal transclival approach. Avoidance of this complication first requires early and accurate identification of the carotid arteries. Preoperative imaging is evaluated to assess for any anatomic variations that may place the carotid artery at increased risk for injury. Intraoperatively, accurate image guidance and the use of a micro-Doppler can facilitate identification of the carotid artery. If a coarse diamond burr is used, it must be first dulled slightly by drilling in other areas before being used to drill over the carotid artery. If carotid injury occurs, large bore suctions are used to control the surgical field and identify the source of bleeding. There are several options for hemostasis, which include bipolar cauterization to weld the defect shut, direct compression, compressive packing, suture repair, or reconstruction using clips (eg, aneurysm clip or Sundt clip graft).[38] Crushed muscle, emergently obtained from the thigh, can be useful to induce thrombosis when placed over the defect under compression. Of note, intra-dural procedures should not be treated with packing alone given that blood will track into the subdural space.[38] Angiography should be performed in the acute and delayed phases to assess the patency of the artery and to rule out pseudoaneurysm formation.

Lastly, there is risk of damage to the lower cranial nerves and lower brainstem. Careful, gentle dissection along with the maintenance of adequate cerebral perfusion pressure is necessary. Intraoperative neuromonitoring is useful to obtain real-time feedback of any unwanted nerve traction or manipulation. In addition, it may be prudent to leave behind anything that is significantly adherent to critical neurovascular structures.

POST-PROCEDURAL CARE

For high-flow CSF leaks, patients are kept on bed rest with the head of bed elevated for 24 hours, after which the patients are aggressively mobilized. Intermittent pneumatic compression stockings are placed on both legs during and after surgery. Patients may be placed on chemoprophylaxis for venous thromboembolism prevention 24 hours after surgery or sooner in high-risk patients. Nasal packings are kept for 5 to 7 days and usually removed in the office. Nasal saline spray is applied several times per day to reduce nasal crusting. Patients are advised to avoid sneezing, bending over, bearing down, or blowing the nose for 4 weeks after surgery.

REHABILITATION AND RECOVERY

For patients with lesions located near the lower cranial nerves, swallow function is tested before a diet is initiated. Patients with existing or new neurologic deficits are assessed for the appropriateness of inpatient or outpatient rehabilitation. Patients are advised of potential sinonasal morbidity including nasal crusting, discharge, and airflow blockage.[39] Most nasal symptoms resolve after 3 to 4 months but may persist in some cases.

Outcomes and Review of the Literature

Surgical outcomes depend on the type of pathologic condition treated and the surgical approach (transclival or odontoidectomy). The most common condition treated with the endoscopic endonasal transclival approach is chordoma. A recent review of the literature comprising 100 cases of endoscopic endonasal treatment of clival chordomas found a gross total resection rate of 70.4%.[40] Rate of postoperative CSF leak was 18.8% of 80 cases reporting on this outcome.[40]

A review of the literature of surgical outcomes for endoscopic endonasal odontoidectomy found 13 studies comprising 92 patients.[12,41–52] Neurologic outcomes after surgery were improved in 94.0%, unchanged in 6.0%, and worse in 0%. Postoperative CSF leak occurred in 5.2%. Tracheostomy was required in 3.4% of patients and dysphagia occurred in 3.6%. Wound infection occurred in 1.9% and meningitis in 4.0%. There were no reported arterial injuries.

SUMMARY

The endoscopic endonasal approach is a direct surgical route that can be used for ventrally located lesions at the CVJ. Lesions with extension lateral to the lower cranial nerves cannot be exclusively treated through an endoscopic endonasal approach. The vascularized nasoseptal flap has dramatically reduced the incidence of postoperative CSF leak, which historically was one of the primary limitations of the endonasal approach. Given that endoscopic endonasal odontoidectomy is performed without retraction of the soft palate, velopalatal insufficiency risk is potential avoidable compared with transoral approaches. Overall, endoscopic endonasal approaches can be performed in appropriate cases safely. A collaborative effort between neurosurgery and otolaryngology is strongly advocated to optimize patient outcomes.

REFERENCES

1. Love JG, Thelen EP, Dodge HW Jr. Tumors of the foramen magnum. J Int Coll Surg 1954;22(1 1):1–17.
2. Stein BM, Leeds NE, Taveras JM, et al. Meningiomas of the foramen magnum. J Neurosurg 1963;20:740–51.
3. Abdullah KG, Schlenk RS, Krishnaney A, et al. Direct lateral approach to pathology at the craniocervical junction: a technical note. Neurosurgery 2012;70(2 Suppl Operative):202–8.
4. Arnautovic KI, Al-Mefty O, Husain M. Ventral foramen magnum meninigiomas. J Neurosurg 2000;92(1 Suppl):71–80.
5. Babu RP, Sekhar LN, Wright DC. Extreme lateral transcondylar approach: technical improvements and lessons learned. J Neurosurg 1994;81(1):49–59.
6. Crockard HA, Sen CN. The transoral approach for the management of intradural lesions at the craniovertebral junction: review of 7 cases. Neurosurgery 1991; 28(1):88–97 [discussion: 97–8].
7. Dasenbrock HH, Clarke MJ, Bydon A, et al. Endoscopic image-guided transcervical odontoidectomy: outcomes of 15 patients with basilar invagination. Neurosurgery 2012;70(2):351–9 [discussion: 359–60].
8. George B, Lot G. Anterolateral and posterolateral approaches to the foramen magnum: technical description and experience from 97 cases. Skull Base Surg 1995;5(1):9–19.

9. Kassam AB, Snyderman C, Gardner P, et al. The expanded endonasal approach: a fully endoscopic transnasal approach and resection of the odontoid process: technical case report. Neurosurgery 2005;57(1 Suppl):E213 [discussion: E213].

10. Kshettry VR, Chotai S, Chen W, et al. Quantitative analysis of the effect of brainstem shift on surgical approaches to anterolateral tumors at the craniovertebral junction. J Clin Neurosci 2014;21(4):644–50.

11. Kshettry VR, Chotai S, Hou J, et al. Successful resection of anterior and anterolateral lesions at the craniovertebral junction using a simple posterolateral approach. J Clin Neurosci 2014;21(4):616–22.

12. Mazzatenta D, Zoli M, Mascari C, et al. Endoscopic endonasal odontoidectomy: clinical series. Spine 2014;39(10):846–53.

13. McGirt MJ, Attenello FJ, Sciubba DM, et al. Endoscopic transcervical odontoidectomy for pediatric basilar invagination and cranial settling. Report of 4 cases. J Neurosurg Pediatr 2008;1(4):337–42.

14. Miller E, Crockard HA. Transoral transclival removal of anteriorly placed meningiomas at the foramen magnum. Neurosurgery 1987;20(6):966–8.

15. Pillai P, Baig MN, Karas CS, et al. Endoscopic image-guided transoral approach to the craniovertebral junction: an anatomic study comparing surgical exposure and surgical freedom obtained with the endoscope and the operating microscope. Neurosurgery 2009;64(5 Suppl 2):437–42 [discussion: 442–4].

16. Rhoton AL Jr. The far-lateral approach and its transcondylar, supracondylar, and paracondylar extensions. Neurosurgery 2000;47(3 Suppl):S195–209.

17. Wolinsky JP, Sciubba DM, Suk I, et al. Endoscopic image-guided odontoidectomy for decompression of basilar invagination via a standard anterior cervical approach. Technical note. J Neurosurg Spine 2007;6(2):184–91.

18. Kassam A, Snyderman CH, Mintz A, et al. Expanded endonasal approach: the rostrocaudal axis. Part II. Posterior clinoids to the foramen magnum. Neurosurg Focus 2005;19(1):E4.

19. Chotai S, Kshettry VR, Ammirati M. Endoscopic-assisted microsurgical techniques at the craniovertebral junction: 4 illustrative cases and literature review. Clin Neurol Neurosurg 2014;121:1–9.

20. Kshettry VR, Benzel EC. Endoscopic-assisted techniques at the craniovertebral junction: understanding indications and limitations. World Neurosurg 2014; 82(6):e711–2.

21. Blitz AM, Macedo LL, Chonka ZD, et al. High-resolution CISS MR imaging with and without contrast for evaluation of the upper cranial nerves: segmental anatomy and selected pathologic conditions of the cisternal through extraforaminal segments. Neuroimaging Clin N Am 2014;24(1):17–34.

22. Atlas G, Lee M. The neural integrity monitor electromyogram tracheal tube: anesthetic considerations. J Anaesthesiol Clin Pharmacol 2013;29(3):403–4.

23. Morera VA, Fernandez-Miranda JC, Prevedello DM, et al. "Far-medial" expanded endonasal approach to the inferior third of the clivus: the transcondylar and transjugular tubercle approaches. Neurosurgery 2010;66(6 Suppl Operative):211–9 [discussion: 219–20].

24. Paulsen F, Tillmann B, Christofides C, et al. Curving and looping of the internal carotid artery in relation to the pharynx: frequency, embryology and clinical implications. J Anat 2000;197(Pt 3):373–81.

25. Pfeiffer J, Ridder GJ. A clinical classification system for aberrant internal carotid arteries. Laryngoscope 2008;118(11):1931–6.

26. Panjabi M, Dvorak J, Crisco J 3rd, et al. Flexion, extension, and lateral bending of the upper cervical spine in response to alar ligament transections. J Spinal Disord 1991;4(2):157–67.
27. Panjabi M, Dvorak J, Crisco JJ 3rd, et al. Effects of alar ligament transection on upper cervical spine rotation. J Orthop Res 1991;9(4):584–93.
28. Little AS, Perez-Orribo L, Rodriguez-Martinez NG, et al. Biomechanical evaluation of the craniovertebral junction after inferior-third clivectomy and intradural exposure of the foramen magnum: implications for endoscopic endonasal approaches to the cranial base. J Neurosurg Spine 2013;18(4):327–32.
29. Perez-Orribo L, Little AS, Lefevre RD, et al. Biomechanical evaluation of the craniovertebral junction after anterior unilateral condylectomy: implications for endoscopic endonasal approaches to the cranial base. Neurosurgery 2013; 72(6):1021–9 [discussion: 1029–30].
30. Ponce-Gomez JA, Ortega-Porcayo LA, Soriano-Baron HE, et al. Evolution from microscopic transoral to endoscopic endonasal odontoidectomy. Neurosurg Focus 2014;37(4):E15.
31. de Almeida JR, Zanation AM, Snyderman CH, et al. Defining the nasopalatine line: the limit for endonasal surgery of the spine. Laryngoscope 2009;119(2): 239–44.
32. Hadad G, Bassagasteguy L, Carrau RL, et al. A novel reconstructive technique after endoscopic expanded endonasal approaches: vascular pedicle nasoseptal flap. Laryngoscope 2006;116(10):1882–6.
33. Kassam AB, Thomas A, Carrau RL, et al. Endoscopic reconstruction of the cranial base using a pedicled nasoseptal flap. Neurosurgery 2008;63(1 Suppl 1): ONS44–52 [discussion: ONS52–3].
34. Peris-Celda M, Pinheiro-Neto CD, Funaki T, et al. The extended nasoseptal flap for skull base reconstruction of the clival region: an anatomical and radiological study. J Neurol Surg B Skull Base 2013;74(6):369–85.
35. Kassam A, Snyderman CH, Carrau RL, et al. Endoneurosurgical hemostasis techniques: lessons learned from 400 cases. Neurosurg Focus 2005;19(1):E7.
36. Schlegel-Wagner C, Siekmann U, Linder T. Non-invasive treatment of intractable posterior epistaxis with hot-water irrigation. Rhinology 2006;44(1):90–3.
37. Stangerup SE, Dommerby H, Siim C, et al. New modification of hot-water irrigation in the treatment of posterior epistaxis. Arch Otolaryngol Head Neck Surg 1999;125(6):686–90.
38. Solares CA, Ong YK, Carrau RL, et al. Prevention and management of vascular injuries in endoscopic surgery of the sinonasal tract and skull base. Otolaryngol Clin North Am 2010;43(4):817–25.
39. Awad AJ, Mohyeldin A, El-Sayed IH, et al. Sinonasal morbidity following endoscopic endonasal skull base surgery. Clin Neurol Neurosurg 2015;130: 162–7.
40. Saito K, Toda M, Tomita T, et al. Surgical results of an endoscopic endonasal approach for clival chordomas. Acta Neurochir 2012;154(5):879–86.
41. Choudhri O, Mindea SA, Feroze A, et al. Experience with intraoperative navigation and imaging during endoscopic transnasal spinal approaches to the foramen magnum and odontoid. Neurosurg Focus 2014;36(3):E4.
42. Duntze J, Eap C, Kleiber JC, et al. Advantages and limitations of endoscopic endonasal odontoidectomy. A series of nine cases. Orthop Traumatol Surg Res 2014;100(7):775–8.
43. Gempt J, Lehmberg J, Grams AE, et al. Endoscopic transnasal resection of the odontoid: case series and clinical course. Eur Spine J 2011;20(4):661–6.

44. Gladi M, Iacoangeli M, Specchia N, et al. Endoscopic transnasal odontoid resection to decompress the bulbo-medullary junction: a reliable anterior minimally invasive technique without posterior fusion. Eur Spine J 2012;21(Suppl 1): S55–60.
45. Goldschlager T, Hartl R, Greenfield JP, et al. The endoscopic endonasal approach to the odontoid and its impact on early extubation and feeding. J Neurosurg 2015; 122(3):511–8.
46. Iacoangeli M, Gladi M, Alvaro L, et al. Endoscopic endonasal odontoidectomy with anterior C1 arch preservation in elderly patients affected by rheumatoid arthritis. Spine J 2013;13(5):542–8.
47. Lee A, Sommer D, Reddy K, et al. Endoscopic transnasal approach to the craniocervical junction. Skull Base 2010;20(3):199–205.
48. Nayak JV, Gardner PA, Vescan AD, et al. Experience with the expanded endonasal approach for resection of the odontoid process in rheumatoid disease. Am J Rhinol 2007;21(5):601–6.
49. Tan SH, Ganesan D, Prepageran N, et al. A minimally invasive endoscopic transnasal approach to the craniovertebral junction in the paediatric population. Eur Arch Otorhinolaryngol 2014;271(11):3101–5.
50. Yen YS, Chang PY, Huang WC, et al. Endoscopic transnasal odontoidectomy without resection of nasal turbinates: clinical outcomes of 13 patients. J Neurosurg Spine 2014;21(6):929–37.
51. Yu Y, Wang X, Zhang X, et al. Endoscopic transnasal odontoidectomy to treat basilar invagination with congenital osseous malformations. Eur Spine J 2013; 22(5):1127–36.
52. Tormenti MJ, Carrau R, Snyderman CH, et al. Endoscopic endonasal resection of the odontoid process: clinical outcomes. 2010 American Association of Neurological Surgeons Annual Meeting. Philadelphia, May 1–5, 2000.

Complication Avoidance in Endoscopic Skull Base Surgery

Peleg M. Horowitz, MD, PhD[a,1], Vincent DiNapoli, MD, PhD[a,b,1], Shirley Y. Su, MD[c], Shaan M. Raza, MD[a,c],*

KEYWORDS

- Endoscopic skull base surgery • Complications • Diabetes insipidus
- Panhypopituitarism • CSF leak • Vascular injury • Cranial nerve injury

KEY POINTS

- Expanded endoscopic resection of pituitary and complex skull base pathology requires an understanding of medical and surgical complications unique to these surgical techniques.
- Common medical complications include anterior and posterior pituitary dysfunction and meningitis; other medical complications such as venous thromboembolism or pneumonia are rare.
- Common surgical complications include vascular injury, cerebrospinal fluid fistula owing to reconstruction failure, cranial nerve injury, and infection/meningitis.

INTRODUCTION

The use of endoscopic endonasal approaches (EEA) to the skull base pathology has evolved significantly over the past 2 decades. Development of the 2-surgeon collaboration between neurosurgery and otolaryngology physicians for the endoscopic resection of pituitary adenomas has led to significant innovation and expansion of this approach to various skull base pathologies. As indications have expanded, surgeons have begun to define the expected incidence of common complications and adopted techniques to avoid or manage these adverse outcomes. With expansion of endoscopic approaches to more challenging tumors (ie, malignancies, intradural pathology), it is imperative that fundamental skull base principles are not short

[a] Department of Neurosurgery, The University of Texas M.D. Anderson Cancer Center, 1500 Holcombe Blvd, Houston, TX 77030, USA; [b] Department of Neurosurgery, The Mayfield Clinic, University of Cincinnati, 260 Stetson Street, Suite 2200, Cincinnati, OH 45267, USA; [c] Department of Head and Neck Surgery, The University of Texas M.D. Anderson Cancer Center, 1500 Holcombe Blvd, Houston, TX 77030, USA
[1] Both authors contributed equally to this article.
* Corresponding author. Department of Neurosurgery, 1500 Holcombe Boulevard, Unit 442, Houston, TX 77030.
E-mail address: smraza@mdanderson.org

Otolaryngol Clin N Am 49 (2016) 227–235
http://dx.doi.org/10.1016/j.otc.2015.09.014
0030-6665/16/$ – see front matter © 2016 Elsevier Inc. All rights reserved.
oto.theclinics.com

changed for the sake of performing an approach. In this article we review the complications and common pitfalls of the EEA for complex cranial base pathology.

ENDOCRINOLOGIC COMPLICATIONS

The most frequent postoperative systemic complications relate directly to the manipulation or disruption of the normal hypothalamic–pituitary axis. Diabetes insipidus (DI), the syndrome of inappropriate antidiuretic hormone release, and panhypopituitarism consequently occur almost exclusively in those populations of patients in which the pituitary gland, stalk, or hypothalamus are involved in either the pathology or the surgical corridor. These can be classified further pathophysiologically as perturbations of anterior gland (secretory function) or posterior gland (osmostat function).

Many studies have suggested equivalent rates of postoperative sodium dysregulation in microscopic and endoscopic pituitary surgery, approximating 11% to 14% in a recent metaanalysis.[1] Risk factors for developing postoperative DI (either transient or permanent) include tumor size, young age, and pathology involving the posterior gland or stalk, that is, Rathke's cleft cyst or craniopharyngioma.[2,3] Pars intermedia tumors and cystic adenomas likely confer an intermediate increase in risk, as does surgical exploration of the posterior gland and intraoperative traction on the pituitary stalk. These perturbations often manifest within the first 48 to 72 hours after surgery. However, delayed postoperative hyponatremia occurs in approximately 15% of cases, peaking between 1 and 2 weeks after surgery, leading to readmission in 6.4% of cases.[4]

Management of postoperative sodium fluctuations starts with vigilant attention to laboratory values, often by checking serum sodium and urine specific gravity every 6 hours for the first 2 to 3 days after surgery, and checking serum sodium on a postoperative clinic visit. The syndrome of inappropriate antidiuretic hormone release is most often mild and managed by fluid restriction and free water deprivation; rare refractory or severe cases may require hypertonic infusion. DI may likewise be mild and managed by drinking free water to thirst, or may require desmopressin by various routes. By carefully educating patients on the signs and symptoms of sodium imbalance and the avoidance of excessive free water on discharge, it may be possible to reduce the incidence of delayed postoperative hyponatremia requiring readmission. Last, the surgeon must be mindful of the possibility of the so-called triple phase response, which encompasses the syndrome of inappropriate antidiuretic hormone release, transient DI, and delayed postoperative hyponatremia.[5]

Hypopituitarism after pituitary surgery likewise has not been shown to differ significantly between microscopic and endoscopic approaches, in approximately 3% to 6% of cases.[1] Adrenal crisis after such surgery can be fatal, although this can be avoided easily with judicious use of preoperative, intraoperative, and postoperative steroid administration. Preoperative low fasting morning cortisol should alert the surgeon that stress dose steroid administration on induction of anesthesia and subsequent taper to a maintenance dose may be indicated. Fasting morning cortisol should likewise be monitored while patients are in house, with cortisol repletion in cases where it is low. Any clinical suspicion for adrenal crisis should prompt swift response to administer steroids because a delay could be life threatening. After cortisol, repletion of thyroid hormone may also be considered, though the longer half-lives of thyroid hormone and other anterior gland hormones make their administration less critical in the immediate postoperative period.

PERIOPERATIVE ANTIBIOTICS AND MENINGITIS

The use of perioperative antibiotics for EEA to skull base and pituitary tumors has been carried over from data relating to open skull base procedures.[6] As the use of the EEA becomes more widely adopted, data specific to these populations are beginning to emerge. Intuitively, one would expect the majority of infections to arise from the repetitive passage of surgical instruments via the nonsterile nasal passageways. As such, the organism most commonly isolated in culture-positive sinusitis is *Staphylococcus aureus* and suggests that the perioperative usage of narrow spectrum antibiotic coverage of gram-positive bacteria is prudent. A study looking at perioperative infections in a population undergoing EEA for various skull base pathologies demonstrated no cases of postoperative meningitis when giving cefazolin or vancomycin (penicillin allergic patients) in the 24-hour perioperative period.[7]

A quantitative analysis of 2005 patients undergoing expanded EEA, excluding transsellar approached for pituitary adenomas, revealed an incidence of postoperative meningitis of 1.8%.[8] In the subgroup experiencing a postoperative cerebrospinal fluid (CSF) leak, the incidence increased to 13%. This was compared with 0.1% of those without postoperative leak ($P<.01$).[8] Independent risk factors for postoperative infection include male sex, history of prior craniotomy or endonasal surgery, ventriculoperitoneal shunt and higher complexity intradural procedures.

These data suggest that the overall rate of postoperative meningitis in patients undergoing EEA to the skull base is low. Additional precautions may be taken for those patients with these risk factors, including use of broader spectrum perioperative coverage, tight control of perioperative glucose for diabetics, preoperative nasal cultures to reveal resistant organisms, and inclusion of antibiotics in operative irrigation solution.

OTHER MEDICAL COMPLICATIONS

Expanded endoscopic endonasal surgery is generally well-tolerated, with shorter operating room times, duration of stay, and lower rates of medical complications than transcranial approaches.[9] Patients with Cushing's disease undergoing surgical treatment are at higher risk for many systemic complications, likely because of the far-reaching adverse effects of long-term hypercortisolemia on the body.[10] In general, postoperative medical complications not directly related to the surgery itself (ie, endocrinopathies) are uncommon.

Venous thromboembolism (VTE) is rare in the population of patients undergoing EEA, and is more likely to occur in patients who are older or have underlying coagulopathy or peripheral vascular disorders.[11] Postoperative neurologic complications, CSF leak, electrolyte imbalances, and cardiopulmonary complications are also associated with VTE, likely because these increase patient immobility and hospital duration of stay. Mechanical prophylaxis with sequential compression boots and early and frequent ambulation are used in most cases unless contraindicated. The use of chemoprophylaxis is controversial, and surgeons must consider the risk of VTE against the risk of postoperative hematoma; as such, it is usually reserved for patients with Cushing disease or other conditions that place them at higher risk.

The incidence of pneumonia is similarly lower after endoscopic approaches to the sellar region than transfrontal approaches, occurring in fewer than 0.6% of patients overall.[12] There is, as expected, an association with older age and presence of congestive heart failure or chronic pulmonary disease. Incentive spirometry can be used to reduce the risk of pneumonia in these populations.

CRANIAL NEUROPATHIES

Incurring a neurologic insult from EEA surgery can increase duration of stay, immobility, and lead to further medical complications. A large series of 800 patients undergoing EEA for skull base pathology demonstrated a low overall risk for transient (2.5%) and permanent (1.8%) worsening of neurologic deficit.[13] Ultimately, ideal approach selection (ie, transcranial vs EEA for paramedian skull base pathology) along with thoughtful and meticulous microsurgical dissection ensure optimal cranial nerve outcomes with any skull base resection.

Patients harboring anterior cranial fossa, sellar, and parasellar skull base lesions often present with visual deficits. Studies examining resection of pituitary lesions with preexisting visual complaints demonstrate equivalent postoperative outcomes, comparing microscopic approaches with EEA, with respect to stability or improvement of visual symptoms. There was no demonstrable increased risk for worsening vision.[14,15] Key factors to preservation and improvement of vision include minimizing nerve manipulation, relieving mechanical pressure at any tethering points, and preservation of vascular supply. Often a neglected artery, the superior hypophyseal branches of the supraclinoid internal carotid artery (ICA) provide arterial supply to the optic chiasm and cisternal segments of the optic nerve. Understanding the arachnoidal relationship of these branches to the growth pattern of the target lesion is critical to avoiding ischemic injury to the optic apparatus.[16] With regard to the management of relief of mechanical pressure of the nerves, lessons learned from the surgical resection of tuberculum meningiomas are useful. Several studies have demonstrated that unroofing of the optic canal by transcranial approach[17] or decompression via EEA[18] leads to improvement of visual symptoms in a majority of cases, and is a critical step in surgically managing tuberculum sellae or planum sphenoidale meningioma with intracanalicular extension into the optic canal. Typically, early canal decompression during the course of the operation provides optimal immediate postoperative outcomes. A review article by Raza and colleagues[16] indicates roles for both endoscopic and transcranial skull base approaches in providing optimal visual outcomes and rates of resection depending on the size of tumor, involvement of the anterior communicating artery perforators, and pattern of optic canal extension (ie, superior vs inferior to the nerve).

Extension of EEA laterally as performed in medial cavernous sinus, transclival, petrous apex and Meckel's cave and infratemporal fossa approaches can carry additional risk to the VIth cranial nerve. Detailed anatomic knowledge of the relationship of the 6th nerve to the cavernous carotid as the nerve transitions through its intracranial (interdural, gulfar, and cavernous) segments (**Fig. 1**) can help to avoid inadvertent injury.[19] Specific landmarks such as the vertebrobasilar junction for transclival approach, the lateral segment of the ICA and sellar floor for medial petrous apex approach, and V2 for Meckel's cave approach allow for reliable localization. Intraoperative electromyographic monitoring of the VIth cranial nerve has been described and can provide additional warning during exposure and dissection.[20]

In the authors' experience, anatomic relationships of tumors to cranial nerves can be predicted to some degree by common sites of tumor origin, tumor consistency, and propensity for growth into a certain area. For example, pituitary adenomas originate within the sella, and tend to push the cranial nerves within the cavernous sinus lateral and the abducens nerve inferolateral if the tumor extends via the retrocarotid space into the cavernous sinus. For disease extending into the cavernous sinus anterior to the cavernous carotid artery, the abducens nerve is displaced superiorly. Chondrosarcomas, contrarily, commonly originate at the petroclival synchondrosis and

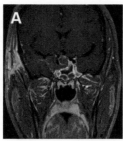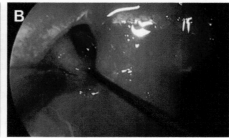

Fig. 1. Cavernous sinus resection with identification of cranial nerve VI. T1-weighted coronal MRI with contrast (*A*) showing a growth hormone–secreting pituitary adenoma invasive into the lateral cavernous sinus. Previous biopsy at an outside hospital indicated this to be a World Health Organization grade II adenoma. An expanded endoscopic endonasal approach was performed to resect the sellar and lateral cavernous sinus components of the tumor. (*B*) Intraoperative view with the Kartush stimulator on the sixth cranial nerve as it transitions from the cavernous sinus to the superior orbital fissure. (*Courtesy of* University of Texas M.D. Anderson Cancer Center, Houston, TX; with permission.)

tend to push the abducens nerve superoromedial. Accounting for these expected anatomic relationships could help in avoiding inadvertent nerve injury during dissection.

MANAGEMENT OF POSTOPERATIVE CEREBROSPINAL FLUID FISTULA

No different from any open skull base resection, of additional importance during any endoscopic resection is avoiding excessive intraoperative CSF egress. There have been several case reports regarding immediate complications related to excessive CSF egress during EEA resections, including symptomatic pneumocephalus, acute subdural hemorrhage, cerebellar sag resulting in intraparenchymal hemorrhage, and traction on the abducens nerves.[21] Such complications can be avoided by ensuring that the lumbar drain (if placed) is clamped during surgery and maintaining the patient at normocapnia (particularly for older patients with age-related cerebral atrophy).

An increasingly rare event, in cases of postoperative CSF leak, the initial workup consists of intracranial imaging to assess for possible graft displacement and pneumocephalus. Often, postoperative nasal drainage owing to residual surgical irrigation in the paranasal sinuses is confused for a CSF leak. The presence of pneumocephalus around the graft site on computed tomography imaging is highly predictive for a CSF fistula.[22] For low-flow leaks with no evidence of intracranial pneumocephalus, the initial treatment is lumbar drainage for 3 to 5 days. For high-flow leaks, these patients are taken back to the operating room for an immediate repair. During such repairs, it is imperative that all layers of the reconstruction are examined thoroughly and any vascularized flaps previously used are assessed for ischemia. Additionally, intrathecal fluorescein can be useful for inspecting adjacent areas of the resection should be assessed for previously unrecognized skull base defects as a source of the leak.

VASCULAR INJURY

ICA injury is a severe but rare complication of both open and endoscopic skull base approaches to invasive cranial base pathology, and carries with it significant morbidity and mortality. In transsphenoidal surgeries performed for pituitary adenomas, published rates of ICA injury range from 0.2% to 1.4%.[23–25] In a large series of 2015 patients undergoing EEA for various skull base pathologies, an overall incidence of ICA injury was reported at 0.3%. This series reported the highest rate of injury for chondroid tumors (chondrosarcoma and chordoma) with an incidence of 2%, which the authors attributed to greater ICA exposure, anatomy obscured by tumor, and more aggressive oncologic goals. Low rates were reported for the pathologies of pituitary adenoma (0.3%), malignancy (0.5%), and meningioma (0.8%). The authors also reported a correlation with the type of approach, which increased in transclival or transpterygoid approaches (0.9%).[26]

The rate of ICA sacrifice after intraoperative injury was 57%, with no patients experiencing new neurologic sequelae.[26] A single mortality (17%) was reported in this group owing to cardiac ischemia related to operative blood loss. These results suggest a very low overall incidence of ICA injury during EEA to ventral skull base pathologies. Knowledge of typical ICA anatomy and course (**Fig. 2**), along with a 2-surgeon, 4-handed technique are suggested as the best preventative measures.[26] Additionally, standard microsurgical dissection techniques using sharp and blunt dissection with

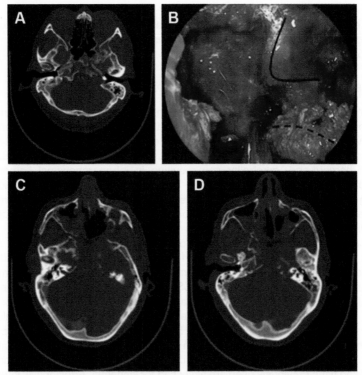

Fig. 2. Extensive recurrent chordoma involving the left internal carotid artery. (*A*) Preoperative computed tomography (CT) angiogram shows circumferential involvement of the horizontal petrous and paraclival segments of left internal carotid artery by calcified tumor. (*B*) Intraoperative picture with involved arterial segments fully skeletonized (*solid black line,* paraclival and lateral internal carotid artery segments; *dashed black line,* superior aspect of the Eustachian tube). (*C, D*) Postoperative CT angiogram imaging demonstrating full extent of carotid exposure. (*Courtesy of* University of Texas M.D. Anderson Cancer Center, Houston, TX; with permission.)

particular attention to arachnoid planes should be used in dealing with intradural pathology (**Fig. 3**).

Preoperative studies, including a computed tomography or conventional angiogram, can guide the management of vascular involvement or intraoperative injury. Such studies provide information with regard to the patient's vascular collateralization and reserve in the situation of an ICA injury. The presence of sufficiently sized anterior communicating artery and posterior communicating arteries suggest an adequately developed circle of Willis. The presence of isolated A1/2 and M1/2 arterial segments indicate a high risk of symptomatic postoperative ischemia in the event of vascular injury. When preoperative studies suggest either circumferential involvement or adventitial invasion (ie, the presence of luminal irregularity) of the ICA, then a balloon test occlusion (BTO) should be done with temporary occlusion across the concerning segment of the vessel. In situations where there is inadequate vascular reserve (ie, the development of clinical symptoms or perfusion mismatch on a Diamox challenge computed tomography perfusion during BTO), then either role of surgery should be reassessed or a vascular bypass performed. Above all, it is important to recognize that, in general, there are few data to support elective carotid resection for the purposes of achieving negative margins.

The intraoperative management of a lacerated ICA starts with the immediate objective of establishing hemostasis and preserving cerebral circulation. One must adhere to standard vascular principles of obtaining proximal/distal control and adequately exposing and visualizing the injury. This may involve exposure of the cervical ICA, via a separate incision, if the horizontal/vertical petrous or parapharyngeal ICA is involved. Techniques of intraoperative management have been reported to include clip reconstruction, bipolar electrocautery, packing, and ICA sacrifice. The most common scenario is that of packing followed by immediate transfer of the patient to the endovascular suite for angiographic investigation. The injured vessel is examined thoroughly for luminal irregularity, dissection, pseudoaneurysm, or subintimal or transadventitial contrast extravasation. Management is contingent upon clinical and radiographic findings of a BTO. An understanding of the evolving array of endovascular techniques, such as stents and flow diverters, is also important to optimal management. In situations where the BTO has failed and a pseudoaneurysm or dissection is present, then a flow diverter with coiling can be a feasible option. If this is not possible, then a high-flow vascular bypass with clip sacrifice of the injured segment provides the

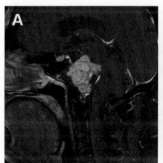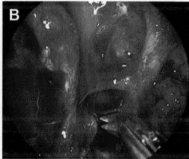

Fig. 3. Chordoma involving middle and lower clivus with intradural extension. (*A*) Sagittal T1-weighted MRI with contrast depicting a chordoma with brainstem compression and involvement of the vertebrobasilar arterial system. (*B*) Sharp dissection to preserve the anterior inferior cerebellar and basilar arteries as tumor is resected. (*Courtesy of* University of Texas M.D. Anderson Cancer Center, Houston, TX; with permission.)

next best option. When the vessel wall has been lacerated, then the management options are either parent vessel sacrifice (if a BTO is passed) or vascular bypass with parent vessel sacrifice (when a BTO is failed). A final important consideration is when the initial postinjury angiogram shows no vessel abnormality. When there is an high index of suspicion, repeat vascular imaging should be performed in 7 to 10 days to rule out a developing traumatic pseudoaneurysm.

SUMMARY

Medical complications related to endoscopic skull base surgery are uncommon, and relate most often to the surgical pathology and nearby structures at risk. Rates of endocrinopathies are similar to those after microscopic transsphenoidal and trans-basal approaches, whereas rates of unrelated medical complications such as VTE and pneumonia are lower in endoscopic approaches. The maturation of endoscopic approaches to the skull base has also led to a significant decrease in CSF leakage with the application of vascularized nasoseptal flaps. However, vascular injury remains a rare but catastrophic complication of this approach.

Overall, complication rates have decreased to a level equivalent to those observed in open anterior craniofacial approaches. Studies have shown improved quality of life and decreased morbidity associated with EEAs.[27,28] A multidisciplinary team including physical and rehabilitative medicine, otology, head and neck surgery, plastic surgery, oromaxillofacial surgery, endocrinology, and neurosurgery physicians is essential in obtaining optimal outcomes and selecting the best surgical plan for each patient. As in all skull base surgeries, success is dictated by proper patient selection, detailed anatomic knowledge, and anticipating common pitfalls.

REFERENCES

1. Gao Y, Zhong C, Wang Y, et al. Endoscopic versus microscopic transsphenoidal pituitary adenoma surgery: a meta-analysis. World J Surg Oncol 2014;12:94.
2. Staiger RD, Sarnthein J, Wiesli P, et al. Prognostic factors for impaired plasma sodium homeostasis after transsphenoidal surgery. Br J Neurosurg 2013;27:63–8.
3. Schreckinger M, Walker B, Knepper J, et al. Post-operative diabetes insipidus after endoscopic transsphenoidal surgery. Pituitary 2013;16:445–51.
4. Hussain NS, Piper M, Ludlam WG, et al. Delayed postoperative hyponatremia after transsphenoidal surgery: prevalence and associated factors. J Neurosurg 2013;119:1453–60.
5. Kristof RA, Rother M, Neuloh G, et al. Incidence, clinical manifestations, and course of water and electrolyte metabolism disturbances following transsphenoi-dal pituitary adenoma surgery: a prospective observational study. J Neurosurg 2009;111:555–62.
6. Horowitz G, Fliss DM, Margalit N, et al. Association between cerebrospinal fluid leak and meningitis after skull base surgery. Otolaryngol Head Neck Surg 2011;145:689–93.
7. Brown SM, Anand VK, Tabaee A, et al. Role of perioperative antibiotics in endoscopic skull base surgery. Laryngoscope 2007;117:1528–32.
8. Lai LT, Trooboff S, Morgan MK, et al. The risk of meningitis following expanded endoscopic endonasal skull base surgery: a systematic review. J Neurol Surg B Skull Base 2014;75:18–26.
9. Villwock JA, Villwock MR, Goyal P, et al. Current trends in surgical approach and outcomes following pituitary tumor resection. Laryngoscope 2015;125:1307–12.

10. Svider PF, Raikundalia MD, Pines MJ, et al. Inpatient complications after transsphenoidal surgery in Cushing's versus non-Cushing's disease patients. Ann Otol Rhinol Laryngol 2015. [Epub ahead of print].

11. Spinazzi EF, Pines MJ, Fang CH, et al. Impact and cost of care of venous thromboembolism following pituitary surgery. Laryngoscope 2015;125:1563–7.

12. Desai SV, Fang CH, Raikundalia MD, et al. Impact of postoperative pneumonia following pituitary surgery. Laryngoscope 2015;125:1792–7.

13. Kassam AB, Prevedello DM, Carrau RL, et al. Endoscopic endonasal skull base surgery: analysis of complications in the authors' initial 800 patients. J Neurosurg 2011;114:1544–68.

14. Cappabianca P, Cavallo LM, Solari D, et al. Endoscopic endonasal surgery for pituitary adenomas. World Neurosurg 2014;82:S3–11.

15. Wang Q, Lu XJ, Ji WY, et al. Visual outcome after extended endoscopic endonasal transsphenoidal surgery for tuberculum sellae meningiomas. World Neurosurg 2010;73:694–700.

16. Raza SM, Schwartz TH. How to achieve the best possible outcomes in the management of retroinfundibular craniopharyngiomas? World Neurosurg 2014;82:614–6.

17. Mahmoud M, Nader R, Al-Mefty O. Optic canal involvement in tuberculum sellae meningiomas: influence on approach, recurrence, and visual recovery. Neurosurgery 2010;67:ons108–18 [discussion: ons118–9].

18. Attia M, Kandasamy J, Jakimovski D, et al. The importance and timing of optic canal exploration and decompression during endoscopic endonasal resection of tuberculum sella and planum sphenoidale meningiomas. Neurosurgery 2012;71:58–67.

19. Barges-Coll J, Fernandez-Miranda JC, Prevedello DM, et al. Avoiding injury to the abducens nerve during expanded endonasal endoscopic surgery: anatomic and clinical case studies. Neurosurgery 2010;67:144–54 [discussion: 154].

20. Grabb PA, Albright AL, Sclabassi RJ, et al. Continuous intraoperative electromyographic monitoring of cranial nerves during resection of fourth ventricular tumors in children. J Neurosurg 1997;86:1–4.

21. Kerr EE, Prevedello DM, Jamshidi A, et al. Immediate complications associated with high-flow cerebrospinal fluid egress during endoscopic endonasal skull base surgery. Neurosurg Focus 2014;37:E3.

22. Banu MA, Szentirmai O, Mascarenhas L, et al. Pneumocephalus patterns following endonasal endoscopic skull base surgery as predictors of postoperative CSF leaks. J Neurosurg 2014;121:961–75.

23. Dolenc VV, Lipovsek M, Slokan S. Traumatic aneurysm and carotid-cavernous fistula following transsphenoidal approach to a pituitary adenoma: treatment by transcranial operation. Br J Neurosurg 1999;13:185–8.

24. Fukushima T, Maroon JC. Repair of carotid artery perforations during transsphenoidal surgery. Surg Neurol 1998;50:174–7.

25. Laws ER Jr. Vascular complications of transsphenoidal surgery. Pituitary 1999;2:163–70.

26. Gardner PA, Tormenti MJ, Pant H, et al. Carotid artery injury during endoscopic endonasal skull base surgery: incidence and outcomes. Neurosurgery 2013;73:ons261–9 [discussion: ons269–70].

27. Castelnuovo P, Lepera D, Turri-Zanoni M, et al. Quality of life following endoscopic endonasal resection of anterior skull base cancers. J Neurosurg 2013;119:1401–9.

28. Patel KS, Raza SM, McCoul ED, et al. Long-term quality of life after endonasal endoscopic resection of adult craniopharyngiomas. J Neurosurg 2015;123:1–10.

Injury of the Internal Carotid Artery During Endoscopic Skull Base Surgery

Prevention and Management Protocol

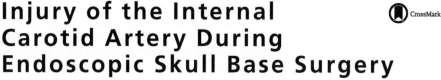

AbdulAziz AlQahtani, MD[a], Paolo Castelnuovo, MD[b],
Piero Nicolai, MD[c], Daniel M. Prevedello, MD[d,e],
Davide Locatelli, MD[f], Ricardo L. Carrau, MD[d,e,*]

KEYWORDS

- Internal carotid artery • Hemorrhage • Complications • Skull base
- Endoscopic surgery

KEY POINTS

- Preoperative planning and the identification of potential risk factors are crucial in preventing an internal carotid artery injury and minimizing its consequences.
- An effective plan of action during the catastrophe relies on a previously established protocol, availability of proper instruments and devices, and an experienced multidisciplinary team.
- Intraoperative hemostasis should be followed by an angiography and endovascular treatment whenever possible.
- Close clinical and radiologic monitoring is important to prevent early and late complications.

INTRODUCTION

Skull base surgery has undergone a remarkable metamorphosis over the past two decades, precipitated in great part by the introduction of the extended endonasal approaches (EEA).[1] Endoscopic endonasal techniques represent just one component

Conflict of Interest: The authors have nothing to disclose.
[a] Department of Otolaryngology–Head and Neck Surgery, Prince Sultan Military Medical City, Riyadh, Saudi Arabia; [b] Department of Otorhinolaryngology, University of Insubria, Varese, Italy; [c] Department of Otorhinolaryngology, University of Brescia, Brescia, Italy; [d] Department of Neurosurgery, Wexner Medical Center at the Ohio State University, Columbus, OH, USA; [e] Department of Otolaryngology–Head and Neck Surgery, Wexner Medical Center at the Ohio State University, Columbus, OH, USA; [f] Department of Neurosurgery, University of Insubria, Varese, Italy
* Corresponding author. The Ohio State University Medical Center, Starling Loving Hall, Room B221, 320 West 10th Avenue, Columbus, OH 43210.
E-mail addresses: carraurl@gmail.com; Ricardo.carrau@osumc.edu

Otolaryngol Clin N Am 49 (2016) 237–252
http://dx.doi.org/10.1016/j.otc.2015.09.009
0030-6665/16/$ – see front matter © 2016 Elsevier Inc. All rights reserved.

oto.theclinics.com

of a larger philosophic and technical shift toward minimally invasive and minimal access strategies to reduce some of the risks and complications associated with traditional open skull base surgery.[2] However, despite the fact that EEAs are effective and less invasive than traditional techniques, some surgeons consider that the risk of injury and inability to control, or repair, a major vascular injury is a significant surgical limitation of the technique.[3] Although this statement is controversial and refutable for properly selected cases, the need to expose and manipulate the internal carotid artery (ICA) within the operative field, irrespective of the approach, often dictates the extent of the surgery and may even force the surgeon to abort the surgical procedure, deeming the tumor "unresectable."[4] Therefore, the relationship of the ICA to the surgical corridor and the target lesion is an important consideration that affects the entire perioperative planning.

Rather than a rare event, encountering the ICA in one form or another is extremely common during endoscopic endonasal skull base surgery. The lateral wall of the sphenoid sinus has an intimate relationship with the ICA and a transphenoidal route is the keystone of most EEAs. A bulging ICA and dehiscence of its bony canal are found respectively in 70% and 22% of patients, therefore compounding the difficulty of a wide range of sinonasal and skull base surgeries.[5] In addition, multiple clinical situations, including the management of advanced sinonasal, middle, and posterior cranial fossa lesions, may require exposure and mobilization of the ICA. Furthermore, lesions within the petrous apex, cavernous sinus, infratemporal fossa, and parapharyngeal space require the identification of pertinent segments of ICA as a critical step.[6]

Injury to the ICA and the resultant bleeding may lead to catastrophic complications that include permanent disabilities and death. Therefore, the prevention and management of such an injury is of paramount importance. The incidence of accidental injury of the ICA during traditional skull base surgery ranges from 3% to 8%.[7] Although the rate of ICA injury during endoscopic sinus surgery is rare (<1%) and has been documented mostly as case reports, the incidence during EEAs is 10-fold higher. EEAs need a wide exposure and aim for more extensive resection; thus, it is logical that they are associated with a higher incidence (4%–9%) of ICA injury.[8,9] Nonetheless, a review of the literature suggests that its incidence is rare, being reported mostly as part of retrospective studies and case reports.[10] One must consider, however, that the incidence of this challenging surgical scenario is likely to be underestimated because many cases are not reported or the calculation of its incidence may include cases that are not at risk (eg, lesions in the anterior skull base).

There is scant literature regarding the comprehensive management of an ICA injury and hemorrhage. This article provides a panorama including a discussion of risk factors that help to recognize those patients at risk for an ICA injury, strategies to prevent the injury, and perioperative management strategies to yield the best possible outcome in case the ICA is injured. Suggested is a plan of action based on the available literature and the authors' experience. The discussion pivots around the management of bleeding from an accidental ICA injury during an EEA, where two surgeons are involved; however, the expounded principles are applicable to other clinical scenarios.

RISK FACTORS

Prevention is best; therefore, each clinical scenario and specific patient circumstances should be appraised during the perioperative period. Preoperative identification of risk factors is paramount to avoid or minimize the risk of ICA injury, to establish a surgical plan in case the vessel is injured intraoperatively, and to consider postoperative strategies that decrease the risk of morbidities related to the vascular accident or its treatment. Risk factors may be cataloged into anatomy related, pathology related, surgeon related, or institution related (**Table 1**). However, one should consider that multiple factors are usually in play during any major surgical complication. A catastrophic complication is rarely the result of an isolated circumstance.

Anatomic Risks

The anatomic relationship between the ICA and the sphenoid sinus has been extensively described. Dehiscent bone over the ICA is found in 4% to 22% of anatomic specimens.[11] Therefore, an incomplete bony cover or the presence of very thin bone over the ICA should be presumed and the mucoperiosteum and bone over the ICA should be dissected with care. Similarly, bulging of the ICA within the sphenoid sinus has been noted in 8% to 70% of patients. This variation and its frequency are subject to the degree of sinus pneumatization. Similarly, the average distance between the cavernous segments of the ICAs is 12 mm; however, it can be less than 4 mm.[12] A close distance between the ICAs places both vessels at risk during the surgical exposure. Furthermore, intersinus septations commonly attach to the internal carotid and optic nerve canals.[13] Bony septations need to be removed gently, avoiding aggressive manipulation that could result in fracturing a septum attached to the ICA canal, thus creating torsion or a sharp edge with a subsequent vascular injury. Strong septations that are resistant to true-cut forceps or rongeurs are best removed using a high-speed drill with coarse or hybrid diamond burrs.

Vascular abnormalities contribute directly to the incidence of ICA injury with subsequent catastrophic perioperative bleeding. Presence of aneurysms, pseudoaneurysms, or carotid-cavernous fistulae has been reported as a contributing factor for inadvertent internal carotid injury. Noticeably, around 10.6% of all intracranial aneurysms are located in the cavernous segment of the ICA.[14]

Ectasia or displacement of the ICA by a tumor may place the vessel at risk by shifting its position into the path of the surgical corridor. Relatively common clinical scenarios include the presence of an ectatic ICA posterior to the median nasopharynx in a patient requiring a transodontoid approach and the anterior displacement of the petrous and paraclival segments in patients with chondrosarcoma.

Table 1 Risk factors for ICA injury	
Category	**Factors**
Anatomy-related	Dehiscent ICA canal
	Sphenoid septa with attachments to the ICA canals
	Short distance between ICAs
	Vessel wall abnormalities
	ICA displacement by the lesion
Pathology-related	Adherence of the lesion to ICA
	Previous extended surgery
	Previous radiotherapy
	Previous bromocriptine therapy
Skills and resource-related	Inexperience in skull base surgery
	Lack of adequate instruments and equipment
High-risk	Radical resection of an adherent lesion
	Encasement of ICA
	Need for wide exposure ($\geq$2 segments of ICA)

Pathology-Related Risks

Tumors in intimate contact with the ICA could obscure or obliterate the plane of dissection leading to a devastating injury of the vessel during their resection. In general, the probability of a tumor invading the ICA wall, and consequently leading to a surgical injury during the tumor dissection, is proportional to the degree of tumor encirclement and its adherence to the vessel. Encirclement of the vessel is ascertained with preoperative imaging, whereas adherence could be hard to predict (it should be expected in previously operated or irradiated patients). Tumor histology may contribute to the risk of a transmural injury through the degree of invasiveness and infiltration of the ICA wall. Gardner and colleagues[15] suggested that chondroid tumors (chordomas and chondrosarcomas) harbor a higher risk for ICA rupture than other pathologies because of the need for greater exposure of multiple segments of ICA and displacement of the vessel out of the anatomic position. We believe that these tumors may destroy the periosteum that normally protects the cavernous sinus and petrous segments of the ICA, thus making it more vulnerable to surgical trauma.

Previous surgery, previous external radiotherapy (risk may be higher after proton or stereotactic radiation), or chemoradiotherapy, and prior treatment with bromocriptine for pituitary tumors also have been linked to ICA injury.[15,16] Increased fibrosis, adhesions, and loss of the surgical landmarks could explain this relationship. Raymond and colleagues[17] found that 30% of patients who suffered an ICA injury have had prior bromocriptine therapy, 30% were revision cases, and 23% had previous radiation therapy.

The site of origin and extension of the lesion also play a significant role in the surgical threat to the ICA. Endoscopic sinus surgery and endoscopic approaches to the anterior cranial fossa carry a meager risk of injuring the ICA.[15] Conversely, middle and posterior cranial fossa approaches carry a considerable risk because the course of ICA is closely related to the surgical corridor and area of resection.

Skills and Resource-Related Risks

Advanced endoscopic endonasal skull base surgery requires a highly qualified team with reasonable experience in managing vascular challenges and reconstructive techniques. Similarly, using inappropriate instrumentation during exposure or dissection of the ICA could lead to an accidental injury. A variety of manual and powered instrumentation including (but not excluding others) rongeurs, forceps, drills (coupled with cutting or aggressive burrs), microdebriders, ultrasonic aspirators, and monopolar electrocautery (blade, needle, or suction tipped) have been implicated in various ICA injuries. In general, powered instruments are best avoided during a dissection close to the ICA, with the exception of high-speed drills that are required to remove bone around the vessel. In addition, dealing with complex or high-risk cases in insufficiently equipped institutions is unwise (eg, no intensive care unit, no endovascular neurosurgeon or interventional radiologist).

High-Risk Factors

As a whole, the previously mentioned problems and concerns are relative factors and any single issue is rarely the culprit of an accidental injury. The likelihood of vascular injury increases exponentially with the amalgamation of multiple risks. For example, the authors consider the following scenarios as high-risk factors:

1. Radical resection with curative intent for lesions that are adherent to the carotid wall.
2. Tumors encircling the ICA greater than 120°.

3. Lesions that require wide exposure of the carotid (ie, exposing one or more segments of the carotid or mobilization of the ICA).
4. Previously irradiated lesions that are attached to the ICA (especially if proton, neutron, or intensified radiotherapy regimens have been used).

Identifying patients at risk helps in patient's counseling, preoperative work-up, appropriate multispecialty consultation, intraoperative preparation, and postoperative follow-up. Furthermore, these patients may require preemptive surgical or endovascular control of the ICA.

PREOPERATIVE WORK-UP

Advanced endoscopic endonasal skull base surgery should be performed in a multidisciplinary environment that provides adequate resources to attend to this complex clinical scenario. The surgical plan must be discussed among the members of the core team, consisting of a skull base otolaryngologist (ie, rhinologist or head and neck surgeon), a skull base neurosurgeon, neuroradiologist, and neuroanesthesiologist. In patients at high risk for an ICA injury the discussion should include a neurointerventional radiologist or endovascular neurosurgeon. Preemptive decisions, such as the need to assess the brain collateral circulation or to sacrifice the ICA as part of the tumor resection, are discussed at this time. Other specialties, such as medical oncologists, radiation oncologists, neuro-ophthalmologists, and endocrinologists, are consulted based on the needs of each case. Furthermore, complex skull base lesions are best managed in comprehensive medical facilities with appropriate diagnostic and therapeutic capabilities.

Imaging is highly valuable not only as a diagnostic tool but also in planning the most appropriate surgical approach and providing detailed anatomy of the ICA course. Consequently, it allows the team to identify patients at risk, thus fostering the required precautions (**Fig. 1**). It has been shown that preoperative imaging decreases the complication rate of endoscopic sinus surgery.[18] Computed tomography (CT) and MRI, with and without contrast, provide complementary information and are customary in the primary evaluation of skull base lesions. Other imaging modalities, such as CT angiogram, MR angiogram, and/or digital subtraction angiogram provide a detailed evaluation of vascular structures and their relationship to the surgical corridor, tumor, and planned resection.

High-risk cases ought to be discussed thoroughly with the neurointerventional radiologist or endovascular neurosurgeon. A balloon test occlusion (BTO) of the ICA is required to assess the adequacy of the collateral cerebral blood flow, and therefore evaluate the potentially deleterious effect of losing one's ICA (see **Fig. 1**). A BTO, even when performed under neurologic surveillance as the only parameter, considerably reduces the incidence of postoperative stroke compared with indiscriminate ICA sacrifice.[19,20] The addition of objective measurements of cerebral blood flow by xenon CT, transcranial Doppler, scintigraphy, or other methods increases the sensitivity of the technique and categorizes the risk for an ischemic stroke. However, even the best BTO is associated with a 5% to 10% false-negative rate resulting in a delayed stroke after therapeutic ICA occlusion, and cannot predict embolic phenomena.[21,22] Additionally, a BTO is associated with a 3% to 4% procedural risk related to intimal damage resulting in arterial dissection and/or pseudoaneurysm formation and consecutive thromboembolism.[21] The benefits of an elective BTO should be weighed against the risks of the procedure and the rate of false-negative findings. Therefore, the procedure is reserved for those patients who carry a high risk of ICA injury (see **Fig. 1**).

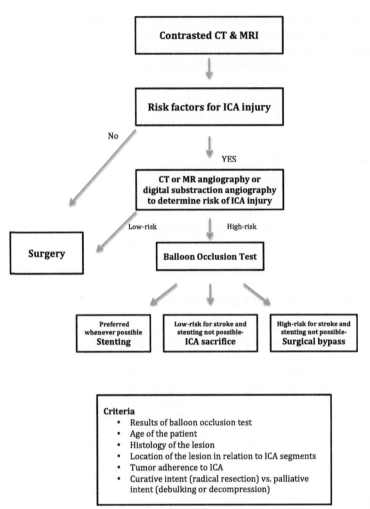

Fig. 1. Surgical planning algorithm based on the risk of injury to the ICA. CT, computed tomography.

Preoperative preparations should also include the optimization of medical comorbidities and cessation of drugs that may increase the tendency for bleeding. Preoperative counseling and informed consent are obligatory steps. Operative risks and expected complications and the possible need for further endovascular treatment should be thoroughly explained. Additionally, the patient should be informed regarding the possibility of using external approaches to manage unforeseen situations. Furthermore, all available treatment options and the goal of the surgery should be discussed in a multispecialty tumor board or planning conference setting. This is especially advocated for patients at high-risk for injury, for whom alternative therapies must be weighed against surgery.

INTRAOPERATIVE
Sign-In and Time-Out Protocol

Paramount preparations that should be completed in the operating theater before starting the surgery include a thorough discussion of the nuances of the case with the anesthesiologist (before induction of anesthesia). The role of the anesthesiologist in avoiding adversity during a catastrophic ICA injury cannot be overemphasized. An estimate of the anticipated blood loss should be discussed and arrangements for replacement must be completed. Ideally, cross-matched blood and blood products should be available in the operating theater (**Table 2**).

In high-risk patients it is prudent to insert two large intravenous catheters for rapid infusion (ie, 16–12 gauge) along with an arterial line for direct arterial blood pressure monitoring. One must consider that during the management of a major intraoperative bleeding it is difficult to insert lines for resuscitation or monitoring. The diminished intravascular volume makes it more difficult to cannulate the vessels, thus wasting precious time. Although controversial, patients at high-risk for an ICA injury can be prepared with a femoral artery cannulation as a pre-emptive measure. Advantages regarding timesaving in case of an emergency vary significantly among institutions and their ability to perform the angiography in the operating room rather than transporting the patient to an angiography suite; thus, whether or not this will be advantageous must be decided by consensus with the interventional radiologist or endovascular neurosurgeon.

For high-risk patients, sterile prepping and draping of the surgical field should include the neck for possible emergency transcervical (external) access or pre-emptive control of the common, internal, and external carotid arteries. In patients with tumors that approach the parapharyngeal ICA, the surgeons can dissect this segment of the vessel via a transcervical approach and leave colored or textured material to separate the vessel from the endonasal dissection. Furthermore, preparation of the abdomen or the thigh is prudent for the harvesting of muscle or fat that may be used to control the ICA injury. As previously stated, any high-risk patient should be discussed with the neurointerventional radiologist or endovascular neurosurgeon. Communication leads to an optimal surgical plan and promotes better coordination, thus minimizing the time spent transferring the patient to the angiography suite after an ICA injury.

The operating room staff should be aware of the risks and critical aspects of the case, and the staff (ie, scrub and circulating nurses) must be experienced. Having a scrub nurse that is unfamiliar with the procedure or the specialized instruments, or a

Table 2 Intraoperative checklist	
Anesthesia	Available packed red blood cells (eg, 4 U) Two large-bore intravenous lines (12–16 gauge) Arterial line +/- Femoral artery cannulation
Instruments and materials	Bipolar electrocautery 3 large-bore suctions (12F catheter) Hemostatic agents Instruments of proper length and angle Endoscopic lens-cleansing system High-speed diamond drill
Devices	Image guidance system Acoustic Doppler ultrasound Somatosensory evoked potentials monitoring
Surgical	Neck, abdomen, and thigh preparation and drape 2 nostrils/4 hands technique Ensure wide exposure Secure the local flap in a safe position

circulating nurse that cannot anticipate and fulfill the emergent needs may present an insurmountable obstacle at the time of a catastrophic complication.

Preoperatively, the staff must check the adequacy of the electrical devices and electric connections (eg, electrocautery), and provide a minimum of three different suction lines connected to an adequate suction system and the potential to equip them with 12F catheter (or larger) suction tips. In addition, the suction canisters should be evacuated from time to time to avoid a full canister and suspended suction in the middle of catastrophic bleeding (ie, suctioning provides visualization and control of the injury). It is prudent to inquire about the condition of the canisters before starting the dissection of the ICA and at regular intervals thereafter. A specific time interval may be decided to automatize the safety inspection of the canisters and lines. Different hemostatic agents and packing materials, in proper quantities, should be available in the operative room so that the circulating nurse does not have to leave the operating suite to chase these materials. Furthermore, one must check the availability of critical instruments, such as suction tips, hemostatic paste or clips and their respective applicators, bipolar electrocautery, and so forth.

Straight and angled instruments, of a length that is adequate to reach the targeted area, are crucial for the efficient and safe manipulation of the deep spaces. A dry surgical field aids with visualization; thus, electrical or radiofrequency bipolar coagulators are valuable because they can control vessels of small to moderate diameter. However, it is important to have bipolar devices that are long, angled, and capable to work in narrow areas.

A carefully calibrated image guidance system is beneficial in confirming major landmarks and the position of the petrous and paraclival ICA bony canals during the procedure. However, anatomic knowledge is fundamental in interpreting the surgical field and correlating it with the preoperative imaging. Different imaging modalities can be uploaded and navigated depending on the available system and software. CT angiogram with or without MRI fusion sequences is useful to delineate bony and vascular structures. Nevertheless, the surgeon should always question the accuracy of the image guidance system, continually confirm its accuracy and anticipate margins of error.

Many skull base lesions distort the bony anatomic landmarks and become intimately associated with the ICA. Acoustic Doppler ultrasonography provides an audible flow signal that represents an accurate and real-time detection of the ICA or any other major vessel.[23,24] This device is extremely useful when the vessels are displaced from their preoperative position after debulking of the tumor and collapsing the adjacent soft tissue, thus changing the anatomy and nullifying the accuracy of the navigation system. However, direct positioning of the probe over the internal carotid segment is necessary to get accurate results.

Diagnostic ultrasonography can image structures deep to the surgical field providing an accurate estimate of their depth and distances. In addition, it can use the Doppler effect to identify vessels and the direction of their flow with a visual image and an audible signal (ie, differentiating arteries from venous sinuses). It provides, however, a very narrow band of visualization and the current probes are somewhat cumbersome to use through an endonasal corridor.

Intraoperative neurophysiologic monitoring of somatosensory evoked potentials can detect parenchymal hypoperfusion following a vascular insult.[25,26] Somatosensory evoked potentials monitoring plays an important role in managing intraoperative blood pressure and maintaining adequate cerebral perfusion during the procedure. However, its role becomes more significant during the management of an ICA injury. Somatosensory evoked potentials monitoring is applied routinely during endoscopic endonasal skull base surgery in some centers; however, because of its availability and cost it could be reserved for high-risk patients.

Any major bleeding during endoscopic endonasal skull base surgery could compromise the visualization and obscure the surgical field. Manual irrigation or the use of endoscopic lens-cleansing systems helps to maintain a clear view and minimize the wasted time needed for the removal and cleansing of the endoscope lens. Manual irrigation is an acceptable alternative but it occupies one of four available hands.

The previously mentioned measures should be discussed during the sign-in and timeout periods and before skin incision (**Fig. 2**). A well-organized plan saves valuable time and focuses and coordinates the efforts by all team members.

Surgical Preparations

The surgical plan should provide a wide corridor that allows unhindered instrumentation and proper exposure of the targeted zone. Anatomic obstacles that lead to displacement and crossing of the instruments in a narrow space restrict any attempt to control the bleeding; thus, they should be eliminated or minimized as much as possible.

Skillful bimanual sharp dissection and careful tissue handling are absolute requirements around danger zones. The paradigm of having two surgeons operating through two nostrils using a three to four hands technique (ie, bimanual dissection) is advantageous to complete complex dissections and control bleeding.[27] Nonetheless, the surgical team should be well integrated and experienced before tackling a high-risk case, thus optimizing steady action during any unexpected event.

Minimizing traction of intracranial tumor or neurovascular structures and the use of customized sharp instruments help to avoid inadvertent avulsion of the surrounding

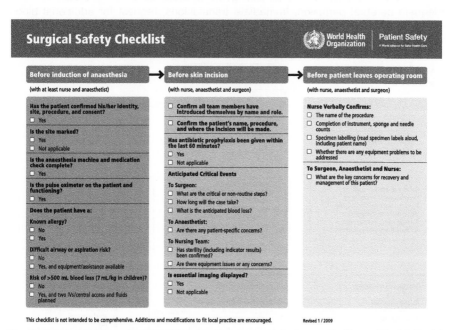

Fig. 2. Surgical safety checklist (sign-in, time-out, and sign-out). (*From* World Health Organization. Surgical safety checklist. Available at: http://www.who.int/patientsafety/safesurgery/checklist/en/. Accessed August 27, 2015; with permission.)

vessels. Use of a high-speed drill to obtain a wide exposure is common practice during extended approaches. However, one should note that using cutting burrs to remove the ICA canal could cause direct damage even in experienced hands. Diamond burrs generate heat that can be transmitted to the wall of the vessel, thus leading to immediate or delayed hemorrhage. Therefore, coarse or hybrid diamond burrs seem to offer the best compromise of attributes, providing adequate control while remaining effective to remove bone. However, coarse diamond burrs of larger diameter (4.5 mm or larger) may have large diamond fragments ("spikes") that can reach far from the visualized spinning core of the burr. This may mislead the surgeon regarding the depth of penetration and to potentially injuring the vessel wall during ICA canal drilling.

During the Catastrophe

Catastrophic bleeding is likely to obscure the injury site and soil the lens resulting in complete loss of visualization. The degree of bleeding is proportional to the extent of the injury; however, initially it could even be indistinguishable from arteries of lesser caliber or even venous sinus bleeding (ie, partial transmural). As soon as it is recognized that the ICA has been injured, the surgeons should clearly and loudly command the attention of all operating room staff and should inform them about the critical situation. One should keep everybody focused but calm, eliminate chatter, and initiate the previously established plan of action through a pre-established chain of commands (**Fig. 3**).

Concomitantly, the surgeons have to work in concert with the anesthesiologist to immediately and effectively exercise resuscitation measures and stop the blood loss.[28] Efforts should be directed to fluid and blood replacement, preventing hypovolemic shock in parallel with maintaining the appropriate blood pressure to keep adequate cerebral perfusion. Immediate transfusions, request for additional blood

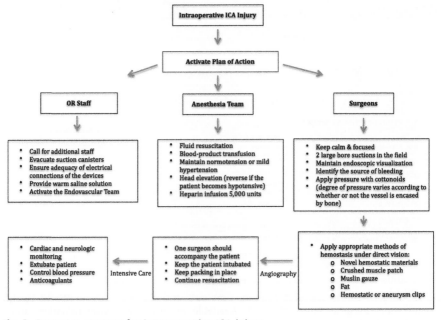

Fig. 3. Response strategy for intraoperative ICA injury.

products, and fast-drip fluid replacement are paramount. Although effective to facilitate the control of small vessel bleeding during extracranial surgery, hypotensive anesthesia is neither effective nor desirable to reduce blood loss or to improve the surgical field visualization during catastrophic bleeding from the ICA. Hypotension and the resulting hypoperfusion with the potential for ischemic brain injury negate any potential benefit.[29] Kassam and colleagues[3] advocate a normotensive or even a controlled hypertensive state to maintain the cerebral perfusion provided by the contralateral ICA. Limited head elevation may help to gain control of concomitant capillary and venous bleeding.

A counterintuitive but important measure is the intravenous administration of 5000 U of heparin. One would instinctively avoid anticoagulants in the presence of hemorrhage; however, heparin helps to prevent embolic phenomena arising from intimal injury.

The surgical team should focus on the surgical field and control of the bleeding. It is important to maintain a clear view to identify and seal the exact location of the injury. Endoscopic visualization is preserved and the bleeding controlled applying the following principles:

- Use a bimanual technique with a two-nostrils/four-hands approach.
- Insert the endoscope in the nasal side with less blood flow (ie, usually nostril opposite to the injury).
- Use two large-bore suction cannulas keeping the endoscope away from the blood stream while the suctions tips face the injured carotid.
- Keep the suction tips hovering directly over the site of injury and not pressing on the vessel wall or adjacent tissue, because this plugs the suction tip allowing the rapid accumulation of blood and leading to loss of visualization.
- If the site of injury is well visualized, the initial control may be achieved exerting pressure with the shaft of the suction or by directly applying pressure with cottonoids.
- A lens-cleansing system with foot-control frees the cosurgeon second hand (fourth hand on the field) to use an instrument or a third suction, and helps to clean the endoscope without having to remove it out of the field. Alternatively, one surgeon pilots the endoscope and irrigates warm saline solution (40°C) while the other surgeon uses two suctions tips to overcome the pooling of the blood and clear the field.
- The operating room staff should maintain the suction lines and canisters functional and activate the angiography suite team.

Digital compression or surgical control of the ipsilateral cervical carotid has been advocated to decrease the blood flow, therefore improving visualization and ease to control the injury.[29,30] However, retrograde bleeding may nullify the effectiveness of this maneuver (ie, it is unreliable and surgical control takes longer to execute than the harvesting and application of a muscle patch). In addition, the difficulty and logistics of bringing a third surgeon in to a very small and hectic field should not be underestimated.

It is prudent to secure the nasoseptal flap away from the targeted area within the nasopharynx, the maxillary sinus, or against the lateral wall of the nose because it tends to float toward the suction. If the flap obstructs the suction, thus becoming a burden, then it may be sacrificed and removed.

The primary measure to control the bleeding is focal packing, applying the least amount of pressure needed to stop the bleeding under direct visualization. Packing the entire nasal cavity is a feasible alternative when facing extracranial pathology, especially if the vessel is still covered by a bony canal. Under these circumstances the nasal packing applies hemostatic pressure without compressing the lumen, thus allowing blood flow and decreasing the chance of cerebral hypoperfusion. In addition, nasal packing can be hastily inserted in a single-surgeon scenario where the lack of a cosurgeon does not allow launching those measures that require three to four hands. However, nasal packing is contraindicated during an intradural approach because blood follows the path of least resistance into the cranial cavity.

Furthermore, blind packing during an intracranial approach (even extradural) harbors the risk of complete occlusion of the ICA or other major blood vessel, such as the basilar and middle cerebral arteries. Major complications, such as stroke and death, are often associated with this forceful packing. Raymond and colleagues[17] reported on 12 patients who suffered an ICA injury and were treated with nasal packing followed by angiography. In 8 of the 12 patients the nasal packing completely occluded the ICA and one patient suffered occlusion of the middle cerebral and basilar artery. The remaining four patients had partial occlusion of the ICA. Furthermore, the nasal packing controlled the bleeding in only nine patients, of whom one died from the basilar artery compression.

Valentine and colleagues,[31] using a sheep model, developed or confirmed the effectiveness of many of the principles that were previously listed and elegantly showed that applying a crushed muscle patch over the injured carotid produced effective hemostasis. They recommended holding the muscle patch in direct contact over the ICA but without compression of the vessel for several minutes. A muscle patch can be harvested quickly from the lateral thigh (preferred site) or abdominal wall. Others have advocated harvesting muscle from the sternocleidomastoid, temporalis, or even tongue muscles. Harvesting of these muscles requires accommodating a third surgeon around the field, which as expressed previously, brings some daunting logistics during an emergency. Harvesting of tongue muscle is even more difficult because of the proximity to the surgical field, and is also associated with contamination by oral flora and potential functional deficits.

Other measures, such as the use of bipolar electrocautery, biologic and synthetic glues, and thrombin/gelatin matrix paste, are ineffective and potentially dangerous.[3,29–32] In a verbal communication (Rhinology 2013, Sao Paulo, Brazil), the skull base surgery team at the University of Pittsburgh Medical Center reported the inadvertent injection of hemostatic paste into the ICA resulting in thrombosis of the ipsilateral intracranial circulation. Hemostatic clips[33] (ie, aneurysm clips) or suturing are effective. However, the injured segment of the ICA has to be fully exposed (ie, mobilized from its bony canal for proximal and distal control); the significant difficulty of this repair requires significant expertise; and even under the best circumstances, it is time consuming. Although the repair is completed the patients may lose a significant volume of blood and the risk of uncontrolled bleeding remains.

External transcervical control of the common, internal, and external carotid arteries is an alternative, albeit with the difficulty of crowding the surgical space. In addition, permanent closure of the carotid system is associated with major complications, such as stroke and death.[34] Furthermore, it blocks the access for endovascular assessment and management.

POSTOPERATIVE RESCUE

Following intraoperative control of the bleeding, the patient needs to undergo an immediate angiography, possibly followed by BTO and, ultimately, endovascular treatment. It is of paramount importance to keep the patient intubated during the transfer and angiography, even if the bleeding has been controlled. In addition, a surgeon should be immediately available and any packing is kept in place throughout the procedure (see **Fig. 3**).

Angiography is performed to identify the site and extent of the injury, to evaluate the efficacy of the primary control, and to evaluate the patency of cross-circulation from the side opposite to the injury. However, BTO is highly recommended to better evaluate the contralateral circulation and to estimate the risk of stroke if the injured ICA would be occluded. BTO, however, is not infallible. One needs to consider that 5% to 10% of patients that pass BTO are still at risk for a delayed infarction.[35] In addition, BTO cannot predict embolic phenomena, or the adequacy of the cross-circulation under duress, such as hypoxia or hypotensive episodes.

Definitive treatment options include vessel sacrifice by embolization, transluminal endovascular stenting, and surgical bypass. Each option has its own advantages and caveats. In general, preserving the ICA using a stent or pipeline is the treatment of choice whenever possible. The safety and effectiveness of stenting are well established[36,37]; notwithstanding, there are certain situations that preclude the use of stent, such as the presence of severe kinking of the ICA, injury at the cavernous segment of ICA, and stenosis of the vessel. Insertion of the stent under these circumstances is technically difficult and might lead to carotid rupture.[37] Remaining treatment options are considered taking into account the result of the balloon occlusion test, presence and histopathology of remaining tumor, and the age of the patient. If it is not possible to use a stent, then embolization and occlusion should be carried out providing that the patient tolerated BTO. Otherwise, an extracranial-to-intracranial surgical bypass is required.

After endovascular treatment the patient could be transferred back to the operating theater provided that his or her general condition allows. Potentially, one could remove the packing and complete the tumor resection. However, this is rarely executed because most patients have undergone significant fluid resuscitation and have probably received anticoagulation. In addition, one must note that endovascular detachable balloons are not approved by the Food and Drug Administration; therefore, sacrifice of the ICA in the United States is most often performed with coils. Coils require several days to stabilize and actuate a full thrombosis of the ICA; thus, manipulation of the injury site and removal of any nasal packing needs to be delayed by an appropriate lapse of time. This is also true for many of the stents and pipelines, which also require several days to seal the injury. Furthermore, they also require antiplatelet therapy for a minimum of 4 weeks.[37]

Most commonly the patient is transferred to the intensive care unit for further observation and monitoring of vital signs, cardiac, and neurologic status. In the intensive care unit, the patient may be awakened and extubated to better monitor neurologic functions. The patient is maintained slightly hypertensive for 2 to 3 days, as recommended by Higashida and colleagues.[38] A postoperative CT scan is routinely done to exclude any intracranial complications, but only after the patient is deemed stable.

Delayed complications, such as pseudoaneurysm or a caroticocavernous sinus fistula, could pass unnoticed for some time leading to major morbidity.[15,28] Therefore, a second angiography should be repeated 1 to 2 weeks after the initial intervention for the early detection of these complications. However, the timing for a second angiography is empirical and not universally accepted. A pseudoaneurysm can develop within hours or months later.

SUMMARY

An ICA injury during endoscopic endonasal procedures is a perilous scenario. Identifying potential risk factors and preoperative planning are crucial in preventing its occurrence and minimizing its consequences. Execution of an effective plan of action during the catastrophe relies on a well-prepared protocol, availability of proper instruments and devices, and an experienced multidisciplinary team. Stabilizing the hemorrhage intraoperatively should be followed by an angiography and endovascular treatment whenever possible. Close clinical and radiologic monitoring of the patient is important to prevent early and late complications.

REFERENCES

1. Nicolai P, Battaglia P, Bignami M, et al. Endoscopic surgery for malignant tumors of the sinonasal tract and adjacent skull base: a 10-year experience. Am J Rhinol 2008;22(3):308–16.
2. Castelnuovo P, Dallan I, Battaglia P, et al. Endoscopic endonasal skull base surgery: past, present and future. Eur Arch Otorhinolaryngol 2010;267(5):649–63.
3. Kassam A, Snyderman CH, Carrau RL, et al. Endoneurosurgical hemostasis techniques: lessons learned from 400 cases. Neurosurg Focus 2005;19:E7.
4. Sanna M, Piazza P, DiTrapani G, et al. Management of the internal carotid artery in tumors of the lateral skull base: preoperative permanent balloon occlusion without reconstruction. Otol Neurotol 2004;25(6):998–1005.
5. Renn WH, Rhoton AL Jr. Microsurgical anatomy of the sellar region. J Neurosurg 1975;43:288–98.
6. Kassam AB, Gardner P, Snyderman C, et al. Expanded endonasal approach: fully endoscopic, completely transnasal approach to the middle third of the clivus, petrous bone, middle cranial fossa, and infratemporal fossa. Neurosurg Focus 2005;19(1):E6.
7. Inamasu J, Guiot BH. Iatrogenic carotid artery injury in neurosurgery. Neurosurg Rev 2005;28(4):239–47.
8. Frank G, Sciarretta V, Calbucci F, et al. The endoscopic transnasal transsphenoidal approach for the treatment of cranial base chordomas and chondrosarcomas. Neurosurgery 2006;59:ONS50–57 [discussion: ONS50–57].
9. Gardner PA, Kassam AB, Snyderman CH, et al. Outcomes following endoscopic, expanded endonasal resection of suprasellar craniopharyngiomas: a case series. J Neurosurg 2008;109:6–16.
10. Valentine R, Wormald PJ. Carotid artery injury after endonasal surgery. Otolaryngol Clin North Am 2011;44:1059–79.
11. Fujii K, Chambers SM, Rhoton AL Jr. Neurovascular relationships of the sphenoid sinus. A microsurgical study. J Neurosurg 1979;50:31.
12. Rhoton AL Jr. The sellar region. Neurosurgery 2002;51(4 Suppl):S335–74.
13. Fernandez-Miranda JC, Prevedello DM, Madhok R, et al. Sphenoid septations and their relationship with internal carotid arteries: anatomical and radiological study. Laryngoscope 2009;119(10):1893–6.
14. Ujiie H, Sato K, Onda H, et al. Clinical analysis of incidentally discovered unruptured aneurysms. Stroke 1993 Dec;24(12):1850–6.
15. Gardner PA, Tormenti MJ, Pant H, et al. Carotid artery injury during endoscopic endonasal skull base surgery: incidence and outcomes. Neurosurgery 2013;73(2 Suppl Operative):ons261–9 [discussion: ons269–70].
16. Hatam A, Greitz T. Ectasia of cerebral arteries in acromegaly. Acta Radiol Diagn (Stockh) 1972;12:410.
17. Raymond J, Hardy J, Czepko R, et al. Arterial injuries in transsphenoidal surgery for pituitary adenoma; the role of angiography and endovascular treatment. AJNR Am J Neuroradiol 1997;18:655.

18. Kantarci M, Karasen RM, Alper F, et al. Remarkable anatomic variations in para-nasal sinus region and their clinical importance. Eur J Radiol 2004;50:296–302.
19. Gonzalez CF, Moret J. Balloon occlusion of the carotid artery prior to surgery for neck tumors. AJNR Am J Neuroradiol 1990;11:649–52.
20. Mathis JM, Barr JD, Jungreis CA, et al. Temporary balloon test occlusion of the internal carotid artery: experience in 500 cases. AJNR Am J Neuroradiol 1995; 16:749–54.
21. Tarr RW, Jungreis CA, Horton JA, et al. Complications of preoperative balloon test occlusion of the internal carotid arteries: experience in 300 cases. Skull Base Surg 1991;1:240–4.
22. Linskey ME, Jungreis CA, Yonas H, et al. Stroke risk after abrupt internal carotid artery sacrifice: accuracy of preoperative assessment with balloon test occlusion and stable xenon-enhanced CT. AJNR Am J Neuroradiol 1994;15:829–34.
23. Dusick JR, Esposito F, Malkasian D, et al. Avoidance of carotid artery injuries in transsphenoidal surgery with the Doppler probe and micro-hook blades. Neuro-surgery 2007;60(4 Suppl 2):322–8 [discussion: 328–9].
24. Yamasaki T, Moritake K, Nagai H, et al. Integration of ultrasonography and endos-copy into transsphenoidal surgery with a "picture-in-picture" viewing system. Technical note. Neurol Med Chir (Tokyo) 2002;42:275–8.
25. Bejjani GK, Nora PC, Vera PL, et al. The predictive value of intraoperative somato-sensory evoked potential monitoring: review of 244 procedures. Neurosurgery 1998;43(3):491–8 [discussion: 498–500].
26. Thirumala PD, Kassasm AB, Habeych M, et al. Somatosensory evoked potential monitoring during endoscopic endonasal approach to skull base surgery: anal-ysis of observed changes. Neurosurgery 2011;69(1 Suppl Operative):ons64–76 [discussion: ons76].
27. Castelnuovo P, Pistochini A, Locatelli D. Different surgical approaches to the sellar region: focusing on the "two nostril four hands technique" [review]. Rhinol-ogy 2006;44(1):2–7.
28. Gadhinglajkar SV, Sreedhar R, Bhattacharya RN. Carotid artery injury during transsphenoidal resection of pituitary tumor: anesthesia perspective. J Neurosurg Anesthesiol 2003;15(4):323–6.
29. Pepper JP, Wadhwa AK, Tsai F, et al. Cavernous carotid injury during functional endoscopic sinus surgery: case presentations and guidelines for optimal man-agement. Am J Rhinol 2007;21:105–9.
30. Weidenbecher M, Huk WJ, Iro H. Internal carotid artery injury during functional endoscopic sinus surgery and its management. Eur Arch Otorhinolaryngol 2005;262(8):640–5.
31. Valentine RJ, Boase S, Jervis-Bardy J, et al. The efficacy of hemostatic tech-niques in the sheep model of carotid artery injury. Int Forum Allergy Rhinol 2011;1:118.
32. Cappabianca P, Esposito F, Esposito I, et al. Use of a thrombin-gelatin haemo-static matrix in endoscopic endonasal extended approaches: technical note. Acta Neurochir (Wien) 2009;151:69–77 [discussion: 77].
33. Valentine R, Wormald PJ. Controlling the surgical field during a large endoscopic vascular injury. Laryngoscope 2011;121(3):562–6.
34. Chaloupka JC, Putman CM, Citardi MJ, et al. Endovascular therapy for the ca-rotid blowout syndrome in head and neck surgical patients: diagnostic and managerial considerations. AJNR Am J Neuroradiol 1996;17:843.
35. Segal DH, Sen C, Bederson JB, et al. Predictive value of balloon test occlusion of the internal carotid artery. Skull Base Surg 1995;5:97.

36. Shawl F, Kadro W, Domanski MJ, et al. Safety and efficacy of elective carotid artery stenting in high-risk patients. J Am Coll Cardiol 2000;35(7):1721–8.

37. Maras D, Lioupis C, Magoufis G, et al. Covered stent-graft treatment of traumatic internal carotid artery pseudoaneurysms: a review. Cardiovasc Intervent Radiol 2006;29:958–68.

38. Higashida RT, Halbach VV, Dowd C, et al. Endovascular detachable balloon embolization therapy of cavernous carotid artery aneurysms: results in 87 cases. J Neurosurg 1990;72:857.

Comprehensive Postoperative Management After Endoscopic Skull Base Surgery

Duc A. Tien, MD[a], Janalee K. Stokken, MD[b],
Pablo F. Recinos, MD[a,c], Troy D. Woodard, MD[a,c],
Raj Sindwani, MD[a,c],*

KEYWORDS

- Endoscopic skull base surgery • Endoscopic skull base reconstruction
- Postoperative management • Postoperative complications
- Postoperative debridement • Postoperative infection • CSF leak
- Quality of life outcomes

KEY POINTS

- The presence and type of cerebrospinal fluid (CSF) leak (low-flow or high-flow) encountered largely dictates early postoperative management strategies.
- Generally, patients should avoid maneuvers that increase intracranial pressures (eg, Valsalva) for at least 4 weeks when a CSF leak is encountered intraoperatively.
- Patients should receive postoperative prophylactic antibiotic coverage for at least 1 week owing to risk of toxic shock syndrome when packing is used.
- To minimize nasal crusting, patients start nasal saline sprays and antibiotic ointment immediately postoperatively; saline irrigations are instated 1 to 2 weeks afterward to facilitate nasal cleansing.
- Skull base patients are seen frequently for endoscopic debridement; once the sinonasal cavity is well-healed, follow-up visits are guided by the need for tumor surveillance.

Funding Sources: None.
[a] Section of Rhinology, Sinus and Skull Base Surgery, Head and Neck Institute, Cleveland Clinic Foundation, Cleveland, OH, USA; [b] Department of Otolaryngology, Head and Neck Surgery, Mayo Clinic, Rochester, MN, USA; [c] Minimally Invasive Cranial Base and Pituitary Surgery Program, Rose Ella Burkhardt Brain Tumor & Neuro-Oncology Center, Neurological Institute, Cleveland Clinic, Cleveland, OH, USA
* Corresponding author. Head & Neck Institute, Cleveland Clinic Foundation, 9500 Euclid Avenue #A-71, Cleveland, OH 44195.
E-mail address: sindwar@ccf.org

INTRODUCTION

Endoscopic endonasal skull base reconstruction has evolved considerably over the past few decades with improved surgical techniques and sophisticated technological advancements of surgical instrumentation. To maximize the success of the skull base defect reconstruction, it is important that the postoperative course is equally insightful to reduce complications such as postoperative cerebrospinal fluid (CSF) leak and meningitis. Despite its critical importance, a standardized regimen for the management of patients after endoscopic skull base surgery is unavailable, and evidence for "optimal postoperative care" is lacking in the current literature. This article reviews the described methods and evidence on the postoperative management of patients after endoscopic skull base reconstruction.

INTRAOPERATIVE CONSIDERATIONS

It should be noted that a smoother postoperative recovery with less crusting and fewer issues can be encouraged by certain intraoperative maneuvers. The primary goal of skull base reconstruction is to reestablish a barrier between the sinonasal cavities and the central nervous system. However, a nearly important secondary goal is to use mucosal preservation techniques, similar to the management of inflammatory sinus disease, that maintain ostial patency and prevent scar formation. Meticulous attention to the native sinonasal anatomy preserve function and translate to improved quality of life (QOL) as patients return to their baseline nasal function more quickly.[1,2] Mucosal stripping is avoided except in areas immediately surrounding the skull base defect to allow the skull base reconstruction to directly adhere to the bony skull base. It is important to medialize the middle turbinates at the end of the case to prevent middle meatal obstruction, and minimizing repetitive trauma to the middle turbinate decreases the risk of scarring.

If a nasoseptal flap (NSF) is harvested and not used as a rotational flap, it should be repositioned to the septal cartilage and bone to decrease the amount of postoperative crusting. When the mucosa is used as a rotational flap several techniques have been described to remucosalize the exposed septum. The mucosa from a resected middle turbinate can be removed and used,[3] or mucosa from the contralateral septum can be folded over.[4] However, in most pituitary tumor cases, an intraoperative CSF leak is not expected but may be encountered. In these cases, a "rescue" flap can be raised, which consists of partially harvesting the most superior and posterior aspect of the flap to protect its pedicle and provide access to the sphenoid face during the trans-sphenoidal approach.[5] The rescue flap can be harvested fully if the resultant defect is larger than expected or if an unexpected CSF leak is encountered. Minimizing exposed bone and cartilage can reduce greatly the extent of crusting experienced postoperatively.

GENERAL POSTOPERATIVE COURSE AND CARE AFTER ENDOSCOPIC SKULL BASE SURGERY

Postoperatively, most patients are admitted to a neurologic nursing floor. Patients with large skull base defects who require a flap are admitted to a monitored unit (in our practice we use a neurologic step down unit or neurologic intensive care unit) for closer monitoring for at least 1 night. A face tent with mist humidification can provide the patient with comfort. Nasal cannulas are strictly avoided to reduce drying of the nasal mucosa and to prevent the theoretic possibility that applied nasal airflow may cause pneumocephalus.[6] The patient's head is kept elevated at 30°, and systolic blood pressure is tightly regulated to be less than 140 mm Hg, if tolerated. On the first postoperative day, the patient is started on nasal sprays (2 sprays of 0.9% saline on each side at least 4 times daily) and antibiotic ointment applied to the nose several times a day to maintain a moist nasal environment and minimize crusting. A bladder catheter is left in place overnight and removed the following day to permit ambulation (removed immediately postoperatively if no leak). The patient should avoid maneuvers that place undue pressure on the reconstruction. CSF leak precautions are reinforced to the patient (avoid bearing down, avoid nose blowing, avoid drinking from a straw, and sneeze with mouth open) and a soft bowel regimen is instituted for a period of 4 to 6 weeks. At our institution, the otolaryngology team largely dictates when the patient can resume normal activities in the postoperative period.

The schedule for follow-up nasal debridement in endoscopic skull base surgery is lacking and most authors use a schedule based on data from studies in endoscopic sinus surgery.[6,7] Long-term follow-up is dictated in our practices by disease pathology. Early after surgery, we believe that skull base patients should be seen frequently and endoscopic debridement performed at regular intervals, and increased as needed. This is important to ensure proper healing and to evaluate for complications such as infection and CSF leak. These visits are also useful to outline next steps in management (eg, starting adjuvant radiation therapy, when to return to work, how long to continue CSF leak precautions) and allow us to comfort and educate the patient and their family through the next phase of their recovery.

Patients are seen for their first debridement about 7 days after surgery. During the initial debridement, nasal crusting is carefully removed from the anterior portion of the nasal cavity. In patients who had no evidence of intraoperative CSF leak or small skull base defect with a low-flow leak, the packing directly overlying the reconstruction can also be gently removed at this initial visit. Patients with large skull base reconstruction do not undergo debridement meticulously in the office initially and care is taken to avoid disturbing the mucosal edges.

Saline irrigations can be instated shortly after surgery (approximately 1–2 weeks), once the initial phase of flap healing has occurred to facilitate more aggressive cleansing of nasal crusting and mucus. At the second postoperative visit, usually 3 to 4 weeks after surgery, the patient undergoes a more complete debridement where the remainder of any crusting is diligently removed. At this time, the entire flap should be visualized and seen to be grossly incorporated into the surrounding mucosa. The patient should continue saline irrigations twice daily, particularly if there is still crusting in the nasal cavity. Additional follow-up visits may be required in cases with persistent crusting. We recommend following the patient endoscopically until the health of their nasal cavity (minimal or no crusting, nonedematous well-healed mucosa, no CSF leak) is clearly established. Once the sinonasal cavity is well-healed (**Fig. 1**), future follow-up visits are guided by the surveillance required for the disease process being managed, which may include interval imaging studies.

EARLY POSTOPERATIVE CARE STRATEGIES DEPENDING ON CEREBROSPINAL FLUID LEAK TYPE AND RECONSTRUCTION

The primary goals after skull base surgery are to return the patient to normal functioning as soon as possible and to ensure that the wound is well-healed. The type of skull base reconstruction and the presence and type of CSF leak (low flow or high flow) encountered largely dictate early postoperative management strategies. High-flow CSF leaks, as defined by Patel and colleagues,[8] are an instance when there is violation of a cistern or ventricle. In general, a multilayered approach for skull base

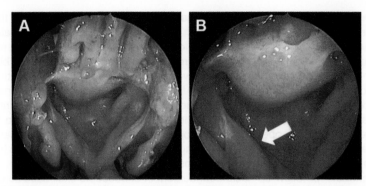

Fig. 1. (*A*) Postoperative endoscopy showing healthy sinonasal cavity 3 months postoperative. (*B*) Close up of well-incorporated margins and pedicle (*arrow*) of a pedicled nasoseptal flap.

reconstruction larger than 3-cm reduces the risk of exposed dura, CSF leak, and meningitis, but for small defects less than 1 cm without a CSF leak, the reconstruction can use a single layer or no graft at all.[9]

POSTOPERATIVE CARE WHEN THERE IS NO CEREBROSPINAL FLUID LEAK

There are several options available for reconstructing a skull base defect when there is not an intraoperative CSF leak. This type of closure is done to promote remucosalization of the sellar face and sphenoid sinus cavity and does not have to include multiple layers or extensive packing. The options include, but are not limited to, a free mucosal graft, which can be obtained from a resected middle turbinate or cadaveric acellular tissue (eg, Alloderm, Lifecell, Inc, Branchburg, NJ) followed by Surgicel (Ethicon, New Brunswick, NJ).

We most often use an epidural inlay DuraMatrix graft (Stryker, Kalamazoo, MI) followed by a tissue sealant (Tisseal [Baxter, Deerfield, IL] or Duraseal [Medtronic, Minneapolis, MN]) that is applied around the edges of the graft. This is then followed by placement of a dissolvable hemostatic packing (eg, Surgicel Fibrillar, Ethicon) to further seal the edges of the defect, cover the defect, and provide hemostasis. Some authors have advocated that tissue sealant may be redundant and an unnecessary expense.[10] When no graft is chosen as the method of closure, a small amount of hemostatic dissolvable packing is placed within the sphenoid cavity. This is the simplest form of skull base patient to manage postoperatively as the care is similar to that for routine sinus surgery: no nose blowing, heavy lifting, or straining for 1 week, and the first postoperative visit is at 1 week. Saline irrigations are started immediately after surgery.

POSTOPERATIVE CARE WHEN THERE IS LOW-FLOW CEREBROSPINAL FLUID LEAK

A low-flow leak is considered to be any leak that does not involve violation of a cistern or ventricle. The closure in this setting is not dissimilar to the type of closure used in repairing a CSF leak for an encephalocele or iatrogenic defect created after a sinus surgery misadventure. Typically, this includes placement of an underlay graft followed by an overlay graft supported by nasal packing. Options for the underlay graft, which is typically placed in the epidural space, include bone, cartilage, or dural substitutes (such as DuraMatrix). A free mucosal graft, which can be obtained from a resected middle turbinate, the septum, the inferior turbinate, or the nasal floor, are good choices for an overlay graft. The use of autologous abdominal fat and cadaveric acellular tissue (eg, Alloderm, Lifecell, Inc) have also been described for anterior and middle cranial fossa skull base defects.[11] An NSF can also be used.

Tissue sealant (eg, Tisseal or Duraseal) can be applied around the edges of the graft followed by a dissolvable hemostatic packing (eg, Surgicel Fibrillar, Ethicon) to further seal the edges of the defect and hold it against the exposed bone. Some authors advocate placing the Surgicel Fibrillar before the tissue sealant to promote an inflammatory response and encourage scaring of the graft to the underlying bone. To further bolster the reconstruction against the bone, we like to place absorbable packing, such as Nasopore (4- or 8-cm, Polyganics, Groningen, The Netherlands) followed by a nonabsorbable packing (eg, Merocel, Medtronic). If feasible, we allow adequate nasal airway beneath the packing for patient comfort postoperatively. The nonabsorbable packing is typically removed at approximately 5 days postoperatively. The patient is started on frequent saline nasal sprays and antibiotic ointment immediately postoperatively while in hospital and is seen in follow-up at about 1 week for debridement. At that time, saline irrigations are usually instituted as well to further cleanse the nasal cavity more aggressively. These are recommended at least until all crusting resolves and the nose is healthy.

POSTOPERATIVE CARE WHEN THERE IS A HIGH-FLOW CEREBROSPINAL FLUID LEAK OR A LARGE COMPLEX SKULL BASE DEFECT

Patients with high-flow CSF leaks generally have more advanced or complex disease and are more challenging to manage postoperatively. All patients with intraoperative high-flow CSF leaks and some patients with complicated or larger defects, particularly those with an exposed carotid artery, warrant the use of a vascularized mucosal flap for the skull base reconstruction. This has been shown to decrease significantly the rate of postoperative CSF leak.[8,12] Like the majority of skull base repairs, reconstruction with a vascularized flap occurs in a multilayered fashion. There are several vascularized options to reconstruct the skull base that have been described in the literature, including inferior turbinate flap, middle turbinate flap, NSF, pericranial flap, palatal flap, and temporoparietal fascia flap.[8] Each flap has its own set of advantages and limitations. When feasible, we generally harvest the NSF and place this in an onlay fashion over an inlay graft, such as abdominal fat and/or a dural substitute (eg, DuraMatrix, Stryker).

Fascia lata gasket seal closure[13] or fascia lata button graft[14] have also been described for high-flow CSF leak repair. These are modifications to the fascia lata graft that place the autologous graft in direct contact with the native dura. The button graft uses fascia lata to create both an inlay and onlay graft.[14] The onlay graft is then centered and sutured on the inlay graft, roughly 0.5 cm circumferentially from the edge of the smaller onlay graft. The authors of this technique compared this closure in 20 cases with 20 prebutton graft cases and found a significant CSF leak reduction from 45% to 10% leak rate ($P<.03$).[14]

The mucosal edges of the vascularized flap are secured to the exposed sphenoid bone using a dissolvable hemostatic packing (eg, Surgicel Fibrillar, Ethicon) followed by a tissue sealant (eg, Tisseal, Baxter) followed by in a similar fashion as described. Covering sinonasal mucosa under a free graft or pedicled graft can result in mucocele formation and should be avoided. One review[15] and an additional case report[16] identified a mucocele formation rate of 8% (12/144 cases) after endoscopic skull base surgery. Therefore, meticulous care should be taken to avoid this complication. A nondissolvable nasal pack (eg, Merocel, Medtronic) is always placed to further bolster the reconstruction. This is left in place for about 5 to 7 days. If a lumbar drain is used as part of the management strategy, CSF is drained at a rate of 5 to 10 mL per hour for 36 to 48 hours, and is clamped for at least 12 hours before being removed.

SPECIAL POSTOPERATIVE CONSIDERATIONS
Postoperative Imaging

The role and timing of postoperative computed tomography and MRI in patients after endoscopic skull base surgery remains unclear. Some authors have advocated routine imaging postoperatively to assess for postoperative sequelae such as subdural hematomas and early tension pneumocephalus that can present without significant neurologic symptoms until patients suffer a catastrophic event.[17] Others have moved away from the routine use of early postoperative imaging after endoscopic skull base surgery; these authors argue that, in the absence of neurologic symptoms, findings on early postoperative imaging did not have an impact on the clinical management of these patients but did contribute to overall health care costs.[18,19] We typically image on the first postoperative day to evaluate for complications and to obtain a baseline scan (**Fig. 2**). Subsequent imaging is individualized and performed based on factors including the pathology and extent of tumor resection obtained (gross total vs subtotal resection). For benign pathology, this is anywhere between 6 and 12 months, whereas imaging is performed sooner and more frequently for malignancies.

The ideal imaging study is also debated. We obtain preoperative MRI with a constructive interference in steady state protocol, which we find better delineates cranial nerves in relation to a tumor and surrounding structures such as dura. Repeat imaging is warranted when there is concern for residual disease. The equivalent protocol — fast imaging employing stead state acquisition — can also be used.[20]

Antibiotic Prophylaxis in Endoscopic Skull Base Surgery

The data on antibiotic prophylaxis in endoscopic skull base surgery are limited in the literature and the need for postoperative antibiotic prophylaxis is controversial. Brown and colleagues[21] prospectively reviewed their series of 90 endoscopic skull base cases. Cefazolin was used in 88% of patients, vancomycin in 9% of patients, and clindamycin in 3% of patients. There were no cases of intracranial infections or meningitis

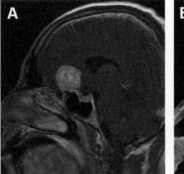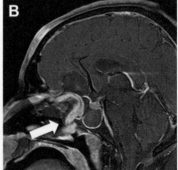

Fig. 2. Sagittal MRI of large planum sphenoidale meningioma resected endoscopically. (*A*) Preoperative and (*B*) postoperative day 1 with pedicled nasoseptal flap repair (*arrow*).

in either group. Furthermore, no antibiotic-related complications occurred during the study. Prior reports of antibiotic use in skull base surgery generally involved malignant pathology and vascularized flaps for reconstruction.[22]

De Almeida and colleagues[23] studied antibiotic prophylaxis in open cranial base surgery and found a decreased incidence of infectious complications in patients treated with a minimum of 24 hours of antibiotics but with no additional effect after 48 hours. Furthermore, there was no significance in the surgical approach, type of reconstruction, duration of surgery, and use of drains for postoperative wound infection. The reconstructive technique for endoscopic skull base surgery involves placement of free tissue grafts and tissue sealants through a "contaminated" field, representing a theoretic source of infection, yet risk for postoperative infection is exceedingly low. There is a paucity of data regarding the use of antibiotic prophylaxis in endoscopic skull base surgery. In our experience, patients receive intraoperative antibiotics and antistaphylococcal coverage for 7 days to reduce the risk of toxic shock syndrome while packing is in place.

Role of Intranasal Balloon Catheter and Nonabsorbable Packing

Although the location of the skull base defect has not been shown to be a risk factor for postoperative CSF leak,[24–26] we still advocate additional measures to reinforce reconstructions in complex defects or those in unusual anatomic locations. For routine transsellar or transtubercular approaches, we recommend a standard multilayered approach, as discussed. Owing to the anatomic nuances and gravitational dependency of the anterior skull base in transplanar or transcribriform approaches, we advocate additional measures to bolster these types of reconstruction. A Foley catheter may be considered when additional support to the reconstruction along the anterior skull base is deemed necessary and may allow the graft to incorporate under less tension. Care should be taken to avoid overinflation of the balloon, which may compromise blood flow to the vascularized flap. The Foley balloon is usually left inflated for approximately 5 days and the patient must be monitored in the hospital. The patient is then observed for several hours to confirm the absence of CSF leak before the balloon is removed. Alternative support strategies also include a finger cot (cut glove finger with a Merocel pack inside of it), traditional Merocel packs, or Vaseline gauze. As with the placement of all nonabsorbable packing materials in the nose, antibiotic prophylaxis against toxic shock is mandatory for the duration of the packing.

Pediatric Patients

Although initially developed to treat adult pathology, endoscopic skull base surgery has proven to be a safe and feasible approach for the management of a variety of pediatric skull base pathologies.[27–29] The anatomic limitations of the pediatric patient can make skull base reconstruction uniquely challenging. Complications in the pediatric skull base population have been reported as high as 28%.[28] Special attention should be made when placing grafts because of an increased rate of mucocele formation.[15] The principles of skull base reconstruction as discussed remain true for the pediatric patient. Depending on the age of the patient, compliance with postoperative care may be difficult. Most children tolerate saline sprays and some may even tolerate gentle irrigations as well if explained enthusiastically by parents. In some cases, a planned surgical debridement under general anesthesia is considered postoperatively.

Postoperative Complications

Postoperative CSF leak is the most common complication after endoscopic skull base surgery. Techniques to address intraoperative CSF leak have become very sophisticated with the implementation of vascularized pedicled flaps. Postoperative CSF leak occurs at a rate of approximately 1.6%[30] to 15.9%.[31] Most CSF leak failures present before hospital discharge. Most authors advocate managing CSF leak initially by diverting CSF with a lumbar drain.[8,30,31] The ideal duration of CSF drainage is not well-described, but most authors recommend 2 to 3 days.[30,31] In a series of 800 patients who underwent endoscopic skull base surgery, a total of 127 patients (15.9%) developed a postoperative CSF leak.[31] Only 23.6% of these patients were treated with a lumbar drain only; endoscopic repair (with or without a lumbar drain) was performed in the remaining three-quarters of patients (76.4%). This study demonstrates that the majority of patients with postoperative CSF leak require reoperation to identify the leak source, but an initial trial of CSF diversion is indicated. In addition, early exploration for CSF leaks have been advocated to avoid infectious complications, such as meningitis and intracranial abscesses, which are well-recognized but rare complications of skull base surgery. Postoperative meningitis occurs in 0.3% to 5.5% of patients undergoing microsurgical transsphenoidal surgery.[31] Kassam and colleagues[31] reported an infection rate of 1.8% and a meningitis rate of 1.3% in their series of 800 patients. The use of CSF diversion via a lumbar drain in the perioperative setting remains controversial, and this topic is discussed extensively elsewhere.

Nasal Morbidity and Quality of Life After Endoscopic Skull Base Surgery

The spectrum of nasal morbidity after endoscopic skull base surgery has been well-described in the literature.[6,15,23,31] These include nasal crusting, nasal discharge, anosmia, nasal obstruction, taste disturbances, headache, and midface and teeth numbness. In a prospective cohort study of 63 patients, the authors found that the most common morbidity is nasal crusting, which was present in 98% of patients with nearly 50% of patients having moderate to severe crusting at 1 month postoperatively.[23] The median time to absence of nasal crusting in this cohort was 101.0 days. Patient who had a more complex approach had a significantly longer time to absence of nasal crusting compared with a simple approach (105.0 vs 93.0 days; $P = .033$). The median time to remucosalization for patients with NSF was 89.0 days (95% CI, 72.7–105.3). It is important to understand the timeline of these changes to provide education to patients about the expected postoperative course.

QOL assessment is an important outcome measure in patients with skull base tumors owing to the complexity of surgery and associated significant morbidity. Several questionnaires and tools have been introduced and used in clinical studies of endoscopic skull base surgery to assess QOL morbidity and sinonasal outcomes. These include Short Form-36 (SF-36),[32] Anterior Skull Base Questionnaire,[1] Anterior Skull Base Nasal Inventory-12,[33] Rhinosinusitis Outcome Measure (RSOM)-31,[32] and Sinonasal Outcome Test (SNOT)-20,[34] and SNOT-22,[35,36] among others. However, because there is no standardized definition for QOL, it is inherently difficult to compare different studies. Several studies show that QOL scores decline the greatest within the first few months after surgery but approaches baseline scores by 3 to 9 months postoperatively.[33–37] Alobid and colleagues[32] reported that patients who undergo expanded endonasal approached with an NSF had more sinonasal symptoms as evident by significantly poorer SF-36 and RSOM-31 scores at 3 months after surgery. A systemic review of QOL after anterior skull base surgery found that QOL of patients undergoing endoscopic surgery is greater and improves earlier compared with open surgery.[37] The authors also reported that there were no clear, long-term deleterious effects on sinonasal outcomes after endoscopic surgery compared with open surgery.

Although several QOL studies suggest that the majority of patients return to baseline function, the current literature is conflicting on long-term olfactory outcomes after endoscopic skull base surgery. Olfactory neuroepithelium lines the cribriform plate, superior turbinate, superior septum, and some areas of the middle turbinate.[38] Portions of neuroepithelium must be removed permanently during the approach to the sella and anterior skull base, yet several studies have published that patients report a temporary, although significant, decrease in olfaction initially followed by a return to baseline functioning several months later.[36,39–42] On the contrary, other studies have shown decreased olfactory outcomes after endoscopic skull base surgery.[2,42] Georgalas and colleagues[2] showed a greater rate of hyposmia in patient with expanded approaches. Tam and colleagues[42] randomized 20 patients undergoing endoscopic skull base surgery to either undergo NSF or no flap and reported a significant reduction in olfaction at 6 months after surgery in patients who had an NSF.

SUMMARY

This article summarizes our experience and reviews the current literature on postoperative management after endoscopic skull base surgery. The primary goals after skull base surgery are to return the patient to normal functioning and to ensure that the wound is well-healed and healthy. The type of skull base reconstruction and the presence and type of CSF leak encountered intraoperatively guide postoperative management. Early postoperative care is focused on recognizing complications and minimizing nasal crusting through nasal saline sprays and irrigations as well as endoscopic debridement. Most recommendations in the literature for management after endoscopic skull base surgery are based on weak, anecdotal evidence. Higher quality evidence is needed to determine optimal postoperative care and to identify factors which are important in reducing morbidity and improving outcomes after skull base surgery.

REFERENCES

1. Abergel A, Cavel O, Margalit N, et al. Comparison of quality of life after transnasal endoscopic vs open skull base tumor resection. Arch Otolaryngol Head Neck Surg 2012;138(2):142–7.
2. Georgalas C, Badloe R, van Furth W, et al. Quality of life in extended endonasal approaches for skull base tumours. Rhinology 2012;50(3):255–61.
3. Kimple AJ, Leight WD, Wheless SA, et al. Reducing nasal morbidity after skull base reconstruction with the nasoseptal flap: free middle turbinate mucosal grafts. Laryngoscope 2012;122(9):1920–4.
4. Kasemsiri P, Carrau RL, Otto BA, et al. Reconstruction of the pedicled nasoseptal flap donor site with a contralateral reverse rotation flap: technical modifications and outcomes. Laryngoscope 2013;123(11):2601–4.
5. Rivera-Serrano CM, Snyderman CH, Gardner P, et al. Nasoseptal "rescue" flap: a novel modification of the nasoseptal flap technique for pituitary surgery. Laryngoscope 2011;121(5):990–3.
6. Nyquist GG, Rosen MR, Friedel ME, et al. Comprehensive management of the paranasal sinuses in patients undergoing endoscopic endonasal skull base surgery. World Neurosurg 2014;82(6):S54–8.
7. Bugten V, Nordgård S, Steinsvåg S. The effects of debridement after endoscopic sinus surgery. Laryngoscope 2006;116(11):2037–43.
8. Patel MR, Stadler ME, Snyderman CH, et al. How to choose? Endoscopic skull base reconstructive options and limitations. Skull Base 2010;20(6):397–404.

9. Kim GG, Hang AX, Mitchell CA, et al. Pedicled extranasal flaps in skull base reconstruction. Adv Otorhinolaryngol 2013;74:71–80.

10. Eloy JA, Choudhry OJ, Friedel ME, et al. Endoscopic nasoseptal flap repair of skull base defects: is addition of a dural sealant necessary? Otolaryngol Head Neck Surg 2012;147(1):161–6.

11. Lorenz RR, Dean RL, Hurley DB, et al. Endoscopic reconstruction of anterior and middle cranial fossa defects using acellular dermal allograft. Laryngoscope 2003;113(3):496–501.

12. Hadad G, Bassagasteguy L, Carrau RL, et al. A novel reconstructive technique after endoscopic expanded endonasal approaches: vascular pedicle nasoseptal flap. Laryngoscope 2006;116(10):1882–6.

13. Garcia-Navarro V, Anand VK, Schwartz TH. Gasket seal closure for extended endonasal endoscopic skull base surgery: efficacy in a large case series. World Neurosurg 2013;80(5):563–8.

14. Luginbuhl AJ, Campbell PG, Evans J, et al. Endoscopic repair of high-flow cranial base defects using a bilayer button. Laryngoscope 2010;120(5):876–80.

15. Awad AJ, Mohyeldin A, El-Sayed IH, et al. Sinonasal morbidity following endoscopic endonasal skull base surgery. Clin Neurol Neurosurg 2015;130: 162–7.

16. Vaezeafshar R, Hwang PH, Harsh G, et al. Mucocele formation under pedicled nasoseptal flap. Am J Otolaryngol 2012;33(5):634–6.

17. Carrau RL, Weissman JL, Janecka IP, et al. Computerized tomography and magnetic resonance imaging following cranial base surgery. Laryngoscope 1991; 101(9):951–9.

18. Nadimi S, Caballero N, Carpenter P, et al. Immediate postoperative imaging after uncomplicated endoscopic approach to the anterior skull base: is it necessary? Int Forum Allergy Rhinol 2014;4(12):1024–9.

19. Diaz L, Mady LJ, Mendelson ZS, et al. Endoscopic ventral skull base surgery: is early postoperative imaging warranted for detecting complications? Laryngoscope 2015;125(5):1072–6.

20. Blitz AM, Choudhri AF, Chonka ZD, et al. Anatomic considerations, nomenclature, and advanced cross-sectional imaging techniques for visualization of the cranial nerve segments by MR imaging. Neuroimaging Clin N Am 2014;24(1): 1–15.

21. Brown SM, Anand VK, Tabaee A, et al. Role of perioperative antibiotics in endoscopic skull base surgery. Laryngoscope 2007;117(9):1528–32.

22. Kraus DH, Gonen M, Mener D, et al. A standardized regimen of antibiotics prevents infectious complications in skull base surgery. Laryngoscope 2005; 115(8):1347–57.

23. De Almeida JR, Snyderman CH, Gardner PA, et al. Nasal morbidity following endoscopic skull base surgery: a prospective cohort study. Head Neck 2011; 33(4):547–51.

24. Mehta GU, Oldfield EH. Prevention of intraoperative cerebrospinal fluid leaks by lumbar cerebrospinal fluid drainage during surgery for pituitary macroadenomas. J Neurosurg 2012;116(6):1299–303.

25. Gruss CL, Al Komser M, Aghi MK, et al. Risk factors for cerebrospinal leak after endoscopic skull base reconstruction with nasoseptal flap. Otolaryngol Head Neck Surg 2014;151(3):516–21.

26. Ivan ME, Bryan Iorgulescu J, El-Sayed I, et al. Risk factors for postoperative cerebrospinal fluid leak and meningitis after expanded endoscopic endonasal surgery. J Clin Neurosci 2015;22(1):48–54.

27. Massimi L, Rigante M, D'Angelo L, et al. Quality of postoperative course in children: endoscopic endonasal surgery versus sublabial microsurgery. Acta Neurochir (Wien) 2011;153(4):843–9.
28. Chivukula S, Koutourousiou M, Snyderman CH, et al. Endoscopic endonasal skull base surgery in the pediatric population. J Neurosurg Pediatr 2013;11(3):227–41.
29. Rastatter JC, Snyderman CH, Gardner PA, et al. Endoscopic endonasal surgery for sinonasal and skull base lesions in the pediatric population. Otolaryngol Clin North Am 2015;48(1):79–99.
30. Esposito F, Dusick JR, Fatemi N, et al. Graded repair of cranial base defects and cerebrospinal fluid leaks in transsphenoidal surgery. Neurosurgery 2007; 60(4 Suppl 2):295–304.
31. Kassam AB, Prevedello DM, Carrau RL, et al. Endoscopic endonasal skull base surgery: analysis of complications in the authors' initial 800 patients. J Neurosurg 2011;114(6):1544–68.
32. Alobid I, Enseñat J, Mariño-Sánchez F, et al. Expanded endonasal approach using vascularized septal flap reconstruction for skull base tumors has a negative impact on sinonasal symptoms and quality of life. Am J Rhinol Allergy 2013;27(5): 426–31.
33. Little AS, Kelly D, Milligan J, et al. Predictors of sinonasal quality of life and nasal morbidity after fully endoscopic transsphenoidal surgery. J Neurosurg 2015; 122(June):1458–65.
34. Balaker AE, Bergsneider M, Martin NA, et al. Evolution of sinonasal symptoms following endoscopic anterior skull base surgery. Skull Base 2010;20(4):245–51.
35. Pant H, Bhatki AM, Snyderman CH, et al. Quality of life following endonasal skull base surgery. Skull Base 2010;20(1):35–40.
36. Zimmer LA, Shah O, Theodosopoulos PV. Short-term quality-of-life changes after endoscopic pituitary surgery rated with SNOT-22. J Neurol Surg B Skull Base 2014;75(4):288–92.
37. Kirkman M, Borg A, Al-Mousa A, et al. Quality-of-life after anterior skull base surgery: a systematic review. J Neurol Surg B Skull Base 2013;75(2):73–89.
38. Doty RL. Olfaction. Annu Rev Psychol 2001;52:423–52.
39. Hart CK, Theodosopoulos PV, Zimmer LA. Olfactory changes after endoscopic pituitary tumor resection. Otolaryngol Head Neck Surg 2010;142(1):95–7.
40. Kim S-W, Park KB, Khalmuratova R, et al. Clinical and histologic studies of olfactory outcomes after nasoseptal flap harvesting. Laryngoscope 2013;123(7): 1602–6.
41. Bedrosian JC, McCoul ED, Raithatha R, et al. A prospective study of postoperative symptoms in sinonasal quality-of-life following endoscopic skull-base surgery: dissociations based on specific symptoms. Int Forum Allergy Rhinol 2013;3(8): 664–9.
42. Tam S, Duggal N, Rotenberg BW. Olfactory outcomes following endoscopic pituitary surgery with or without septal flap reconstruction: a randomized controlled trial. Int Forum Allergy Rhinol 2013;3(1):62–5.

Index

Note: Page numbers of article titles are in **boldface** type.

Otolaryngol Clin N Am 49 (2016) 265–271
http://dx.doi.org/10.1016/S0030-6665(15)00200-5
0030-6665/16/$ – see front matter © 2016 Elsevier Inc. All rights reserved.

oto.theclinics.com

Moving?

Make sure your subscription moves with you!

To notify us of your new address, find your **Clinics Account Number** (located on your mailing label above your name), and contact customer service at:

Email: journalscustomerservice-usa@elsevier.com

800-654-2452 (subscribers in the U.S. & Canada)
314-447-8871 (subscribers outside of the U.S. & Canada)

Fax number: 314-447-8029

**Elsevier Health Sciences Division
Subscription Customer Service
3251 Riverport Lane
Maryland Heights, MO 63043**

*To ensure uninterrupted delivery of your subscription, please notify us at least 4 weeks in advance of move.

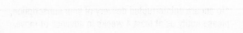

Printed and bound by CPI Group (UK) Ltd, Croydon, CR0 4YY

03/10/2024

01040395-0010